Competency Exam Prep & Review for Nursing Assistants

Third Edition

Barbara Acello, MS, RN
Barbara M. Kast, RN, BA

Delmar
Thomson Learning™

Africa • Australia • Canada • Denmark • Japan • Mexico • New Zealand • Philippines
Puerto Rico • Singapore • Spain • United Kingdom • United States

NOTICE TO THE READER

Delmar Staff:
Health Care Publishing Director: William Brottmiller
Acquisitions Editor: Doris Smith
Development Editor: Marjorie A. Bruce
Executive Editor: Cathy L. Esperti
Executive Marketing Manager: Dawn F. Gerrain
Marketing Coordinator: Karen Summerlin
Project Editor: Stacey Prus
Production Coordinator: John Mickelbank
Art/Design Coordinator: Mary Colleen Liburdi
Cover Design: TDB Publishing Services

For more information, contact Delmar, 3 Columbia Circle, PO Box 15015, Albany, NY 12212-0515; or find us on the World Wide Web at http://www.delmar.com

International Division List

Asia:
Thomson Learning
60 Albert Street, #15-01
Albert Complex
Singapore 189969
Tel: 65 336 6411
Fax: 65 336 7411

Japan:
Thomson Learning
Palaceside Building 5F
1-1-1 Hitotsubashi, Chiyoda-ku
Tokyo 100 0003 Japan
Tel: 813 5218 6544
Fax: 813 5218 6551

Australia/New Zealand:
Nelson/Thomson Learning
102 Dodds Street
South Melbourne, Victoria 3205
Australia
Tel: 61 39 685 4111
Fax: 61 39 685 4199

UK/Europe/Middle East:
Berkshire House
168-173 High Holborn
London
WC1V 7AA United Kingdom
Tel: 44 171 497 1422
Fax: 44 171 497 1426
Thomas Nelson & Sons Ltd.
Nelson House
Mayfield Road
Walton-on-Thames
KT 12 5PL United Kingdom
Tel: 44 1932 252211
Fax: 44 1932 246574

Latin America:
Thomson Learning
Seneca, 53
Colonia Polanco
11560 Mexico D. F. Mexico
Tel: 525-281-2906
Fax: 525-281-2656

Canada:
Nelson/Thomson Learning
1120 Birchmount Road
Scarborough, Ontario
Canada M1K 5G4
Tel: 416-752-9100
Fax: 416-752-8102

Spain:
Thomson Learning
Calle Magallanes, 25
28015-Madrid
ESPANA
Tel: 34 91 446 33 50
Fax: 34 91 445 62 18

International Headquarters:
Thomson Learning
International Division
290 Harbor Drive, 2nd Floor
Stamford, CT 06902-7477
Tel: 203-969-8700
Fax: 203-969-8751

Library of Congress Cataloging-in-Publication Data
Acello, Barbara.
    Competency exam prep and review for nursing assistants / Barbara Acello, Barbara M. Kast.--3rd ed.
        p. ; cm.
    Kast's name appears first on the earlier edition.
    Includes bibliographical references and index.
    ISBN 0-7668-1429-7
        1. Nurses' aides--Outlines, syllabi, etc. 2. Nurses' aides--Examinations, questions, etc.
I. Kast, Barbara M. II. Title.
    [DNLM: 1. Nurses' Aides--Examination Questions. 2. Nurses' Aides--Outlines. 3.
Clinical Competence--Examination Questions. 4. Clinical Competence--Outlines. 5.
Nursing Care--methods--Examination Questions. 6. Nursing Care--methods--Outlines.
WY 18.2 A173c 2000]
RT84 .k37 2000
610.73'06'98--dc21   00-022703

Dedication

To Shari Allen, CNA, Janine Anderson, AIN/CNA and Patti Green, CNA for their high standards of excellence in nursing assisting. These assistants freely give their love, support, and dedication to residents and other staff, insisting on thorough, high quality care. They are committed to their chosen profession and set a positive example for others. I am grateful for their inspiration, professionalism, and support.

Barbara Acello, MS, RN
June 2000

Brief Contents

Contents

Performance Procedures

Preface

INTRODUCTION

This training manual was developed to comply with the guidelines set by the Department of Health and Human Services in compliance with Public Law 100-203, referred to as the Omnibus Reconciliation Act of 1987 (OBRA). This law requires that nursing assistants (nurse aides) have, at a minimum, 75 hours of training and a complete competency evaluation program.

This manual was designed to serve as a guide to the competency evaluation program. Included in this course is the content required to successfully complete the written and the manual skills components of the examination.

Cardiopulmonary resuscitation (CPR) is not included in this curriculum. It is strongly recommended by the author that the CPR and Clearing Obstructed Airway components be taught by a certified CPR instructor.

ORGANIZATION OF TEXT CONTENT

Chapters 1 through 7 serve as the initial training. By OBRA standards, this initial training must consist of at least 16 hours. The author feels 16 hours can provide only an overview of the content of chapters 1 through 7. Reinforcement of the content in these chapters can be given in succeeding lessons.

This manual is a very basic "need-to-know" text. It is assumed that the instructor will draw upon professional experiences involving care of the elderly to provide the "nice-to-know" content. Throughout the entire content of this manual, the intent of the OBRA law is supported. This ensures that residents in the long-term care facilities are treated with care, dignity, and respect, while assisting residents to attain and maintain the highest possible level of independence.

More than 40 basic nursing procedures are included in this text. These procedures are included in the competency examination evaluation program in many states. The procedures were selected based on the OBRA guidelines, as well as suggestions by the manuscript reviewers. There are common steps at the beginning and end of all nursing procedures. These steps are listed on the inside covers of your text to emphasize the importance of handwashing, communication, safety, and respecting the resi-

dent's right to privacy. As students become proficient in clinical skills, these procedures become automatic.

This exam review can be used with other Delmar resources to create a complete training program.

TRAINING PACKAGE USING DELMAR RESOURCES

Several texts and a video series were developed to meet training needs leading to the certification of nursing assistants for jobs in the long-term care industry.

Video Series

Nursing Assisting Video Series, 3rd edition, is a series of twenty-two videos. The videos contain 138 segments relating to specific skills. The instructor can start skills training immediately using these high-quality video demonstrations. Medical professionals developed the videos based on requests from our textbook users. The procedural steps coordinate with all Delmar competency-based texts for nursing assistants. The procedures and activities shown on the videos recognize the nursing assistant as a skilled paraprofessional who works as an important member of the interdisciplinary team under the supervision of a licensed nurse.

Geriatric long-term care is a specialized segment of the health care industry. The focus of nursing assistant training must reflect the specific health care needs of long-term care residents, the significance of establishing a personal relationship with the resident, and the vulnerability of the elderly person suddenly placed in an institutional environment. To that end, the videos were produced to be current in light of the OBRA legislation and accurate in reflecting the "real" environment in a long-term care facility. Special emphasis is placed on the fact that the nursing facility resident is a real person with a unique identity and a personal life history. We are highly aware that the nursing assistant is also a complex person with goals and problems that affect his or her daily approach to life. Consequently, we have tried, beyond providing guidelines for nursing procedures and a message of compassion for our residents, to develop a program that will instill a sense of pride and self-worth in the student.

Text Packages

Essentials for the Nursing Assistant in Long-Term Care is a complete text for any 75- to 120-hour curriculum. This text starts with 16 hours of initial training and then covers basic and intermediate procedures. It is designed to enhance learning for "average" and "special needs" learners and for those who speak English as a second language. An Instructor's Manual is available, providing program management support and learning resources.

Competency Exam Prep & Review for Nursing Assistants, 3rd edition, can be used with the video series and Hegner's *Assisting in Long-Term Care.* This combination of learning aids is ideal for the 100- to 150-hour program.

For multicompetency programs, the instructor may choose from any of the following texts:

- *Nursing Assisting: Essentials for Long-Term Care* by Barbara Acello

- *Nursing Assistant: A Nursing Process Approach,* 8th edition, by Hegner, Caldwell and Needham
- *Assisting in Long-Term Care,* 3rd edition, by Hegner, Caldwell and Needham

The Delmar program provides a complete collection of materials for all levels of nursing assistant education, from basic to advanced.

Competency Exam Prep & Review was designed to provide exposure to test-taking using multiple choice questions in a simulation of the certification examination. A chapter is provided on test-taking techniques to help the learner build confidence to take the certification exam and succeed.

Competency Exam Prep & Review for Nursing Assistants is part of the most comprehensive and flexible training system available. It is hoped these extensive resources will contribute to quality assurance and to job satisfaction and self-esteem for long-term care paraprofessionals. The author and publisher hope their efforts may also improve the quality of life for long-term care residents.

About the Authors

ABOUT THE AUTHORS

Barbara Kast is an instructor of nursing assistants and health occupations, Northeast Metro Technical College, White Bear Lake, Minnesota. Ms. Kast has been project consultant for the state of Minnesota Department of Vocational Technical Education in the design and implementation of the nursing assistant curriculum.

Barbara Acello is an independent nurse consultant and educator. She has many years of experience in nursing assistant education in the public and private sectors. She is an approved RN Program Director in the state of Texas and a contributor to the Texas Curriculum for Nurse Aides.

Contributors

CONTRIBUTORS

Eloise Sampson, RN, BSN, MPH, is an instructor at Northeast Metro Technical College. Ms. Sampson contributed to the review quizzes at the end of each chapter as well as the practice exam in this book.

Larry J. Bailey is a professor of vocational education studies, Southern Illinois University, Carbondale, Illinois. He contributed to Appendix B: Test-Taking Methods and Guidelines.

Acknowledgments

The authors would like to thank Doris Smith, acquisitions editor, and Marjorie Bruce, developmental editor, of Delmar Thomson Learning for their ongoing encouragement, assistance, and support. Dennis Clarkson, CNA, and Laura Fowler, CNA, provided invaluable insights into the needs of the nursing assistant and helped to make the art meaningful. Catherine Johnson, LVN was most helpful in sharing the strengths and needs of student classroom materials. Although too numerous to mention, the authors wish to thank their friends, families, and coworkers for their patience and support throughout the development of this manuscript.

The authors also would like to thank the reviewers whose insightful comments were very helpful in preparing the first and final drafts of the manuscript.

Cynthia A. Bean, RN, MS
Consultant NYSED, Erie 1 Boces
West Seneca, NY

Sally Winkler Flesch, PhD, RN
Professor and Department Chair/Allied Health
Department
Black Hawk College Moline, IL

Helen Hutton, RN
Nursing Assistant/Home Health Aide Instructor and
Competency Examination Coordinator
Century College
White Bear Lake, MN

Laura Logan, RN, BSN, CCRN
Program Coordinator, Health Careers Department,
Community Services Division
Angelina College
Lufkin, TX

Barbara Pollack, RN, BS, OCN
President, Nursing Unlimited, Inc.
North Miami Beach, FL

Barbara L. Swanson, RN,C
Director of Education
Maplewood Care Center
Maplewood, MN

Dorothy A. Watson, MSN, RN
Associate Professor of Nursing
Roane State Community College
Harriman, TN

The Role and Responsibilities of the Nursing Assistant

OBJECTIVES

In this chapter you will learn about your role and responsibilities as a member of the health care team. After reading this chapter, you will be able to:

- Spell and define key terms.
- Describe the role of the nursing assistant.
- List the responsibilities of the nursing assistant.
- Describe the nursing assistant's role in the health care delivery system.
- Describe the purpose and intent of the OBRA legislation.
- Identify members of the interdisciplinary health care team.
- Describe ethics for the nursing assistant.
- Identify legal issues the nursing assistant must be aware of.
- Describe the purpose of the individualized resident care plan.
- Explain why individualized care is important.
- Define restorative care and explain why this type of care is important.
- Identify normal changes that occur during the aging process.

KEY TERMS

abuse: doing physical or mental harm to the resident, or threatening the resident with harm

acute illness: an illness that occurs quickly and does not last very long

aiding and abetting: seeing someone do something wrong and not reporting it

assault: trying to or threatening to touch a resident's body without permission

attitude: how you present yourself; an outward reflection of your feelings

battery: touching someone without permission

care plan: an individualized plan that lists the problems, needs, strengths, and goals for the resident

and describes what care and interventions should be done

charge nurse: the person responsible for supervising the resident's care and assignments during a certain work period

chronic illness: an illness that lasts for a long time, perhaps for life

clergy: a minister of the gospel, a pastor, priest, or rabbi

client: the individual cared for in the home

continuity of care: the process by which the care of a resident continues uninterrupted, using the same methods and approaches by all caregivers to meet the resident's goals

dependability: being trustworthy; reliable

dignity: the state of being respected or held in honor or esteem

disease: a state in the body in which normal functions are disturbed and do not perform as they should

ethics: rules of moral, responsible conduct that guide a person's behavior

etiquette: being polite, courteous, and kind toward others

false imprisonment: restricting someone's movement without permission

geriatrics: related to the aged or the aging process and diseases of the elderly

health: a state in which the body functions normally and is free from disease

interdisciplinary team: a group of individuals working and cooperating to help the resident attain the highest level of function possible

invasion of privacy: failure to keep resident information confidential or exposing the resident's body during caregiving

involuntary seclusion: isolating a resident as a form of punishment

job description: a list of duties and responsibilities for a particular job

long-term care facility: a nursing home or place where people with longstanding or chronic disabilities are cared for

licensed practical nurse (LPN) or **licensed vocational nurse (LVN):** one who has completed a 12- to 18-month nursing program and passed a state licensing examination for practical nurses

negligence: carelessness; failing to give the care needed in the way you were trained

nursing assistant (NA), nurse aide (NA), nurse assistant, state registered (NASR), state tested nurse assistant (STNA): a person who works under the supervision of a licensed nurse to provide personal care and nursing-related services to persons in health care facilities

OBRA 1987: Omnibus Budget Reconciliation Act of 1987; a set of laws that govern long-term care facilities and nursing assistant practice

patient: a person in a hospital who needs care

registered nurse (RN): a person who has completed two to four years of nursing school and has passed a state licensing examination for registered

nurses. The RN is responsible for assessing and planning care for residents and supervising other nursing employees.

rehabilitation center: a health care facility whose goal is to help ill or injured persons to function at their highest level of independence

resident: a person living in a nursing home or other long-term care facility

restorative care: care designed to help the resident attain and maintain the highest level of functioning possible

subacute care: highly specialized care for individuals with specific medical problems that require frequent skilled intervention. This care is delivered by highly trained personnel.

theft: taking something that does not belong to you

THE ROLE OF NURSING ASSISTANTS

Welcome to the health care field! You are about to become a member of a growing industry in which your work can give you great personal satisfaction. The most common title for this position is **nursing assistant (NA).** In some states the worker is called a **nurse aide (NA).** In others, the title **nurse assistant, state registered (NASR)** is used. Some states call this position **state tested nurse assistant (STNA).** Regardless of the title of your position, you will help others while achieving personal growth and satisfaction. The nursing assistant works in a health care setting to help the nurse give personal care to a resident, patient, or client (Figure 1-1).

HEALTH CARE FACILITIES

Health care facilities can be separated into two groups: those that give acute care and those that give less acute care, usually for long periods. Hospitals are examples of acute care facilities, where persons usually stay for a short time. Individuals who receive care in hospitals are called **patients.** Patients in hospitals have **acute illnesses** and injuries. An acute illness is one that occurs quickly and does not last very long. Some people receive care in their own home after they are discharged from the hospital. In the home, the caregiver may be called a home health aide (HHA) or home care aide (HCA). The home health aide usually completes a nursing assistant program and learns additional home health applications of the material. The person being cared for is called the **client. Long-term care facilities** are referred to by different names, such as convalescent homes, nursing homes,

Figure 1-1 Being a nursing assistant is a rewarding career for both men and women.

care centers, care facilities, **rehabilitation centers,** skilled nursing facilities, and other names. The people who reside in these long-term care facilities are called **residents.** Many residents in long-term care facilities have **chronic illnesses.** A chronic illness is one that lasts a long time, usually for life. These individuals usually stay for a long time, sometimes for years. The long-term care facility is their home, and you are a visitor in it. Many residents in long-term care facilities are elderly, although younger residents may also reside in the facility because they require daily personal care. Since the term **geriatrics** means care of the elderly, you may be called a geriatric aide. Some long-term care facilities have highly specialized units such as those where care is provided to residents with AIDS or Alzheimer's disease, those who use ventilators for breathing, or those who require **subacute care.** This book is designed to prepare you to work in a long-term care facility.

THE OBRA LEGISLATION

OBRA 1987 means Omnibus Budget Reconciliation Act of 1987. OBRA refers to federal laws that regulate long-term care facilities. In 1987 the OBRA legislation mandated sweeping changes in the long-term care industry. This changed the way that care is given. Before OBRA, care was provided to keep residents comfortable. The OBRA legislation requires long-term care facilities to use all resources available to help residents reach their highest level of function, both physically and mentally. The legislation also requires that care be given in a home-like environment and that residents be given choices and control over their care and routines.

Another change resulting from the OBRA legislation requires all states to develop a process for the training and competency testing of nursing assistants. The law requires training for nursing assistants in long-term care facilities specifically, but most health care agencies also require nursing assistant training for their employees.

The OBRA legislation requires specific content for the nursing assistant course and states that the course must be a minimum of 75 hours in length. Individual states may require additional training. After the nursing assistant completes the class, he or she must take and successfully complete a written and performance examination to be entered on the state nursing assistant registry. Only nursing assistants who have passed the examination and are on the state registry may work in long-term care facilities. Some states allow nursing assistants to work if they are enrolled in a training program and will complete their training within four months from their date of hire. In these states, you may perform only skills that you learned in class and for which you have been found proficient by the instructor.

The law also requires that the nursing assistant attend a minimum of 12 hours of continuing education classes a year, although again, individual states can require additional hours and specific subjects. These classes usually are provided by the long-term care facility. It is your responsibility to attend them to maintain your certification.

THE NURSE SUPERVISOR

As a nursing assistant you will be supervised by a licensed nurse. The nurse may be a **registered**

nurse (RN), a **licensed practical nurse (LPN),** or a **licensed vocational nurse (LVN).** The supervising nurse, sometimes called the **charge nurse,** is responsible for making your work assignment. This is the nurse of whom you will ask questions and to whom you will report information about the resident. Your work assignment includes work duties, assignment of the residents you will care for, and extra jobs that must be done on your unit. The nursing assistant is a part of the nursing service department in the long-term care facility.

PERSONAL QUALIFICATIONS

Because your role as a nursing assistant involves giving personal care to others, you must have certain qualities and personal characteristics.

Important Qualities for a Nursing Assistant

Nursing assistants should:

- have a sincere interest in working with people.
- have an **attitude** of respect toward the elderly.
- believe in the **dignity** of each person.
- be able to control their emotions.
- be honest, reliable, and dependable.
- have a positive attitude toward their job and employer.
- show willingness to accept direction and change.
- have a patient, cheerful, and sensitive nature.
- have a clean and neat appearance.
- be in good health without lifting restrictions. A nursing assistant must stand and walk for long periods, and lift and move people.
- be free from communicable diseases.
- be drug- and alcohol-free.

THE RESPONSIBILITIES OF NURSING ASSISTANTS

The responsibilities of the nursing assistant usually are listed in detail in a **job description.** A job description will be given to you by your employer or supervisor. The description details the particular tasks you are expected to do in that facility. This may vary from one health care facility to another. Remember, everything you do is under the supervision of a nurse.

Job Description

Your job description will list the duties and tasks you are expected to do and may include such things as:

- personal care of the resident
  - helping the resident with personal care, such as bathing, mouth care, grooming, dressing, toileting, and skin care
  - helping residents with equipment or devices such as hearing aids, glasses, and dentures
  - caring for the resident who is dying
- assisting residents with nutrition and hydration
  - helping the resident to eat and drink
- care of the environment
  - caring for the resident's environment
  - maintaining safety in the environment
  - helping with unit organization, cleanliness, and efficiency
- infection control
  - practicing measures that prevent the spread of infection
- observation and recording
  - taking and recording vital signs
  - observing and reporting abnormal signs and symptoms
  - measuring height and weight
  - keeping records required by facility policy
  - reporting any suspected or actual resident abuse
- assisting with movement, exercise, and ambulation
  - lifting, moving, turning, and transferring residents
  - helping residents with mobility
  - helping residents with exercise programs
- other responsibilities
  - helping the resident to maintain the rights guaranteed by the Resident's Bill of Rights
  - helping the resident with mental health and emotional needs
  - doing other tasks as assigned by your supervisor within the legal role of the nursing assistant

The policies of facilities vary, but generally you are expected to care for any resident in the facility. Although you may be assigned to a certain group of residents, answering call signals of all residents usually is required. Male and female nursing assistants usually are expected to care for residents of both sexes. If this concerns you, discuss the situation with the employer before accepting the job.

Long-term care facilities usually require nursing assistants to wear a uniform. The type of uniform will be decided by your employer. The purpose of a uniform is to maintain a professional appearance. Some facilities use different color uniforms to identify members of various departments. Another purpose of the uniform is to prevent the spread of infection. It should be worn only once and changed when you get home. The uniform often includes a name tag that lists your name and title. It is your responsibility to follow facility policy regarding the uniform code.

Dependability is an important quality of any employee of a health care facility. It is important that you remain healthy so that you can be depended on to be at work. It is your responsibility to let your employer know well in advance when you are ill and cannot report for work. You should call your supervisor personally and explain the situation. If you do not call until the beginning of your shift or if you do not call at all, replacing you will be very difficult. In some facilities, failure to call in an absence results in dismissal. Dependability also means you are responsible for doing the job that you were hired to do in the manner in which you were trained.

Job Limitations

The nursing assistant has certain job limitations and does not perform certain tasks. These will vary from one health care facility to another, but the following tasks usually are job limitations. Nursing assistants *do not*:

- give medications.
- apply prescription creams or ointments to the resident's skin.
- give reports on residents' medical condition to family members or others.
- take orders from the doctor.
- perform any procedures they have not been taught.
- perform any tasks forbidden by state law or the policies of the institution.

Whenever you are not sure of a task or procedure, always ask the charge nurse for help.

THE INTERDISCIPLINARY HEALTH CARE TEAM

A nursing assistant is a part of the very important **interdisciplinary team.** The goal of the entire staff of the long-term care facility is to provide the best care possible for the residents. This requires the cooperation of staff in all departments. We each may think the service we provide is the most important, but cannot care for the resident unless all of us are doing our jobs. Care provided in the long-term care facility is designed to help the resident maintain the highest level of functioning possible considering the resident's condition. Many individuals work together for the resident's benefit. Every member of the team contributes to the resident's care.

Members of the Interdisciplinary Team

The following individuals make up the interdisciplinary team:

- resident, family, or legal guardian
- physician
- nursing staff
- staff members from the various therapy departments, including physical, occupational, speech, respiratory, and activity therapy
- social workers
- dietary staff
- housekeeping, maintenance, and laundry staff
- office, administrative, and clerical workers
- **clergy**
- other staff from within or outside the nursing facility as required to help meet the residents' needs

ETHICS FOR THE NURSING ASSISTANT

Ethics is part of a moral code that guides the behavior of the health care worker. Ethics involves making judgments about what is right and what is wrong. An ethical nursing assistant is one who:

- promotes health, independence, safety, and quality of life for each resident.
- respects each resident as an individual and treats all residents with respect.
- understands and follows all the principles covered by the Resident's Bill of Rights.
- respects the resident's area as the private space of that resident and treats the personal belongings of the resident with care.
- keeps information about the resident confidential.
- respects the resident's right to privacy.
- maintains a positive attitude toward the facility.
- functions as a member of the health care team working within the limits of the job description, facility policies, and state laws.

- acts as a responsible employee at all times.
- performs procedures only in the manner trained and does not take shortcuts.
- accepts no money, tips, or favors for service to the resident.
- considers the resident's needs to be most important.
- demonstrates **etiquette;** that is, exhibits a polite, courteous, and kind attitude to residents, visitors, and other staff members.

LEGAL ISSUES FOR THE NURSING ASSISTANT

Laws are rules passed by governmental agencies and are to be obeyed by everyone. If you do not obey the law, you could be found liable. If you do things in the manner in which you were taught, you will be following the law. Situations to *avoid* are as follows:

- **Negligence** involves being careless and failing to give the care needed and expected by the resident.
- **Theft** is taking something that does not belong to you.
- **Aiding and abetting** involves seeing someone doing something wrong or stealing something and not reporting it.
- **False imprisonment** is restricting someone's movement without permission; for example, applying restraints without proper authorization.
- **Involuntary seclusion** is isolating a resident as a form of punishment.
- **Assault** means trying to or threatening to touch a resident's body without permission.
- **Battery** means touching the resident without permission.
- **Invasion of privacy** involves failure of the nursing assistant to keep resident information confidential or exposing the resident's body when care is being given.
- **Abuse** means doing physical or mental harm to the resident, or threatening the resident with harm.

THE RESIDENT'S CARE PLAN

Within 21 days of admission to a long-term care facility, a comprehensive written **care plan** is developed. A temporary care plan is usually started to provide guidelines for care until the resident is thoroughly assessed by the interdisciplinary team and the comprehensive care plan is completed. The comprehensive care plan is developed in a staff conference to which the resident and family members of the resident's choosing are invited. The resident's strengths are used as a basis to overcome problems and needs. Long- and short-term goals are defined and agreed upon by everyone present. The care plan lists approaches to help the resident meet the goals within a set period of time and states who is responsible for each approach. The care plan assures that the resident will have **continuity of care.** All staff members are expected to use the care plan as the basis of the care they give, so everyone works toward the same goals and uses the same approaches. As a nursing assistant, you are responsible for knowing what your job is and how it relates to the care plan (Figure 1-2). Ask your supervisor about anything you do not understand. If you notice that certain approaches are not working or if you discover something else that is not listed on the care plan works, inform your supervisor. The care plan is updated quarterly, and whenever there is a change in the resident's condition.

An important responsibility you have as a nursing assistant is to notice any changes in the resident. Any changes, no matter how minor they seem, must be reported to the supervising nurse. When observing and reporting, you must be accurate. Reporting too much is better than forgetting to report something.

INDIVIDUALIZED CARE

The long-term care facility is home to many different types of residents. Because patients stay in hospitals for shorter periods, we are seeing many residents come to the long-term care facility to complete their recovery. Many long-term care facilities are developing special units for these residents. You may find one entire facility that specializes in a certain type of care. Some facilities have separate areas or units that provide specialized care. Many long-term care facilities do not specialize; they admit persons with any type of disability. The reasons for admission to the long-term care facility may vary widely, which emphasizes the importance of individualized care for each resident.

Although the residents' ages may vary, most of the residents are elderly. People are living longer than ever before. As one ages, the resistance to disease, stress, and injury decreases. Therefore, the elderly are more likely to require help in meeting their personal needs. It is important that each resident be treated as an individual. Remember the following when giving individualized care:

- Each resident is a separate person with different wants and needs.

NURSING ASSISTANT CARE PLAN

DIETARY

Diabetic _____ Calorie ☐

Dining Room: (Bkfst) (Lunch) (Dinner)

Room: Bkfst.   Lunch   Dinner

Feeder Room: Bkfst.   Lunch   Dinner

Set Tray Up ☒

Feed ☐

Tube Feeding ☐

Adaptive Equipment

Regular
Diet

House supplement 2p+HS
Nourishment/Supplement/HS Snack

Measure:

Intake ☒

Output ☒

ELIMINATION

Toilet q 2 hrs. ☒

Bedpan/Urinal ☐

Incontinence Bowel ☐

Incontinence Bladder ☐

Catheter

Foley ☐

Supra Pubic ☐

Condom ☐

Leg Bag ☐

Catheter Strap ☐

Ostomy ☐

RESTRAINTS

Vest: When _____ ☐

Waist (soft) When in Chair ☐

Mitts _____ ☐

Geri Chair ☐

Roller Bar: When in W/C ☐

Lap Belt ☐

Other *Self release belt* ☒

Restrain at All Times ☐

SIDERAILS

At All Times ☐

At Night Only ☒

Signed Release: ☐

Do not use any restraint not checked above.
Observe q 30 minutes and release q 2 hours x's
10 minutes for care/exercise.

BATHING

Tub ☐

Shower ☒

Bed ☐

Day: M (T) W (T) F (S) S

AM ☐   PM ☒

Shampoo

Beauty Shop ☐

Staff ☒

AM/PM Care

Self ☒

Staff ☐

Shave by Noon, Remove Facial
Hair. Finger Nail Care on
Bath/Shower Day. Toe Nail Care
as Directed by Nurse.

HEARING

Hard of Hearing:

Right ☐   Left ☒

Hearing Aid:

Right ☐   Left ☒

Look at Resident While
Speaking to Them.

FREQUENCY OF VITAL SIGNS

Weight *weekly*

TPR *monthly*

B/P *monthly*

POSITIONING

Turn q 2 hours ☒

Range of Motion with Cares ☒

Special Mattress/Device

Sheepskin

Positioning Equip.

_____

Braces/Splints/Cones

(R) *Hand splint.*

Follow Turning Schedule.

DRESSING

Self ☐

Assist ☒

Supervise ☐

Total ☐

Adult Brief ☐

Lap robe ☐

All Residents to Wear
Underwear.

SIGHT

Blind:

Right ☐   Left ☐

Poor Vision ☐

Glasses ☒

Contact Lens ☐

Clean Glasses or Contact
Lens with A.M. Care.

ORAL CARE

Self ☐

Assist ☒

Own Teeth ☐

No Teeth ☐

Dentures:

Upper ☒

Lower ☐

Partial ☐

Oral Care in A.M., at
Bedtime and PRN.

MOBILITY

Independent ☐

Cane ☐

Walker ☒

Wheelchair ☒

Own ☐

Other ☐

No Weight Bearing:

Right ☐   Left ☐

Partial Weight Bearing

Right ☐   Left ☐

Gait Belt ☒

Transfer ☐

Hoyer Lift ☐

No. of Assist for Transfers

_____

Other _____

Special Instructions:

*ABL Goals: Wash face,
hands, & chest. Will
put on blouse & button it.
Mobility Goals: Ambulate c̄ gait belt,
Walker, and minimum assist to
dining room for lunch each day.
Encourage independence c̄ selfcare.
Allow the resident to struggle slightly.
but not to the point of frustration.
Praise her efforts, then assist her in
completing the task.*

Room No.: *203-2*   Date: *1/4/97*

Resident: *Wallace, Eleanor*

Figure 1-2 A nursing assistant care plan.

- Help residents to become and remain independent.
- Maintain dignity by treating residents appropriately for their age.
- Allowing residents to do as much as possible and promoting and encouraging independence adds to feelings of dignity and self-worth.
- Offer choices whenever possible. This helps the resident maintain a sense of control and adds to self-esteem.
- If the resident cannot complete a skill independently, compliment him or her for the part he or she was able to complete. Finish the task without complaint.
- Allow residents who are completely unable to perform self-care to direct you in their care. Directing the care verbally gives the resident a sense of control and improves self-esteem.
- Be involved with the resident's family, and be aware of activity programs that include family members.
- Schedule care to allow residents to participate in activity programs.
- Assist residents to meet their physical, psychosocial, and spiritual needs by using the approaches listed on the care plan.

RESTORATIVE CARE

Restorative care is care given to help the resident become as independent as possible, considering the limitations of his or her medical condition. Restorative care is highly individualized based on the resident's strengths and needs. When providing restorative care, we look at the whole person, not just the disease or diagnosis. The goal of this type of care is to help the resident function at the highest level possible. This includes physical function, mental function, and psychosocial well-being. The care plan will guide the nursing assistant on what restorative measures to take and how to do them. The nursing assistant should maintain a restorative attitude by believing that restorative approaches will help the resident. Maintaining a restorative attitude takes patience. It takes time for residents to learn new skills. Even learning new ways to do previously learned skills does not happen immediately. Patience and a consistent approach from all caregivers will help the resident learn new skills and regain abilities lost due to illness or injury. Doing things for residents that they can do for themselves does not help the resident. Over time, residents lose the ability to perform certain activities if they do not practice them consis-

tently. The nursing assistant's role here is to offer support and encouragement, and allow enough time for the resident to complete tasks independently. If the resident is having difficulty, it is the nursing assistant's responsibility to suggest easier ways of doing the task. If you are not sure, consult the care plan or the charge nurse. Over the long term, providing restorative care is very beneficial to the resident physically and helps the resident to develop healthy self-esteem.

BODY SYSTEMS

The human body is made up of tiny cells. Similar cells group together to form organs. Similar organs group together to form systems. There are 10 body systems. These are the:

- integumentary system
- skeletal system
- muscular system
- endocrine system
- reproductive system
- digestive system
- cardiovascular (circulatory) system
- respiratory system
- urinary system
- nervous system

All systems must function normally for the person to be healthy. One might think that if one system was weak, the other, stronger systems, would make up for it. In fact, the reverse is true. One weak system will affect the resident's entire body and state of health.

NORMAL AGING PROCESS

Because many residents in a long-term care facility are elderly, having a general understanding of the normal aging process is important for the nursing assistant. All nursing care is given to help residents reach their highest state of health, well-being, and independence. When in good **health,** the body functions properly. In **disease,** the body is not functioning as it should.

Body Systems and Normal Aging

All parts of the body are affected by the normal aging process. When studying the body, we look at it as a group of systems that work together. A body system is a group of organs working together to do a particular function. A brief overview of body systems and how the aging process affects each follows.

Integumentary System. The integumentary system includes the skin, hair, and nails. Sweat and oil glands are part of the exocrine glands.

- Changes in normal aging:
  — Skin becomes fragile, tears easily, and loses fatty tissue under skin.
  — Hair thins and grays.
  — Nails thicken and harden.
  — Less natural oil and sweat are produced.
  — Circulation to the skin decreases.

- Results of normal aging:
  — Skin is less sensitive to heat.
  — Skin is less resistant to injury.
  — Skin bruises and tears more readily.
  — Skin becomes drier.
  — Tissues heal slowly.
  — Changes in skin and other systems make body regulation of temperature more difficult. The elderly often complain of feeling cold.

- Nursing assistant responsibilities:
  — Protect residents' skin from injury by padding side rails, arms of chairs, and so on. Long-sleeved clothing also helps protect the skin.
  — Keep residents' skin clean, dry, and free from secretions and excretions.
  — Use lotions as the resident requests and as stated on the care plan.
  — Report any injuries or changes in the appearance of the skin to the charge nurse.
  — Know your facility policy for providing nail care. Some facilities do not allow nursing assistants to trim nails. Most facilities require nursing assistants to clean nails, but some do not allow the use of sharp objects, such as nail files.
  — Prevent pressure sores from developing.

Skeletal System. The skeletal system includes the bones and joints.

- Changes in normal aging:
  — Bones become porous and brittle.
  — The spine becomes less flexible and stable, and is more easily injured.
  — Joints become less flexible.

- Results of normal aging:
  — Fractures occur easily.
  — Loss of height occurs.

- Nursing assistant responsibilities:
  — Monitor the resident's nutrition to be sure that the diet is balanced.
  — Provide a safe environment to prevent injury.
  — Assist the resident to use devices to make ambulation easier, if ordered.

Muscular System.
- Changes in normal aging:
  — Muscles lose strength and bulk.
  — Ligaments become less flexible.

- Results of normal aging:
  — Slower movements.
  — Less strength.
  — Posture may become stooped.

- Nursing assistant responsibilities:
  — Help the resident exercise to prevent contractures, or deformities of the joints.
  — Perform range-of-motion exercises as directed by the care plan.
  — Be patient with the resident. Avoid completing tasks for the resident to save time.

Endocrine System.
- Changes in normal aging:
  — Decreased production of estrogen and progesterone.
  — Insulin production becomes less efficient.

- Results of normal aging:
  — Weight gain.
  — Diabetes mellitus.

- Nursing assistant responsibilities:
  — Monitor the resident for signs and symptoms of diabetes mellitus.
  — If the resident is diabetic, monitor for signs and symptoms of hyperglycemia and hypoglycemia.
  — Monitor weight monthly, or as stated on the care plan.

Reproductive System.

- Changes in normal aging:
  Females:

  — Ovulation and menstruation cease.
  — Vaginal walls become thinner and drier.
  Males:

  — Scrotum enlarges and becomes less firm.
  — Prostate gland may enlarge.

- Results of normal aging:
  Females:

  — Increased risk of injury and infection.
  Males:

  — Difficulty with urination.

- Nursing assistant responsibilities:

  — Assist with cleanliness and personal hygiene by providing proper perineal care.
  — Monitor for signs and symptoms of infection, and report to the nurse.
  — In males, monitor for urinary dribbling, urine retention, difficulty with starting flow of urine, and frequency of urination.

Digestive System.   The digestive system includes the stomach, intestines, and other organs that help digest food.

- Changes in normal aging:

  — Digestive system gradually slows.
  — Appetite decreases.
  — Sense of thirst decreases.
  — Chewing ability is often decreased due to loss of teeth and dental problems.
  — Loss of primary tastebuds of sweet and salt.

- Results of normal aging:

  — Constipation may occur.
  — Residents may consume less food and not take in enough nutrients and fluids in the diet.
  — Residents may increase condiment use at meals.

- Nursing assistant responsibilities:

  — Monitor residents' bowel movements and record them according to facility policy.
  — Report signs of constipation to the nurse.
  — Report dental caries and unusual mouth odors.

  — Check dentures for proper fit.
  — Monitor resident food intake and record it according to facility policy.
  — Offer substitutes if residents do not eat food items on their tray.
  — Eliminate unpleasant sights, odors, and sounds when residents are eating.
  — Make mealtime pleasant and encourage residents to eat. Help them if necessary.
  — Report to the nurse if the resident eats less than 75 percent of a meal.
  — Report changes in weight to the nurse.
  — Pass snacks and supplements; assist and encourage residents to consume them, and record the percentage.

Cardiovascular System.   The cardiovascular system includes the heart and blood vessels. The circulatory system is restricted to the blood vessels.

- Changes in normal aging:

  — Cardiac output is reduced.
  — Blood vessels become less elastic.
  — Inner walls of blood vessels become narrow.
  — Heart disease is common in the elderly.

- Results of normal aging:

  — Residents may need to rest more frequently.
  — Exercise is necessary to stimulate circulation.
  — Blood pressure may be elevated.
  — Heart rate decreases.
  — Fluid may collect in tissues, especially in the lower legs and feet.

- Nursing assistant responsibilities:

  — Monitor vital signs as instructed by the nurse.
  — Report blue color of the skin immediately, especially in the lips and nail beds.
  — Report swollen areas to the nurse.
  — Provide adequate rest periods between activities.
  — Help and encourage the resident to exercise in the manner stated on the care plan.

Respiratory System.   The respiratory system includes the lungs and air passages.

- Changes in normal aging:

  — Exchange of oxygen and carbon dioxide are decreased.

— Lungs lose some elasticity.

— Breathing capacity is decreased.

— Deep breathing is more difficult.

- Results of normal aging:

    — Respiratory infections are more likely.

    — Respiratory changes may make an elderly person more tired.

- Nursing assistant responsibilities:

    — Report difficulty breathing to the charge nurse immediately.

    — Know positions that promote good air exchange.

    — Monitor for and report shortness of breath on exertion.

    — Encourage residents to breathe deeply.

Urinary System.   The urinary system includes the kidneys and bladder. A common word for the elimination process performed by this system is urination or voiding.

- Changes in normal aging:

    — Kidney function is reduced.

    — Bladder elasticity decreases.

    — Men often have prostate enlargement.

- Results of normal aging:

    — Bladder emptying is less efficient.

    — More urinary infections occur.

    — Need to empty the bladder is often urgent and frequent.

    — Coughing and sneezing may cause women to be unable to control urine passage.

    — Men may have trouble urinating.

- Nursing assistant responsibilities:

    — Report changes in color, consistency, amount, and odor of urine.

    — Report painful or burning urination.

    — Toilet residents according to the schedule on the care plan.

    — In mentally confused residents, monitor behavior for clues of the need to toilet.

    — Do not scold residents if accidents occur.

    — Keep residents clean, dry, and odor-free.

    — Assist with bowel and bladder evaluations and programs.

Central Nervous System.   The central nervous system includes the brain and spinal cord. The nervous system involves nerve endings.

- Changes in normal aging:

    — Nerve cells are lost.

    — Reaction time to stimuli is slower.

    — Blood flow to the brain is decreased.

    — Diseases of these systems may cause physical or mental disability.

- Results of normal aging:

    — More time is needed when caring for many elderly residents.

    — Residents may need more time to make choices.

- Nursing assistant responsibilities:

    — Keep the environment safe and free from hazards.

    — Know seizure precautions to follow.

    — Monitor water temperatures with a thermometer before bathing residents.

    — Be patient and allow the resident adequate time to perform activities.

The Senses.   The eyes, ears, nose, and tastebuds of the mouth are part of the senses.

- Changes in normal aging:

    — All senses gradually slow down.

    — Vision and hearing acuity decreases.

- Results of normal aging:

    — Vision, hearing, and agility are reduced.

    — Irritations on skin and feet may go unnoticed due to less sensation or feeling.

- Nursing assistant responsibilities:

    — Know how to communicate with residents who have vision and hearing impairments.

    — Be patient and allow enough time for the resident to answer questions.

    — Keep the environment safe and hazard-free.

    — Report observations about resident skin condition to the nurse.

Becoming aware of these normal changes in the aging process is important. The changes that occur in these body systems will affect the manner of care needed for each resident. For your convenience, aging changes are summarized in Table 1-1.

TABLE 1-1 Aging Changes

Body System	Aging Changes
Circulatory	■ Heart rate slows, causing a slower pulse and less efficient circulation. The resident has less energy and slower responses. He or she tires easily. ■ Blood vessels lose elasticity and develop calcium deposits, causing vessels to narrow. ■ Blood pressure increases because of changes to the blood vessel walls. ■ Heart rate takes longer to return to normal after exercise. ■ Veins enlarge, causing blood vessels close to the skin surface to become more prominent.
Respiratory	■ Lung capacity decreases as a result of muscular rigidity in the lungs. ■ The ability to cough effectively is reduced; this results in pooling of secretions and fluid in the lungs, increasing the risk of infection and choking. ■ Shortness of breath on exertion as a result of aging changes in lungs. ■ Gas exchange in the lungs is less effective, resulting in decreased oxygenation.
Integumentary	■ Skin thins and loses elasticity, wrinkles appear, skin becomes irritated and breaks, cuts, and tears easily. ■ Increased fragility of blood vessels that nourish the skin, causing bruising, senile purpura, and skin tears. ■ Reduced blood flow in vessels that nourish the skin results in delayed healing. ■ Reduced secretion from oil glands that supply the skin causes dryness and itching. ■ Decreased perspiration, resulting in impaired ability to regulate temperature. ■ Subcutaneous fat diminishes, resulting in less protection and complaints of feeling cold. ■ Blood supply to the feet and legs is reduced, increasing risk of injury and ulcers, feeling of coldness. ■ Fingernail and toenail growth slows and nails become brittle. ■ Hair thins and turns gray.
Urinary	■ Bladder capacity decreases, increasing the frequency of urination. ■ Kidney function increases at rest, causing increased urination at night. ■ Weakening of bladder muscles, causing leaking of urine or inability to empty the bladder completely. ■ Enlargement of the prostate gland in the male, causing frequency of urination, dribbling, urinary obstruction, and urinary retention.
Digestive (Gastrointestinal)	■ Decreased saliva production in the mouth, causing difficulty with digestion of starches. ■ Tastebuds on the tongue decrease, beginning with sweet and salt; changes in tastebuds may result in appetite changes and increase in condiment use. ■ Gag reflex is less effective, increasing the risk of choking. ■ Movement of food into the stomach through the esophagus is slower. ■ Slower digestion of food in the stomach, so food remains there longer before moving to the small intestine. ■ Indigestion and slower absorption of fat as a result of decreased digestive enzymes. ■ Food movement through the large intestine is slower, resulting in constipation.
Endocrine	■ Delayed release of insulin, increasing blood sugar level; incidence of diabetes increases greatly with age. ■ Metabolism rate and body function slow, reducing the amount of calories needed for the body to function normally. This increases the risk of overweight and obesity.

(continues)

Reproductive	Changes in the Male
	■ Hormone production decreases, decreasing size of testes and lowering sperm count.
	■ More time required for an erection.
	Changes in the Female
	■ Fewer female hormones are produced.
	■ Vagina becomes shorter and narrower.
	■ Vaginal secretions decrease.
	■ Breast tissue decreases and the muscles supporting the breasts weaken.
Nervous	■ Tasks involving speed, balance, coordination, and fine motor activities take longer because of slowed transmission of nerve impulses.
	■ Balance and coordination problems as a result of deterioration in the nerve terminals that provide information to the brain about body movement and position.
	■ Visual changes result from decreased flexibility in the lens in the eye.
	■ Dryness and itching of the eyes as a result of decreased secretion of fluids.
	■ Difficulty hearing due to a decrease in the nerves and blood supply to the ears.
	■ Risk of injury increases because of decreased ability to feel pressure and temperature changes.
	■ Decreased blood flow to the brain, which may result in mental confusion and memory loss.
Musculoskeletal	■ Loss of elasticity of muscles and decrease in size of muscle mass result in reduced strength, endurance, muscle tone, and delayed reaction time.
	■ Bones lose minerals, become brittle, and break more easily.
	■ Spine becomes less stable and flexible, increasing the risk of injury.
	■ Posture may become slumped over because of weakness in back muscles.
	■ Degenerative changes in the joints cause limited movement, stiffness, and pain.

Generalizations Relating to Normal Aging

You have already learned that each resident is an individual. However, some general statements are true about normal aging:

- All body systems are affected.
- Resistance to injury and disease is decreased.
- People age at different rates.
- All body systems gradually slow down.
- The aging process is affected by lifestyle, heredity, and nutrition; mental, physical, and emotional health; and by attitude.

KEY POINTS IN THIS CHAPTER

▲ The nursing assistant provides personal care while working under the supervision of a nurse.

▲ The person living in a long-term care facility is a resident.

▲ A nursing assistant is part of the nursing service team.

▲ Good health, honesty, dependability, and sincere desire to work with people are required qualities of a nursing assistant.

▲ The job description is a list of tasks and duties you are expected to perform as a nursing assistant.

▲ Your assignment is made by the nurse and may include working with any resident, male or female.

▲ Cooperation with all members of the health care team is an important part of your role.

▲ The care plan is a written plan that describes strengths, weaknesses, interventions, and goals for each resident and directs resident care.

▲ Each resident is an individual and must be treated with respect and dignity.

▲ All body systems gradually slow down.

REVIEW QUIZ

1. Nursing assistants may also be called:
   a. practical nurses.
   b. nurse aides.
   c. nurse helpers.
   d. registered nurses.

2. Persons who live in long-term care facilities are called:
   a. clients.
   b. patients.
   c. residents.
   d. retired.

3. Which term means care of the elderly?
   a. resident
   b. medical
   c. nursing
   d. geriatrics

4. Who is the nursing assistant's supervisor?
   a. licensed nurse
   b. physician
   c. administrator
   d. therapist

5. Which department in the long-term care facility is the nursing assistant a part of?
   a. administration
   b. nursing
   c. dietary
   d. housekeeping

6. Which of the following qualifications are necessary for the nursing assistant?
   a. honesty
   b. dependability
   c. reliability
   d. all of the above

7. The responsibilities of a nursing assistant are listed in a:
   a. job description.
   b. policy manual.
   c. procedure manual.
   d. resume.

8. Some tasks and duties a nursing assistant is expected to do include:
   a. taking doctors' orders.
   b. giving medications.
   c. helping residents with personal care.
   d. all of the above.

9. Male and female nursing assistants:
   a. usually work on separate units of the facility.
   b. work with nursing assistants of the same sex.
   c. are expected to care for residents of either sex.
   d. care for only same sex residents.

10. Part of the uniform you will wear daily includes:
    a. caps or hats.
    b. isolation gowns.
    c. sterile gloves.
    d. a name tag.

11. What should you do if you are not certain of a task assigned to you?
    a. Tell the nurse you are unsure of the task and ask for help.
    b. Ask another nursing assistant to do it.
    c. Forget about doing the task.
    d. Do the task anyway.

12. Which of the following are members of the interdisciplinary team in the long-term care facility?
    a. nursing staff
    b. dietary personnel
    c. social workers
    d. all of the above

13. A written plan listing strengths, needs, goals, interventions, and who is responsible for assisting with specific tasks in the care of the resident is the:
    a. assignment sheet.
    b. care plan.
    c. job description.
    d. team report.

14. Which of the following statements is true regarding the normal aging process?
    a. All body systems slow down with aging.
    b. All elderly residents age at the same rate.
    c. The nervous system is the only system that is visibly affected by aging.
    d. all of the above

15. Ethical behavior for the nursing assistant means to:
    a. practice good body mechanics.
    b. cooperate with others.
    c. know what is right and what is wrong.
    d. all of the above.

16. Mrs. King has asked for pain medication. When you tell the nurse, she is very busy. You should:
    a. offer to take the medication to Mrs. King.
    b. inform the nurse that Mrs. King is requesting pain medication.
    c. do nothing and tell the nurse later.
    d. tell Mrs. King that the nurse is too busy to give her the medicine.

17. The nursing assistant who is assigned to care for Mr. Redman is off the unit on break. Mr. Redman's call signal is on. You should:
    a. ignore the signal.
    b. tell Mr. Redman that his assigned nursing assistant will do what he asks when she returns to the unit.
    c. answer the signal and find out what the resident wants.
    d. inform the nurse that Mr. Redman has his call signal on.

18. A resident speaks with you about a financial matter. She says that she does not want her son to know that she has money in a savings account at Capital Bank. You should:
    a. tell the resident's son about the account.
    b. tell the other nursing assistants about the bank account.
    c. advise the resident to tell her doctor about the account and ask for his advice.
    d. say nothing about the bank account.

19. Mrs. Burns tells you that you are her "favorite nursing assistant." At Christmas, she puts a $20.00 bill in your pocket and insists that you take it. You should:
    a. thank Mrs. Burns and accept the money.
    b. tell Mrs. Burns you will do special favors for her because of the gift.
    c. advise the resident that you cannot accept money from her and that you are happy to care for her without gifts.
    d. tell Mrs. Burns that you can only accept gifts from her family because facility policy prohibits you from accepting gifts from residents.

20. You are assigned to care for Mrs. Beattie. She is in a restorative care program so that she can return to her home when she recovers from her illness and becomes more independent. Her care plan states that she is to wash her face, hands, and chest, then the nursing assistant is to complete her bath. When you hand Mrs. Beattie the washcloth, she tells you that she will not bathe herself. The resident says, "I am paying you to take care of me, so you will do it." You should:
    a. tell the resident that you are not being paid specifically to bathe her.
    b. ask Mrs. Beattie why she feels this way, and tell her why it is important that she do as much of her own care as she can.
    c. begin to wash Mrs. Beattie's face, because this is what she wants.
    d. inform Mrs. Beattie that you are too busy to bathe her, and that you have others to care for who need your help more than she does.

21. Mr. McClure is a resident who yells and complains frequently. He tells you that he will "have you fired" if you do not give him extra sugar packets for his coffee. Mr. McClure is on a diabetic diet. You know that sugar is not allowed on a diabetic diet. You should:
    a. tell the resident that the sugar is not allowed on his diet and that he has no right to threaten you.
    b. give Mr. McClure as much sugar as he wants because you need your job.
    c. offer Mr. McClure a sugar substitute, then notify the nurse of his threats.
    d. pretend that you don't hear Mr. McClure ask for more sugar and leave the room quickly.

CHAPTER 1
CROSSWORD PUZZLE

Directions: Complete the puzzle using these words found in Chapter 1.

acute	dignity	OBRA
attitude	disease	patient
care	ethics	plan
charge	geriatrics	privacy
client	health	resident
dependability	interdisciplinary	restorative
description	negligence	theft

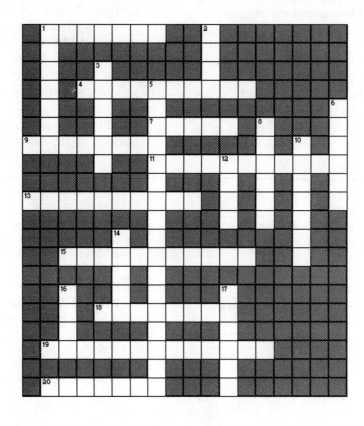

CHAPTER 1
PUZZLE CLUES

ACROSS

1. Exposing the resident's body when giving care is a form of invasion of _____ .
4. Carelessness, failing to give care needed.
7. Taking something that does not belong to you.
9. Your _____ is an outer reflection of your inner feelings.
11. _____ care is designed to help the resident reach his highest level of functioning.
13. Care of the elderly is also known as _____ .
15. A listing of the nursing assistant's responsibilities can be found in the job _____ .
18. The person being cared for in a long-term care facility.
19. Being trustworthy, able to be relied upon.
20. _____ means treating a person with respect and honor.

DOWN

1. The person being cared for in the hospital.
2. Instructions for taking care of the resident are usually found on the care _____ .
3. Freedom from disease, wellness.
5. The _____ team meets to plan the care of the resident based on an assessment of strengths and needs.
6. The person being cared for in the home is usually called the _____ .
8. Your immediate supervisor is usually the _____ nurse.
10. A state of illness when the body does not function properly.
12. Omnibus Budget Reconciliation Act.
14. A hospital is an example of an _____ care facility.
16. The nursing assistant is responsible for helping the resident with personal _____ .
17. Principles, values, rules of moral, responsible conduct.

Basic Human Needs

OBJECTIVES

In this chapter you will learn the importance of basic human needs and ways you can help residents meet these needs. After reading this chapter, you will be able to:

- Spell and define key terms.
- Describe basic needs common to all people and list ways that the nursing assistant can assist residents in meeting their needs.
- Identify developmental tasks associated with the aging process.
- Explain why understanding the resident's culture is important to the nursing assistant.
- List the steps of the grieving process and describe what occurs in each step.
- Identify coping mechanisms for grief and loss.
- Describe changes that occur when the resident is dying and list nursing assistant responsibilities.
- Demonstrate postmortem care.

KEY TERMS

acceptance: the final stage in the grieving process, in which the resident is calmly waiting for death

anger: the second step in the grieving process, in which the resident is angry because of a terminal diagnosis

apathy: indifference, emptiness, lack of feeling or emotion

bargaining: the third stage in the grieving process, in which the resident attempts to buy more time.

coping mechanisms: responses to stress that people use to protect feelings of self-esteem

culture: a pattern or lifestyle of a group of people

denial: refusing to accept something as the truth; also, the first stage in the grieving process, in which the resident refuses to believe the terminal diagnosis

depression: the fourth stage in the grieving process, in which the resident is trying to deal with the loss of everything he or she has

developmental tasks: tasks that must be accomplished in each stage of life if a person is to mature in a healthy manner

grieving process: stages of grief that a dying person and family members go through to move to a point of acceptance of illness and death

personal space: a comfortable distance for communication

physiological needs: physical human needs

postmortem care: care of the body after death

psychological needs (psychosocial needs): the emotional, spiritual, and mental needs of human beings

religion: a formal system of beliefs, including cere-monies and rituals that demonstrate faith

self-actualization: the state of having achieved one's full potential or ability

self-esteem: satisfaction with oneself

spiritual needs: needs concerning one's spiritual or religious beliefs

spirituality: any way that people answer the desire to be connected with the largeness or wholeness of life

stereotyping: placing all members of a group into one category and believing they are all alike

therapeutic: to cure, heal, or preserve health

HUMAN NEEDS

All people have the same basic human needs, de-spite their age, sex, position, or status in life. Some needs, however, come first and must be satisfied be-fore other needs become important. For example, breathing is more important than eating, although both are necessary to live. When our physical needs are met, we move up to higher levels of needs, such as safety and security, and love and belonging (Fig-ure 2-1). These basic needs are what cause people to behave as they do (Figure 2-2).

Figure 2-1 Showing care and concern for residents is an important nursing assistant responsibility.

Knowledge of basic human needs will help you understand and give better care to the resident. The resident who is always calling for attention may need to feel a sense of love and belonging. Many residents in the long-term care facility must have help to meet their needs.

Basic human needs can be grouped into two cat-egories: physical and psychological. Physical needs are called **physiological.** These needs concern the body and are necessary for survival.

Other needs involve the emotional, spiritual, or mental relationships of humans. The terms to de-scribe this emotional type of need are **psychologi-cal** or **psychosocial.**

All the basic human needs are equally important. These needs must be at least partially met for a per-son to be healthy. Learning about ways to meet these needs will help you give quality care to each resident. People from different countries and cul-tures may have different needs and customs. Be sen-sitive to these differences.

Physical Needs and Ways to Help the Resident Meet These Needs

Assist residents to meet physical needs as follows:

* Food
  — Provide adequate lighting and a clean area before serving the meal tray. Eliminate un-pleasant sights and odors.

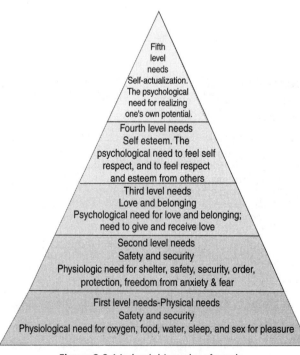

Figure 2-2 Maslow's hierarchy of needs.

— Make mealtime as pleasant as possible.

— Help the resident eat, if needed.

— Position the resident correctly to enable swallowing and prevent choking.

— Thicken liquids on tray as described in the care plan.

— Help the resident with special foods.

— Feed the resident when necessary.

— Provide special utensils if the resident needs them.

— Give the resident oral hygiene before and after meals.

— Assist the resident to use the toilet before and after meals.

— Position the resident close to the table so she does not have to reach for food. The elbows should not be dangling in the air; they should be supported when eating, if this is the resident's preference.

— Ensure that the table height is correct, and not too high for the resident.

• Oxygen, air

— Elevate head of bed for residents who have breathing problems.

— Properly position residents in bed and chairs.

— Make sure clothing or other garments are not too tight.

— Assist with oxygen therapy when necessary. Check the flow meter for accuracy each time you are in the room.

— Know how to perform the Heimlich maneuver.

• Water

— Offer fluids frequently, especially in hot weather.

— Keep fresh water within reach at all times.

— Thicken liquids as described in the care plan.

— Help the resident drink, if needed.

— Monitor intake and output, if ordered.

• Elimination, toileting

— Assist residents with toileting needs.

— Provide privacy during elimination.

— Be calm and unemotional in your response to residents who are unable to control the passage of urine or stool.

— Assist residents with personal hygiene needs after elimination.

• Rest

— Help with bedtime and sleep preparation.

— Let the resident determine bedtime and routines before going to sleep.

— Recognize any changes in sleep patterns.

— Allow the resident to rest during the day, if desired.

• Activity and exercise

— Encourage range-of-motion exercise during routine care and activities of daily living (ADLs).

— Ambulate, transfer, and move residents properly.

— Help residents to ambulate, walk, or exercise frequently as indicated on the care plan.

— Assist residents to participate in activities of choice.

— Remind residents of scheduled activities, plan care around them, and assist residents to activities if needed.

— Encourage residents to be as independent as possible when it is consistent with the care plan.

• Stimulation

— Encourage involvement in facility activities.

— Take time to listen to residents and encourage them to talk and visit.

— Place residents in areas where they can observe activity.

— Do not isolate residents.

— When seating residents, arrange seating to promote socialization.

• Sexuality

— Assist residents with hygiene, cleanliness, and grooming.

— Encourage the use of appropriate clothing, cosmetics, and hair styles to maintain sexual identity (Figure 2-3).

— Compliment the resident on his or her appearance.

— Provide privacy to couples expressing intimacy needs. Knock before entering rooms.

— If a resident is masturbating, respond in a neutral manner. Take the resident to his or her room and provide privacy. Be nonjudgmental, and do not make the resident feel guilty or foolish. Remember, all humans need sexual satisfaction.

Figure 2-3 Sexuality is expressed by attractive appearance and touch. The ability to express sexuality is important to residents of all ages.

Safety and Security Needs and Ways to Help the Resident Meet These Needs

Ways to help residents meet their safety and security needs are as follows:

- Safety

  — Keep the area safe and free of hazards.

  — Keep the call signal and needed personal items within reach of all residents, even those who are mentally confused.

  — Perform your job duties in the manner in which you were trained.

  — If you are unsure of how to perform a task, consult your supervisor and the facility procedure manual.

  — Know which tasks you legally can do.

  — Use lifting aids and transfer belts when indicated.

  — Follow your facility policy for use of side rails and restraints.

  — Always be alert to safety. Think safety first when you enter a resident's room and last when you leave the room.

- Security

  — Respect the resident's belongings and handle them with care.

  — Help the resident adjust to new surroundings, other residents, and staff.

  — Reassure residents, providing physical and mental support.

  — Welcome family and friends.

  — Provide privacy. Knock on doors and wait for response before entering the room.

  — Maintain confidentiality when the resident tells you something.

  — Keep the environment safe and hazard-free.

  — Make the resident feel confident in your ability to do your job.

  — Keep the resident's belongings safe.

Love and Belonging Needs and Ways to Help the Resident Meet These Needs

You can help residents satisfy the needs of love and belonging in these ways:

- Caring about someone

  — Listen to the resident, and do not appear rushed. Encourage residents to talk of the past when appropriate.

  — Show interest in residents' family and experiences.

  — Encourage contact and visits with other residents.

  — Ask the nurse or social worker for information about the resident's past, if this information will help you care for the resident.

  — Realize that some residents may have close friends who are not family members.

- Being cared about

  — Show interest in the resident.

  — Touch residents gently to show that you care.

  — Show kindness and consideration.

  — Be kind and friendly to visitors and family members.

  — Inform and encourage family and friends to attend activities.

  — Family members may be invited to participate in the care conference with the resident's consent.

  — Be patient and understanding when interacting with residents.

  — Treat residents as you would like your family members to be treated.

  — Allow residents to cry if needed. Offer to stay with the resident. Offer support. Occasional crying is a way to relieve built-up stress, but frequent crying may indicate a serious problem that should be reported.

  — Provide a comfortable, homelike environment.

  — Place residents' personal items in a prominent place in the room.

Self-Esteem and Ways to Help the Resident Meet This Need

Residents' **self-esteem** is enhanced when the nursing assistant understands the following:

- Sense of identity and self-esteem

  — Always call the resident by the preferred name. If you are unsure, use Mr., Mrs., or Miss.

  — Include the resident in conversation and decisions about care.

  — Speak with the resident when providing care.

  — Show an interest in the resident's past and present activities.

  — Allow privacy when requested. Knock on doors and wait for a response before entering.

  — Allow choices whenever possible, and give the resident what is requested if it is not against the care plan.

  — If the resident's choice is against the care plan, inform the charge nurse.

  — Respect the resident's choice in clothing if it is appropriate and clean.

  — Respect individual differences in culture, heredity, interests, religion, and values.

  — Offer the resident as much control as possible over his or her personal space.

  — Allow the resident control over daily routines.

- Feeling important and worthwhile

  — Recognize residents' accomplishments and give praise freely.

  — Always acknowledge the resident's presence. Include the resident in your conversation with others in the room.

  — Respect the resident's property and personal items.

  — Talk to residents as adults.

  — Encourage independence as much as possible.

  — Allow residents to do as much as possible.

  — Show interest in family members and past accomplishments and experiences.

  — Be courteous to family members and encourage their continued involvement and visits.

  — Treat residents with dignity and respect.

  — Develop communication skills for vision- and hearing-impaired residents.

Self-Actualization, Religion, and Spirituality and Ways to Help the Resident Meet These Needs

Self-actualization is the state of having reached one's highest potential or ability in life. It is also a feeling of being satisfied with oneself.

Assist the resident to meet these needs as follows:

- Self-actualization

  — Look for the resident's strengths, and offer sincere praise.

  — Support hobbies, interests, and awareness of current events.

  — Encourage and praise accomplishments.

  — Take time to appreciate the history of the resident.

- Spirituality and Religion

  — Listen to the resident's concerns.

  — Respect the resident's religious beliefs (Figure 2-4).

  — Do not try to impose your religious beliefs on the resident.

  — Respect the resident's choice if she chooses not to participate in religious activities.

  — Plan care so that the resident can be involved in religious activities.

  — Provide privacy when clergy are visiting.

  — Respect and handle religious symbols, pictures, or other objects with care.

  — If the resident asks to see a member of the clergy, refer the request to the nurse.

  — Provide for religious and **spiritual needs** and customs.

CULTURAL INFLUENCES ON HEALTH CARE DELIVERY

You will care for residents from many different **cultures.** A culture is a pattern or lifestyle of a group of people. Residents may come from other countries or communities. Their beliefs, values, religion, and health care and hygienic practices may be different from your own. View this as an opportunity to learn more about others. Learn as much as you can about the residents' cultures. This will help you to meet their needs. Avoid **stereotyping** residents. Stereotyping means placing all members of a group into a certain category, believing they are all alike. Treat all residents as individuals, and recognize their individuality.

Figure 2-4 Respecting the resident's spiritual needs is an important responsibility. Spiritual needs may be greater when residents are ill.

Culture may influence the residents' beliefs about illness and care. The best way to find out about someone's beliefs is to ask. Asking is not offensive. It shows that you want to learn, and are trying to find ways of helping the resident.

Cultural Influences on Personal Space

Personal space is a comfortable distance for communication. The preferred distance between parties varies with the culture. In the United States, a comfortable distance is about 18 to 36 inches. Residents from other cultures may be uncomfortable with this distance. Their personal space may be closer or farther away. Be sensitive to residents' needs. If they appear uncomfortable when you are close to them, move back.

People from some cultures will not permit members of the opposite sex to care for them. Saudi Arabians, for example, will not permit a male caregiver to enter the room if a female resident is alone. If you encounter this situation, consult the charge nurse. Avoid offending the resident.

Gestures and Eye Contact

People in the United States make eye contact when speaking. They also use gestures. In some cultures, making eye contact and using gestures is offensive. In some countries, gestures have different meanings than they do in the United States. For example, we nod the head to indicate yes and no. In India, the head motions are the opposite of those in the United States. Thus, nodding the head up and down means

no. Shaking the head from side to side means yes. Monitor your body language, gestures, and eye contact carefully. If your body language makes the resident uncomfortable, avoid doing it.

Cultural Influences on Pain

Residents from other cultures may react differently to pain. In some cultures, residents are very emotional. They may cry, scream, and have dramatic reactions. In others, the resident will show no response, despite having severe pain. In some cultures, displaying pain is a sign of weakness.

Cultural Influences on Personal Hygiene

In the United States, it is normal to bathe and use deodorant daily. Women remove hair from their legs and underarms. Some cultures have different customs. They do not bathe regularly or use deodorant. Some women do not remove body hair. This may be a difficult problem for you to deal with. Do not be offended if the resident's hygiene is different from your own. Consult the care plan for instructions in caring for the resident. If you are having problems accepting cultural differences, speak with the charge nurse or social worker. Table 2-1 lists various cultural preferences for activities of daily living and health practices.

Cultural Influences on Clothing

In some cultures, certain garments have cultural or religious significance. Men may cover their heads. In other cultures, women keep their heads covered. Women in some cultures may not show any skin besides the face and/or hands. The resident may be very uncomfortable during bathing, or while in bed, wearing only a gown. Learn all that you can about the resident's culture. Make accommodations that show you care.

Cultural Influence on Health Practices

People in some cultures believe that certain home remedies will cure their illness. Residents may believe in using wraps, rubs, teas, inhaled herbs and spices, or other folk remedies. Friends and family members may practice these remedies on residents. Some may interfere with the resident's treatment. Consult your charge nurse.

Cultural Influence on Choice of Food

Residents may refuse to eat certain foods because of their beliefs. Some residents believe that eating certain foods will heal their illness. Residents may refuse certain foods or food combinations because of their religious beliefs. In some religions, people fast and do not

TABLE 2-1 Culture and Personal Hygiene Preferences

Culture	Hygienic Practices/ADLs	Clothing/Jewelry	Self-Care
American Indian	Very modest. May not cut hair except for certain health practices when mourning. May save hair clippings. Some tribes do not permit outsiders to touch the hair. May perform ritualistic washing. Navajo may save fingernail clippings.	Avoid touching a medicine bag. Ask resident or family to remove it, if medically necessary. If removed, always keep it in plain sight.	Self-care is expected to the extent the resident is able. Family may participate in care.
Arab American	Very modest. Most bathe daily. Some women believe bathing postmenstrually is harmful. Some avoid bathing when ill, believing it will interfere with their recovery. May believe that washing hair causes colds. Most females wash perineum with water after toileting.	Keep the resident's body covered as much as possible. Prefer long sleeves. Women wear long dresses and pants. Keep body covered when members of opposite sex are present. Many women cover the head with scarves. Some wear blue beads or amulets. These protect them from the evil eye. Some wear amulets when ill.	May expect families and health care workers to care for them, particularly during illness.
Central American	Very modest. Women cover legs. Women may prefer caregiver and physician of the same gender. Some bathe daily, others do not. Some women keep their heads covered. Mayan women may braid hair. Some may resist using urinal or bedpan.	Crosses, rosary beads, and other religious items may be important. Some wear red earrings to protect them from the evil eye. They believe that red is a protective color. May wear a bag of herbs around the neck. Avoid removing it, if possible.	Expect others to care for them during times of illness.
Chinese American	Very modest. Women usually prefer a caregiver of same gender. This culture has very high personal hygiene standards. Bathe daily. They may avoid washing hair when ill. Some may resist using urinal or bedpan.	Believe that wearing jade and some other articles brings them good luck and health. Avoid removing these items, if possible.	Most prefer to complete their own ADLs. Older men may expect family or staff to care for them.
Colombian	Very modest. Usually request a caregiver of same gender. This culture has very high personal hygiene standards. Bathe daily. Women may remove leg and underarm hair daily. Men shave daily.	May wear rosary beads, crosses, or religious items.	May expect family or staff to care for them when ill.

(continues)

Cuban	Very modest. Females will accept a male caregiver, but prefer caregiver of same gender. This culture has very high personal hygiene standards. Bathe and shampoo daily. May shampoo less often if ill. Women may avoid washing hair during menses. Some may resist using urinal or bedpan. Women may prefer peri care with soap and water after toileting.	May wear rosary beads, crosses, or religious items.	May expect family or staff to care for them when ill. Female family members may prefer to perform ADLs for the resident.
Filipino	Very modest. This culture has very high personal hygiene standards. Bathe and shampoo daily. Females may prefer peri care with soap and water after toileting. Some may resist using urinal or bedpan.	May wear rosary beads, crosses, or religious items.	Most prefer to complete ADLs independently. Family members may assist.
Gypsy	Very modest. Strongly believe in separation of sexes and will resist a caregiver of the opposite gender. Very high personal hygiene standards. Gypsies must keep upper and lower body separate. They use a separate washcloth, towel, and soap for the upper and lower body. Shampoo daily. Keeping the head clean is symbolic, and is believed to help keep them pure. Often request a clean pillowcase daily. Avoid touching the head and pillowcase, if possible. May refuse to use the bedpan. Avoid touching the upper body with bedpan.	Many keep an amulet under the pillow, or wear it around the neck. Avoid moving an amulet near the foot of the bed.	Most prefer self-care. If unable, usually prefers to have family members provide care.
Haitian	Very modest. Males may refuse to wear hospital gowns, insisting on keeping the lower body covered. May believe that physicians should be male and nurses female. Hold health care workers in high regard. Most shower daily. At bedtime, females perform peri care with soap and water. Men shampoo daily, women weekly. Women may wear rollers in hair at night. May refuse to use the bedpan or urinal. Many perform peri care with soap and water after toileting.	May wear rosary beads, crosses, or religious items. Some believe in and practice voodoo.	Will follow caregivers' instructions, but most prefer self-care for ADLs. If unable, family may perform ADLs. Family may request permission before assisting.

(continues)

Continued

Iranian	Modesty and hygiene vary with age and adherence to Iranian traditions. Usually very modest. May request a caregiver of same gender. May refuse to bathe when ill. Perform perineal care with water after each urination and bowel movement. May refuse to use the bedpan.	May wear a gold charm around the neck to symbolize Islam.	If ill, may refuse to perform self-care. Some are very resistant to any suggestion of self-care.
Japanese American	Very modest. Prefer a caregiver of same gender. This culture has very high personal hygiene standards. Bathe daily, and shampoo frequently. May request a tub bath in evening.	May wear special prayer beads.	Prefer self-care for ADLs. If unable, family members may assist. May resist caregiver assistance with ADLs.
Korean	Very modest. Men and women usually prefer to wear pants; both may prefer pajama bottoms at night. Elderly may wear thermal undergarments for warmth. This culture has very high personal hygiene standards. Bathe daily, and use many washcloths. Elderly women may shampoo once or twice weekly because of dryness in hair. May perform peri care after each elimination.	May wear rosary beads, crosses, or religious items. Usually wear little jewelry.	Many elderly believe that the family is responsible for performing ADLs. Family may not ask permission; they assume this is their responsibility.
Mexican American	Very modest. Women may prefer a caregiver of same gender. Most have high hygienic standards and bathe and shampoo daily. Female may refuse to use the bedpan due to beliefs about uncleanliness.	May wear rosary beads, crosses, or religious items.	Will perform own ADLs, if asked. Many prefer family or health care workers to perform ADLs. May believe that self-care hinders recovery.
Puerto Rican	Very modest. Most prefer to wear underwear at all times. Men prefer pajama bottoms. Most bathe and shampoo daily, but may refuse bathing during illness. May refuse bedpan; prefer using commode.	May wear amulet as protection against illness and injury. Avoid removing; may require priest to bless it or pray first. May wear crosses, rosary, or other religious items.	Prefer self-care for ADLs. If unable, may prefer family members to assist.

(continues)

Russian	Gender of care provider may not be an issue except for peri care. Some may refuse to bathe when ill; otherwise bathe daily. Avoids washing hair when ill. Will use bedpan, urinal, or commode. Elderly women may request warm or thermal clothing.	Some wear religious medallions, crosses, or pictures of saints.	Some will ask family of opposite gender to leave the room during personal care. May prefer to have nursing assistant or family perform ADLs when ill.
Samoan	Very modest. Prefer to dress in street clothing if out of bed. Women may refuse clothing that exposes the thighs. Shower and shampoo frequently, as often as three times daily. Some women may refuse shampoo during menses. Toileting is very private. May refuse to use bedpan or urinal.	Some wear rosary, cross, or other religious items.	Prefer self-care for ADLs. If unable, prefer to have family assist.
Vietnamese	Very modest. Most bathe daily. Some prefer peri care after each elimination. Believe that going to bed with wet hair causes headaches.	Catholics may wear crosses, rosary, or other religious items. Buddhists may light incense.	Prefer self-care for ADLs. If unable, may prefer family members of same gender to assist.
West Indian	Very modest about private areas of body. Exposing private parts to others is shameful and embarrassing. Avoids personal care by opposite gender. Bathes or showers once or twice daily. May prefer to perform peri care in the evening, instead of bathing. May refuse showers if ill. Shampoos weekly, due to dryness, although some individuals wash hair more frequently. Will use bedpan, urinal, or commode, but demands privacy. Very strict about handwashing after toileting.	May wear religious pin, cross, or picture of saint. Avoid removing them, if possible. Residents believe that these items protect them.	Prefers self-care, but will accept ADL care from staff member of same gender, if unable. May prefer that a family member perform ADL care.

eat on certain days. Consult the charge nurse if a resident does not eat. He may be able to make arrangements for a substitute that the resident will accept.

Language Barriers
Speak English when addressing residents. Speak slowly and gently. Show respect for the resident. If the resident does not speak English, ask if he has a bilingual dictionary, or some other means of communication. If not, try writing or using gestures.

Some residents can read English, although they cannot speak it. Keep each communication simple and clear. Drawing pictures may be useful. Before performing a procedure, demonstrate it. Always ask if the resident understands, or say "Okay?" A smile may not mean that the resident understands. Some people smile to be polite. Caring for a resident who does not speak English will take extra time.

SPIRITUALITY

Spirituality and religion are not the same thing. **Spirituality** is any way that people answer the desire to be connected with the largeness or wholeness of life. Aspects of spirituality include:

- a belief in the goodness of people
- caring for others, and a willingness to listen to others
- an awareness of an inner, reflective life
- attention to what provides balance in our lives and makes us feel whole
- a connection to what really matters to us in life, relationships, and work
- a sense of humor
- a connection with and an appreciation of nature
- a sense of hopefulness
- peace with oneself
- personal integrity

A resident's spirituality will help him through difficult times in life. Spirituality is personal and is expressed in different ways. Elderly residents use their spirituality to help them cope with living in a long-term care facility, facing illness and death, and coping with loss. You use your own spirituality when caring for residents in the long-term care facility. Supporting residents' spirituality is an important responsibility.

RELIGION

Religion is a formal system of beliefs, including ceremonies and rituals that demonstrate faith. Some religions have objects of religious significance, such as rosaries and crosses. Handle religious articles with care. Respect the residents' beliefs, even if you disagree with them. Support residents' beliefs by allowing them to speak openly about these beliefs and practice them. Be a willing listener. Provide privacy during prayer and when members of the clergy are visiting.

DEVELOPMENTAL TASKS

Theorists suggest that as people mature from infancy to old age, they must pass through several stages. **Developmental tasks** that help you grow psychologically must be accomplished in each stage to help you mature and move to the next stage. Realize that this theory is general. People mature in many different ways.

An understanding of the normal adult developmental tasks will help you understand the residents for which you care. The stages and developmental tasks of the adult are grouped into four categories: early adulthood, middle adulthood, late adulthood, and old age.

Early Adulthood—20 to 40 Years

The developmental tasks in this age group are:

- establishing personal and economic independence from parents
- developing a career
- making a commitment in a relationship
- establishing a family

Middle Adulthood—40 to 65 Years

The developmental tasks in this age group are:

- expanding personal and social involvement and responsibility
- adjusting to physiological changes of middle age
- reaching and maintaining satisfaction in one's career
- observing the maturation or growing of children

Late Adulthood—65 to 75 years

The developmental tasks in this age group are:

- adjusting to decreasing strength and stamina
- adjusting to aging changes in the body
- adjusting to losses
- adjusting to chronic medical problems
- adjusting to retirement income and financial concerns
- examination of one's lifetime and accepting one's past

Old Age—75 Years Until Death

The developmental tasks in this age group are:

- adjusting to declining physical health and increasing dependency on others
- realizing and accepting one's own mortality
- dealing with chronic illness and continued loss of friends and family

GRIEF AND LOSS

When a person anticipates or experiences a loss, she goes through the **grieving process.** This process was first described by Dr. Elisabeth Kübler-Ross. You

TABLE 2-2 Stages of Grief

Denial	Resident refuses to accept the truth.
Anger	Resident may act out feelings, directing anger to caregivers and family.
Bargaining	Resident attempts to "make deals" for more livable time.
Depression	Resident comes to full realization that situation cannot change and feels saddened over things that will be left unfinished.
Acceptance	Resident recognizes that death is part of the natural progression of life.

probably have experienced the grieving process if you have lost a pet or moved to a new school. Imagine how much more difficult it is to lose a loved one. The grieving process involves five steps: denial, anger, bargaining, depression, and acceptance (Table 2-2). Because the grieving process varies for each of us, not all persons experience each step. Some people move from one stage to another and back again. Staff, friends, and family members also go through the grieving process. The steps are not always obvious to others. Sometimes we recognize the steps in other people, but fail to recognize them in ourselves.

Completing all the steps in the process may take a very long time. The resident may die before completing the process. During the grieving process, be honest, reassuring, and understanding. Show the resident that you care. Helping a resident die in comfort and dignity is very important.

Denial

The first stage in the grieving process is **denial.** Denial begins when a person learns of the terminal diagnosis. The resident may believe that the diagnosis is wrong. She may display false hope and tell untrue stories. During this period, the resident may refuse to participate in her care, and may not follow the directions of the physician and nursing staff. The resident and family need strong emotional support during this stage. Allow them to talk about their feelings. Do not provide false hope. Spend time with the resident. Show her that she will not be left alone.

Anger

The second stage of the grieving process is **anger.** In this stage, the resident feels angry with herself, the family, staff, the doctor, and her higher power. She may be verbally abusive and refuse care and nutrition. The resident is not angry with you personally. She is angry with her situation. Practice empathy. Let the resident know that you care and that you understand how she feels.

Bargaining

The third stage of the grieving process is **bargaining.** The resident hopes she can live to see a special event, such as a graduation or the birth of a grandchild. The resident may bargain with her higher power. She may make promises, such as attending church every Sunday, in return for more time. The resident is trying to postpone the inevitable. This stage is usually short. Spend as much time as you can with the resident to show that you sincerely care. Listen to the resident. Don't deny what she says. Avoid providing false hope.

Depression

Depression is the fourth stage in the grieving process. During this stage, the resident is dealing with the loss of everything she has. Her physical ability may decline. She may also be feeling regret for things she has said or done in the past. The resident may experience **apathy.** This is an empty feeling. She may also have no interest in others or in the environment. The resident may have decreased concentration, sleeplessness, fatigue, frequent crying, and loss of appetite. During this stage, the resident begins to separate herself from life. Avoid trying to humor or cheer her. Allow her to express her feelings. Visit as often as you can. Sit quietly and provide support.

Acceptance

The final stage in the grieving process is **acceptance.** The resident may feel empty, but peaceful. She is quietly waiting for death. The emotional pain is usually less during this stage. The resident may not want to be alone. Make her comfortable and spend as much time with her as possible. If she does not object, allow the family to assist with care. Helping care for the resident assists family members to work through the grieving process. Communication may be limited in this stage.

Coping Mechanisms

The resident in the long-term care facility has experienced many losses. An understanding of the coping mechanisms people use to deal with losses and stress in life will help you understand your residents.

Coping mechanisms are responses to stress that a person uses to protect feelings of self-esteem. Coping mechanisms develop throughout a person's life. Success or failure in gaining positive coping skills depends largely on how well the developmental tasks of earlier life have been mastered. When a person's coping ability is strained or inadequate, the following reactions may be seen:

- chronic complaining
- angry, irritable behavior
- agitation
- restlessness
- depression
- withdrawal
- weight loss or gain
- sleep disturbances

Residents who react this way may need additional emotional support. Your understanding of basic human needs, normal adult developmental tasks, and coping mechanisms will help you provide quality care for the resident. The following are other ways the nursing assistant can provide this support:

- Use **therapeutic** communication.
- Offer the resident choices whenever possible.
- Realize that angry outbursts are often the result of feelings of hopelessness, losses experienced, or unmet needs. Do not take these outbursts personally.
- Direct the resident's emotional energy in positive ways. Encourage activity programs.
- Report changes in the resident's behavior to the charge nurse.

DEATH AND DYING

You will be working with persons in the long-term care facility who are near death. Remember, death is a part of living. Death comes to all living things. Many persons look at death as a frightening time. Studies of people who had near-death experiences have shown that death is not unpleasant or frightening. Interviews with many elderly persons showed they have little fear of death. As a nursing assistant in a long-term care facility, dealing with death-related issues may be part of your job. Our society as a whole tends to avoid meaningful discussions of death. Discussing your own fears of death may help

you better understand death and dying. Caring for the person when death is near and caring for the body after death probably will be part of your responsibility.

Cultural Beliefs at the Time of Death

Cultural practices and beliefs surrounding death and dying are diverse. Some families express their grief loudly. Others are calm and quiet. Most take comfort in their spiritual and religious beliefs at the time of death. Table 2-3 lists cultural and religious beliefs surrounding death and dying.

Physical Signs Indicating That Death is Near

Some physical changes occur before a person dies. These include:

- Level of responsiveness decreases.
- The lower jaw relaxes and the mouth falls open.
- Skin becomes pale, moist, and cool.
- Lips and fingertips take on a dusky color.
- Pulse becomes rapid, weak, and thready.
- Breathing becomes slow, labored, irregular, noisy.
- Blood pressure decreases.
- Discharge of urine and feces is involuntary.
- Eyes stare, and pupils do not respond to light.
- Skin takes on a blue or dusky appearance, beginning in the lower extremities and moving upward.

Nursing care for the dying resident is a continuation of care that shows dignity and respect. Some other points to remember while caring for the dying resident are:

- Check the care plan for special instructions, or ask the nurse.
- Respect the religious beliefs of the resident and family.
- Keep the resident clean and comfortable.
- Moisten the lips and mouth as directed, and give frequent oral care.
- Touch and continue to talk to the resident as you normally would.
- Say only things you want the resident to hear. Explain all procedures before doing them. The sense of hearing may be present even if the resident does not seem aware. Do not say anything that will upset or frighten the resident.
- Support family members. Allow them to be involved in care, if appropriate.

TABLE 2-3 Cultural/Religious Beliefs Affecting Care at the Time of Death

Culture/Religion	Religious Belief
Adventist (Seventh Day, Church of God)	Some believe in divine healing, anointing with oil, and prayer. Believe in prolonging life, but may allow some to die naturally. Most do not believe in withholding care, or euthanasia. Will permit organ donation and autopsy.
American Indian	There are many different tribes, and beliefs vary with each. Some believe an owl is an omen of death. Some tribes have family members prepare the body for burial. Some tribes will not touch the dead person's belongings. Some tribes believe the dead are happy in the spirit world. Others believe the body is an empty shell. Some have extensive preparation of the body and visitation of the deceased. In some tribes, if a member dies at home, the house may be abandoned forever, or may be burned.
Armenian Church	Holy Communion may be given as a form of last rites; laying-on of hands is practiced.
Baptist	Pastor, resident, and family counsel and pray. Resident may be given communion. Some practice healing and laying-on of hands.
Black/African Americans	The deceased is highly respected. Health care providers usually prepare the body. Cremation is usually avoided. May have concerns about organ donation.
Black Muslim	Practices for washing the body, applying the shroud, and funeral rites are carefully prescribed.
Brethren	Anointing with oil is done for physical healing and spiritual guidance.
Buddhist Churches of America	The state of mind of the dying person is believed to influence rebirth. The priest is contacted to provide last rites. Chanting may be done at the bedside after death. Grieving is permitted by family. After death, the body is viewed as an empty shell. Autopsy and cremation are permitted.
Cambodian (Khmer)	Monks recite prayers. Family wants to be present at time of death and may want to care for the resident. Incense may be burned. Death is accepted in a quiet, passive manner. Family and monks may wish to prepare the body. A white cloth is used as a shroud and mourners wear white.
Central Americans	Catholics may want a priest to administer Sacrament of the Sick. Candles may be used if oxygen is not in use in the room. Family members may wish to prepare the body.
Chinese Americans	Family may prefer that resident not be told of impending death, or may prefer to inform the resident themselves. May not want to talk about the terminal illness with anyone. Some believe that dying at home is bad luck. Others believe that the spirit gets lost if the resident dies in the hospital. Family members may place special cloths and amulets on the body. Some prefer to bathe their own family members after death.
Christian Scientist	A Christian Science Practitioner may be called for spiritual support. Euthanasia is forbidden. Will not seek medical assistance to prolong life. Family responsible for disposal of the body. Most will not donate organs.
Church of God	Believes in divine healing through prayer. Speaking in tongues may be used.
Church of Jesus Christ of Latter Day Saints (LDS or Mormon)	Euthanasia forbidden. Request peaceful, dignified death. Body is dressed in white temple clothing before viewing by family members. Cremation is discouraged. Believes in baptism for others who have died and preaching to deceased. Organ donation and autopsy permitted.

(continues)

Continued

Colombians	Catholic prayer and Anointing of the Sick common. Family may practice Catholic prayer at bedside. Family members may cry loudly or become hysterical. All family members may want to see the body before it is taken to the morgue. In Colombia, the deceased are usually buried within 24 to 36 hours. The charge nurse may need to inform them that in the United States the body may not be buried this quickly.
Cubans	Family may not want resident told of impending death. This varies according to Cuban culture. Family members may stay with resident 24 hours a day during terminal phase of illness.
Eastern Orthodox	Last rites are given. Anointing of the sick is performed as a form of healing with prayer. Cremation is discouraged.
Episcopal	Last rites are available, but not mandatory. May practice prayer, communion, and confession.
Ethiopians	Friends are told of death before family so they can be present when family is informed. Female family members are never told first. Great displays of feelings are encouraged at death. They may cry loudly and hysterically. Women may tear their clothing and beat their chests. Men may cry out loud. Some families may want to say goodbye to the deceased before the body is removed from the room.
Filipinos	Head of family is informed away from resident's room. Catholic priest is called to deliver Sacrament of the Sick. Do-not-resuscitate decisions may be made by the entire family. Religious objects may be placed around the resident. Family may pray at the bedside when resident is dying. After death, may cry loudly and hysterically. Family may wish to wash the body. Death is considered a very spiritual event. All family members may say goodbye before body is removed from the room.
Friends (Quaker)	Do not believe in life after death (spiritual afterlife).
Greek Orthodox	The priest should be called while the resident is still conscious. Practices last rites and administration of communion. Believe that life should be preserved until terminated by God.
Gypsies	In general, discussion of death is avoided in this culture. Eldest in authority is informed of death first. A priest may be present for body purification. Family may want the window open at the time of death and afterward so the spirit can leave the room. May ask for special personal items in room at the time of death. An older female relative may remain at the window to keep spirits out of room. The moment of death and the resident's last words are very significant. The body after death may represent a source of spiritual danger to the family. Family may want body embalmed immediately after death to remove blood. They may sit with the body around the clock after death, and will eat and drink at this location.
Haitians	Elaborate rituals after death. When death is imminent, family will cry hysterically and uncontrollably. Family members may bring religious symbols and medallions. They have a deep respect for the dead. Family members may wish to wash the body and participate in postmortem care.
Hindu	Death is the opposite of birth, but not the opposite of life. Both mark passage. Believe that unsatisfied karmic debt will pass into the next life. Believe in rebirth. Euthanasia is forbidden. Specially prescribed rites. Family, friends, and priest may chant continuously before and after death. Priest may tie a thread around wrist or neck and place water in mouth immediately after death. The thread is a blessing,

(continues)

and should not be removed. People in this culture express grief very loudly. The family washes and dresses the body and only certain persons may touch the dead. Autopsy and organ donation permitted. May prefer cremation to burial.

Hmong — Important to wear fine traditional Hmong clothing at the time of death. Family may put amulets on body, which should not be removed. The family usually prepares the body at the funeral home. The body cannot be buried with hard objects, buttons, or zippers against the body.

Iranians — Death is seen as the beginning of a spiritual relationship with God, not the end of life. Family may wish to be present at all times when resident is dying, and may cry and pray at bedside. Family may wish to wash the body.

Islam (Muslim) — Begging forgiveness and confession of sins must be done in presence of family members before death. Believe in judgment after death. There are five steps to prepare the body for burial. The first step involves washing of the body by a Muslim of the same gender. May offer special prayers at bedside to ease pain and suffering; however pain, suffering and illness are viewed as God's will, and are part of paying for sin. Some have spiritual leader give resident holy water to drink prior to death to purify body. After death, arms and legs are straightened and the toes tied together with a bandage. May be opposed to autopsy.

Japanese — Resident and family may be aware of impending death, but will not speak about it. Family may wish to remain at bedside during terminal stage of illness. Cleanliness and dignity of the body are very important.

Jehovah's Witness — Euthanasia forbidden. Practice baptism and communion. May be opposed to autopsy, but acceptable if required by law. Organ donation forbidden.

Judaism (Reform, Conservative, and Orthodox) — Jews believe in the sanctity of life. Medical care is generally expected, and there are no medication restrictions. Most surgical procedures are permitted, but body parts that have been removed are traditionally saved for later burial. For most Jews, medical treatment cannot be stopped once it has been started, but members are not required to use extraordinary measures to prolong life. Expect to die with dignity. May be opposed to prolonging life if resident has irreversible brain damage. However, active euthanasia is forbidden. Traditional Jews use a burial society to care for the body after death. Society members may or may not be members of the deceased's congregation. Would prefer no autopsy, but will permit it if legally required. Embalming is generally discouraged. Burial as soon after death as possible. Cremation discouraged. For traditional Jews, mourning begins with a seven-day period called *shiva,* in which men do not shave, and family and close friends do not read the newspaper or watch television. Mourning extends over a year. Jewish practices and beliefs can be very different from family to family. Asking the resident or family members about their practices is probably best. Asking is not offensive, and shows that you care about and respect the resident's and family's wishes.

Koreans — Chanting, incense, and prayer may be used. Family crying and mourning may be extreme. Family may want to spend time alone with resident after death. Some may wish to wash the body.

Lutheran — Practice prayer. Last rites optional; resident may request anointing of the sick.

Methodist — May request donation of body or body parts to medical science.

(continues)

Continued

Mexican Americans	Entire family may be obligated to visit the sick and dying. Pregnant women may be prohibited from visiting. Spiritual items may be important. May want to die at home because of fear that the spirit will get lost in the hospital. Crying loudly and wailing is culturally accepted and a sign of respect. A Catholic priest is called for the Sacrament of the Sick. A family member may wish to assist with postmortem care. Family will want time alone with the body before it is removed from the room.
Orthodox Presbyterian	Scripture reading and prayer. Full forgiveness is granted for any illness connected with a sin.
Puerto Rican	If death is imminent, family may stay around the clock. Some believe that all immediate family members must be present at time of death. Believe that the body must be treated with great respect.
Roman Catholic	Takes ordinary, but not extraordinary, means to prolong life. May refuse lifesaving care. Euthanasia is forbidden. Sacrament of the Sick is mandatory. Resident or family may request anointing if prognosis is poor. Autopsy, organ donation, and cremation are permitted.
Russian	Family may not want resident to know of terminal diagnosis. Depending on religion, family may wish to wash the body and dress it in special clothes.
Russian Orthodox	Practice prayer, communion, and last rites by priest. Many wear a cross necklace, which should not be removed, if at all possible. After death the arms are crossed and fingers set in the form of a cross. Clothing must be a natural fiber so the body changes to ashes sooner. May be opposed to autopsy, embalming, or cremation.
Samoans	Resident and family prefer to be told of terminal diagnosis as early as possible. Family would prefer to care for resident at home, if possible. Family members usually prefer to prepare the body.
Sikhs	Believe that the soul remains alive after death. Family washes the body and dresses deceased member in new clothing.
Unitarian Universalist	Cremation may be preferred to burial.
Vietnamese	DNR decisions are made by entire family. For Catholic families, religious items are kept close to resident. For Buddhist families, incense is burned. Families prefer time alone with the deceased before body is moved. The body is highly respected, and the family may prefer to wash it. Some may prefer the body left as it is.
West Indians	When death is near, close family and friends wish to remain at the bedside to pray. Family members may wish to view the body exactly as the resident was at the time of death. Most wish to be alone with the deceased.

POSTMORTEM CARE

If you are to prepare the body after death, refer to your facility's policy and procedure for **postmortem care,** or ask the nurse if you have any questions. Some facilities have a morgue to which the body is taken. In other facilities the body will be left in the room until it can be transferred to a mortuary. Assist the roommate to leave the room temporarily.

Always use *standard precautions* (Chapter 6) when providing postmortem care. The body can be infectious after death. Handle the body very gently to prevent bruising. Respect the religious beliefs of the deceased. Beliefs vary, and people of some faiths have special religious requirements for preparation of the body.

PERFORMANCE PROCEDURE

1   Postmortem Care

1   Wash your hands.

2   Gather supplies: shroud kit with gown and identification tags, a basin of warm water, soap, washcloth, towels, swabs for oral care, linen, gown, and gloves.

3   Pull the curtains and close the door for privacy.

4   Treat the body gently and with respect.

5   Apply gloves.

6   Raise the bed to a comfortable working height.

7   Place the resident on her back, with a pillow beneath the head and shoulders in proper body alignment.

8   Close the eyes by gently pulling eyelids down.

9   Provide mouth care using moistened oral care swabs or sponges.

10 Place cleaned dentures in the mouth or in a labeled denture cup. The dentures should be sent to the funeral home with the body.

11 Close the mouth. A rolled-up washcloth may be placed under the chin to keep the jaw closed.

12 Remove all tubing from the body if this is your facility policy. In most facilities this is done by the nurse.

13 Bathe the body, comb hair, and straighten the arms and legs.

14 Apply clean dressings to wounds, if necessary.

15 Place a disposable pad under the buttocks.

16 Put a gown on the body.

17 Attach an identification tag to the body as indicated by facility policy.

18 Replace soiled linen and cover the body to the shoulders with a sheet.

19 Remove gloves and dispose according to facility policy.

20 Wash your hands.

21 Tidy the unit.

22 Wash your hands.

23 Provide privacy and allow family members to be alone with the resident.

24 Collect all belongings, place them in a bag and label them correctly. Usually these are given to the family. If no family members are present, follow facility policy. Complete and sign the inventory sheet if this is your facility policy.

25 After the family leaves, wash your hands and put the shroud on the body. Wear gloves if contact with blood, body fluid, secretions, or excretions is likely.

26 Remove gloves, if worn, and dispose according to facility policy.

27 Follow facility policy to take the body to the morgue, or close the door until the funeral home staff arrives.

28 Notify the nurse when the funeral home staff arrives.

29 Assist the funeral home personnel to move the body if necessary.

30 Strip and clean the unit according to your facility policy after the body has been removed.

KEY POINTS IN THIS CHAPTER

▲ All people have the same basic human needs, though some people may express their needs in different ways.

▲ Physical needs, called physiological needs, refer to the needs of the body.

▲ Psychological or psychosocial needs refer to the emotional or mental needs of the resident.

▲ Developmental tasks at one level must be mastered before moving to the next level.

▲ The resident's culture, spirituality, and religion influence your ability to provide care.

▲ Coping mechanisms are used and developed in life to deal with stresses.

▲ The grieving process is a series of five stages that a person experiences in anticipation of a loss or after suffering a loss.

▲ A resident who is dying must be cared for with the same respect and dignity given to all other residents.

▲ The resident's body must be treated with respect after death.

REVIEW QUIZ

1. Which of the following statements is true?
   a. All people have the same basic human needs.
   b. The basic human needs of people vary according to age.
   c. Men and women have very different basic human needs.
   d. All people express their basic needs in exactly the same way.

2. What are psychological or psychosocial needs?
   a. needs having to do with the physical body
   b. mental and emotional needs
   c. need for food, air, water, and exercise
   d. elimination needs

3. Nursing assistants can help residents to meet the need for food by:
   a. keeping the head of the bed flat at mealtime.
   b. always providing privacy when residents are eating.
   c. keeping the dining area as quiet as possible.
   d. making mealtime as pleasant as possible.

4. Nursing assistants can help residents meet the need for exercise and activity by:
   a. assisting residents to the bathroom at least once a day.
   b. helping residents to ambulate and exercise according to the care plan.
   c. keeping residents in bed as much as possible.
   d. assisting residents to meals.

5. The nursing assistant can help meet the resident's need for sexual expression by:
   a. dressing residents in clothing that is appropriate.
   b. providing privacy for couples who have intimacy needs.
   c. providing privacy for residents who are masturbating.
   d. all of the above.

6. The resident's need for love and belonging can be met by:
   a. keeping the head of the bed up when bathing the resident.
   b. making sure that equipment is working properly.
   c. showing interest and listening closely to the resident.
   d. keeping the resident alone most of the time.

7. What is your best response when the resident you are caring for begins to cry?
   a. Let the resident cry and ask if you can do something to help.
   b. Say nothing. Give the resident a tissue, leave the room, and close the door.
   c. Tell the resident, "Stop crying. Things will get better."
   d. Allow the resident to cry, but call the family immediately.

8. Calling the resident by the name she prefers is one way of meeting the need for:
   a. privacy.
   b. love.
   c. identity.
   d. spiritual growth.

9. How can the nursing assistant help the resident meet her religious needs?
   a. by insisting that the resident attend all religious services in the facility
   b. by treating religious belongings with care and respect

c. by calling your pastor to visit with the resident
d. all of the above

10. A developmental task of late adulthood is:
    a. developing a career.
    b. establishing a family.
    c. making commitments in family life.
    d. accepting one's mortality.

11. Responses persons develop in life to handle stress are called:
    a. coping mechanisms.
    b. grieving process.
    c. developmental tasks.
    d. physiological developments.

12. What is the first step in the grieving process?
    a. anger
    b. denial
    c. depression
    d. acceptance

13. When caring for a resident who is dying, you should:
    a. keep the room dark.
    b. keep family members away from the dying resident.
    c. continue caring for, touching, and talking to the resident.
    d. never let the resident see family members who are crying.

14. Physical signs of approaching death include:
    a. decreasing responsiveness.
    b. pale skin.
    c. weak and rapid pulse.
    d. all of the above.

15. Which of the following is the last sense to be lost by the dying resident?
    a. vision
    b. hearing
    c. smell
    d. taste

16. You are assigned to care for Mrs. Nova, a 67-year-old resident who has been in the long-term care facility for five years. Mrs. Nova is disabled because of severe arthritis, and her ability to care for herself is limited. When you are in the room, the resident talks nonstop and tries to keep you in the room for as long as she can. Mrs. Nova is very demanding and uses the call signal frequently. You have been very busy all morning and are tired of answering her signal for simple requests. Mrs. Nova is probably using the call signal because she has an unmet need. Which of the following best describes the need that is causing her behavior?
    a. safety and security
    b. love and belonging

c. self-actualization
d. physiological needs

17. Mr. Huynh is an 87-year-old resident who is mentally confused. You notice that he is sitting in his wheelchair yelling loudly when you pass by. A few minutes later, when you pass again, he is quiet. You notice a large puddle of urine on the floor near the resident's chair. You go to the utility room to get the mop and the "wet floor" sign, and return to the area. What is the most likely cause of Mr. Huynh's yelling?
    a. He needed safety so that he would not fall on the slippery, wet floor.
    b. He was yelling for no reason.
    c. He needed to go to the bathroom.
    d. He was bored.

18. Mrs. Barnes is an alert resident who raised a large family. Her husband operated a farm and was away from home for long hours most of the time. Mrs. Barnes was the primary caregiver for her children. Now that the resident is in the long-term care facility, she is demanding and unpleasant. She is easily frustrated and yells at you because of minor irritations over which you have no control. Mrs. Barnes may be upset because she has lost control over her environment and routines. A good approach to take with this alert resident is to:
    a. give her choices.
    b. leave her alone when she is upset.
    c. follow very rigid routines.
    d. try to talk to her about her unacceptable behavior.

19. Mr. Joiner is a 65-year-old resident with advanced prostate cancer. The doctor just told Mr. Joiner that his condition is terminal and that further treatment will not help. You go to the resident's room to help him to the dining room. He tells you, "The Doctor told me that I am dying of cancer, but he is wrong. I do not feel sick at all." Mr. Joiner is probably experiencing:
    a. anger.
    b. acceptance.
    c. bargaining.
    d. denial.

20. You answer Mr. Hernandez's call signal and he yells at you for taking too long. He tells you that his breakfast was cold and that his favorite shirt is lost. You know that the call signal has been on for less than a minute, that breakfast was not cold, and that his shirt is in the laundry. He says that these things are "all your fault" and that he will report you to your supervisor because you are not taking proper care of him. You should:
    a. inform the resident that you will not take care of him if he reports you.

b. understand that the resident is frustrated and that you should not take his comments personally.

c. tell the resident that he is imagining things.

d. call the family at once.

21. Mrs. Bellman has been a resident of your facility for as long as you can remember. She has a serious heart condition. When you come on duty, the nurse tells you in report that this resident is dying and that she is not responding to spoken words. When you enter Mrs. Bellman's room, you find that her bed is very wet and you must change all of the linen by using the occupied bedmaking procedure. You know that:

a. Mrs. Bellman is no longer aware of who is in the room or what is being done.

b. you should only change the top bedding so that you do not disturb the resident.

c. you should explain to the resident what you are going to do.

d. all of the above.

CHAPTER 2
CROSSWORD PUZZLE

Directions: Complete the puzzle using these words found in Chapter 2.

acceptance	depression	process
actualization	elimination	psychological
ambulate	esteem	safety
anger	love	security
bargaining	needs	shroud
belonging	oxygen	spiritual
coping	physiological	tasks
denial	postmortem	therapeutic

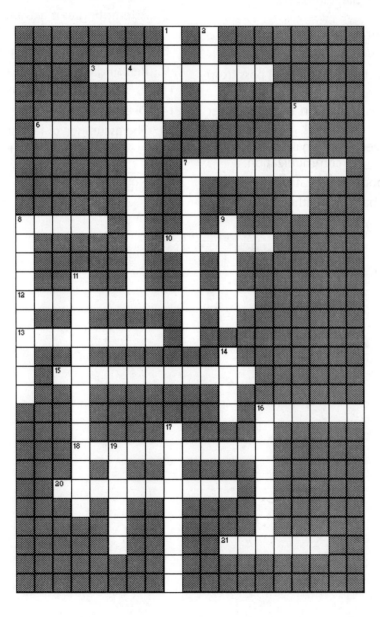

CHAPTER 2
PUZZLE CLUES

ACROSS

3. Feeling very sad and unhappy
6. There are five steps in the grieving _____ .
7. Feeling as if you are a part of something
8. The second stage of the grieving process in which the resident is mad
10. You are practicing _____ when you protect residents from injury by eliminating risks in the environment.
12. Emotional and mental needs
13. To walk
15. The process by which urine and stool pass from the body
16. The covering that is placed on the body after death
18. When residents need emotional support, it is helpful to provide _____ communication.
20. Care given to the body after death is _____ care.
21. _____ is in the air that we breathe.

DOWN

1. All humans have basic _____ for food, water, and oxygen.
2. Developmental _____ must be accomplished if a person is to mature.
4. Concerning the function of the body systems
5. Methods people have of handling stress are _____ mechanisms.
7. Attempting to make a deal with a higher power for more time to live is an example of _____ .
8. The final stage of the grieving process is _____ .
9. Refusing to accept the truth is a form of _____ .
11. Achieving one's full potential is self-_____ .
14. Deep fondness or affection
16. The assurance of feeling safe
17. Praying is a way for the resident to meet her _____ needs.
19. Satisfaction with oneself is self-_____ .

Rights of the Resident

OBJECTIVES

In this chapter you will learn about the importance of the resident's rights. After reading this chapter, you will be able to:

- Spell and define key terms.
- List residents' rights.
- Describe ways to accommodate the resident's right to make choices and explain why this is important.
- Describe your role in helping the resident resolve grievances.
- List ways you can help the resident participate in activities.
- Describe care that maintains a resident's dignity.

KEY TERMS

adaptive equipment: equipment or supplies used to make a task easier

confidentiality: keeping information or facts private

grievance: a complaint

infringe: to violate, remove, take away, or make difficult to attain

neglect: failure to perform needed care for a resident

nontherapeutic: not relating to treatment or therapy

ombudsman: a person who acts as an advocate for the resident

reprisal: an act performed to gain revenge or to punish another

restraints: any device or equipment used to restrict a person's freedom of movement or access to his or her own body

RESIDENTS' RIGHTS

The Resident's Bill of Rights is a federal law. All members of the health care team must respect these rights. The purpose and intent of the law is to make sure that all residents of the long-term care facility are treated with dignity and respect. The law guarantees that residents have the same rights as any other citizen. A copy of these rights is given to each person on admission (Figure 3-1).

Residents have the right to:

- have resident rights explained both verbally and in writing.
- be treated with dignity and respect.
- receive quality care regardless of race, color, ethnic origin, age, religion, marital status, sexual preference, medical condition, or physical disability.
- receive encouragement and support in making personal choices to accommodate individual needs.
- have advance notice if a change in room or roommate is necessary.
- have personal likes, dislikes, and special needs considered in the care and services given by the nursing facility.
- be respected and protected from harm, physically, mentally, and verbally.

RESIDENT'S BILL OF RIGHTS

This facility presents a Resident's Bill of Rights with the expectation that observation of these rights will contribute to more effective resident care and greater satisfaction for the resident, his physician, and the long-term care facility.

This facility enunciates these rights with the commitment that they will be observed and respected by the long-term care facility on behalf of its residents, as an integral part of the healing process. It is recognized that a personal relationship between the physician and the resident is essential for the provision of proper medical care. The traditional physician-resident relationship takes on a new dimension when care is rendered within the organized structure of a long-term care facility. It is in acknowledgment of these facts that this facility affirms these rights. The resident:

1. is fully informed, as evidenced by the resident's written acknowledgment, prior to or at the time of admission and during stay, of these rights and of all rules and regulations governing resident conduct and responsibilities;

2. is fully informed, prior to or at the time of admission and during stay, of services available in the facility, and of related charges including any charges for services not covered under titles XVIII or XIX of the Social Security Act, or not covered by the facility's basic per diem rate;

3. is fully informed, by a physician, of his or her medical condition unless medically contraindicated (as documented, by a physician, in the medical record) and is afforded the opportunity to participate in the planning of his or her medical treatment and to refuse to participate in experimental research;

4. is transferred or discharged only for medical reasons, or for his or her welfare or that of other residents, or for nonpayment for his or her stay (except as prohibited by titles XVIII or XIX of the Social Security Act), and is given reasonable advance notice to ensure orderly transfer or discharge, and such actions are documented in the medical record;

5. is encouraged and assisted, throughout the period of stay, to exercise his or her rights as a resident and as a citizen, and to this end may voice grievances and recommend changes in policies and services to facility staff and/or to outside representatives of the resident's choice. The resident is free from restraint, interference, coercion, discrimination or reprisal;

6. may manage his or her personal financial affairs or be given, at least quarterly, an accounting of financial transactions made on his or her behalf should the facility accept written delegation of this responsibility for any period of time, in conformance with state law;

7. is free from mental and physical abuse, and free from chemical and (except in emergencies) physical restraints except as authorized in writing by a physician for a specified and limited period of time, or when necessary to protect the resident from injury to self or to others;

8. is assured confidential treatment of personal and medical records, and may approve or refuse their release to any individual outside the facility, except, in case of transfer to another health care institution, or as required by law or third-party payment contract;

9. is treated with consideration, respect, and full recognition of dignity and individuality, including privacy in treatment and in care of personal records;

10. is not required to perform services for the facility that are not included for therapeutic purposes in the plan of care;

11. may associate and communicate privately with persons of his or her choice, and send and receive personal mail unopened, unless medically contraindicated (as documented by the resident's physician in the medical record);

12. may meet with, and participate in activities of social, religious, and community groups at his or her discretion, unless initially contraindicated (as documented by the resident's physician in the medical record);

13. may retain and use personal clothing and possessions as space permits, unless to do so would infringe upon rights of other residents, and unless medically contraindicated (as documented by the resident's physician in the medical record); and

14. if married, is assured privacy for visits by his or her spouse; if both are residents in the facility, they are permitted to share a room, unless medically contraindicated (as documented by the attending physician in the medical record).

No roster of rights can guarantee for the resident the kind of treatment he or she has a right to expect. A long-term care facility has many functions to perform, including the treatment of disease and disabilities, rehabilitation of accompanying conditions, the education of both the resident and the resident's family, as well as participating in the education of the health professions. All of these activities must be conducted with a primary concern for the residents and the recognition of their dignity as human beings.

Figure 3-1 The nursing assistant must respect the Resident's Bill of Rights.

- be free from abuse, **neglect,** and involuntary seclusion.
- have privacy during procedures and when requested.
- have **confidentiality** about their medical condition, medical records, personal information, and other details relating to their care.
- be addressed by their preferred name.
- have continuity of care.
- have personal possessions treated with respect and have them safeguarded.
- have assistance, privacy, and confidentiality in personal communication, including mail, telephone calls, and visitors.
- have visits from the **ombudsman,** representatives of state agencies, family, or physician at any reasonable hour. The resident may also choose to prohibit certain people to visit.
- complain about care and services without fear of **reprisal,** or punishment, and to expect a response.
- be informed about services available and their cost.
- refuse treatment. If treatment is refused, an explanation of the likely results of refusal must be given to the resident.
- select another person to make treatment decisions if the resident becomes incapable of making these decisions.
- be free from **nontherapeutic** chemical and physical **restraints.** If a restraint must be used, it should be the least restrictive device available to keep the resident safe.
- wear their own clothing, keep appropriate personal possessions, and be allowed to manage and spend their own money.
- participate in care conferences and give family members permission to attend.
- exercise citizenship rights and vote in elections.
- choose the physician responsible for care.
- live in the same room with their spouse, if married.
- be informed of the procedures for filing confidential complaints and for working out complaints.
- be given information about available resources.
- organize and participate in resident and family councils.
- complain to the state survey agency.
- review state survey findings.
- participate in religious or political activities if these do not infringe on other residents' rights.

These rights give residents the same rights as any citizen. It is part of your role and responsibility to support and help residents exercise their rights. If residents are mentally confused, you are required to protect their rights if they are not able to do so themselves. The reason for this law is to promote the interests and well-being of residents in health care facilities. The long-term care facility and its staff must encourage and help residents to exercise these rights.

Ways the Nursing Assistant Protects Resident Rights

Some ways that you, as a nursing assistant, can take responsibility for seeing that residents' rights are protected are to:

- Give quality care to all residents, regardless of race, color, ethnic origin, age, religion, marital status, sexual preference, medical condition, or physical disability.
- Treat all residents with dignity and respect. Perform your duties to the best of your ability, and do not neglect to care for residents who are assigned to you.
- Give privacy when caring for the resident. Knock on doors and wait for an answer before entering. Pull the privacy curtain and window curtain, if necessary, when doing care. Cover the sitting female resident with a blanket or lap robe so that she is not exposed.
- Give privacy to residents and visitors.
- Keep information learned about residents' medical conditions and personal situations confidential. Do not discuss information learned about phone calls, mail, or visitors. If information learned relates to the resident's condition, tell the nurse.
- Report changes in condition to the charge nurse in a timely manner.
- Call the resident by the name that the resident wants to be called.
- Protect the resident's personal possessions.
- Help the resident make phone calls, write letters, or address envelopes, if requested.
- Report injuries or suspected abuse or neglect immediately.

RESIDENTS' RIGHT TO MAKE CHOICES

It is frustrating when you are physically unable to do the things you want to do. This inability affects your self-esteem. Giving a resident choices is a way to show respect for the resident's opinion and give the resident a measure of control over routines and the environment. Making choices has a positive effect on the resident's self-esteem (Figure 3-2).

The Resident's Bill of Rights gives the resident the right to make personal choices. As a nursing assistant, you have the most contact with residents in the facility. Therefore, you have the most opportunities to assist the resident to make choices. Help residents make choices in the following ways:

- Offer options whenever possible.
- Accommodate the resident's requests as to when to do certain procedures.

Figure 3-2 Offering the resident choices shows that you value her opinion.

- Take the time to talk to the resident so you can learn personal preferences.
- Talk with the family to learn the resident's interests.
- Report resident preferences to the nurse.

A study of long-term care facilities showed that there are differences in what residents and staff feel is important. This study supports the fact that residents need to be asked what and when they want things done. Remember, this is encouraged by the Resident's Bill of Rights.

RESOLVING GRIEVANCES

A **grievance,** or complaint, may be filed when the resident feels his rights have been **infringed** upon. The Resident's Bill of Rights gives the resident the right to voice grievances without fear of reprisal, or punishment. The policy of your facility will describe how this procedure is to be carried out. Usually your responsibility is to report the resident's grievance to the nurse, making sure that what you report is accurate (Figure 3-3). Some facilities have a social worker who is responsible for helping resolve grievances. Always know and follow the procedure of your facility.

RESIDENTS' PARTICIPATION IN ACTIVITIES

The activity department of the long-term care facility has a special function. It plans recreational and social functions for the residents. Activities combat

Figure 3-3 Residents have the right to voice grievances without fear of reprisal.

boredom and promote positive self-esteem. These functions are a form of therapy for the resident. Your role is to cooperate with the activity department. Some ways you can help the residents participate in activities are:

- Plan your work so that residents can attend activities of choice.
- Review the activity calendar and be aware of the activities planned for the day.
- Tell all residents what activities are scheduled and encourage them to attend.
- Help residents dress properly, but remember to allow the resident to do as much self-care as possible.
- Inform residents' family or friends about activities.
- Escort residents to and from activity programs if necessary.
- Talk to residents about their activities, and praise their accomplishments.

MAINTAINING THE RESIDENT'S DIGNITY

There are many ways you can help maintain the resident's dignity. Dignity means treating a person with respect. Maintaining the resident's dignity at all times is important.

Long-term care residents have had to make many difficult adjustments. The resident has suffered many losses and may be angry and frustrated. Re-

member, the resident once was a younger, active person. Treat the resident as you would want a member of your family treated.

The nursing assistant can help maintain the resident's dignity by doing the following:

- Call residents by their preferred name.
- Treat all residents with respect.
- Help the resident be as independent as possible. Let the resident do as much for himself as possible, if consistent with the care plan.
- Encourage residents to be involved in their care and make choices.
- Assist and teach the resident to use **adaptive equipment** to enable her to be as independent as possible.
- Handle the resident's personal possessions with care and security. Do not throw personal items away without permission.
- Always explain what you are going to do before you do it, and obtain the resident's permission and cooperation.
- Become familiar with the resident's care plan so that you can provide individualized care.
- Be alert to safety concerns.
- Protect residents from abuse, mistreatment, and disrespect.
- Report any instances of poor care, abuse, or neglect to the proper person.

KEY POINTS IN THIS CHAPTER

▲ The Resident's Bill of Rights is a law that must be respected by all members of the health care team.

▲ The Resident's Bill of Rights guarantees that residents will be treated with dignity and respect.

▲ The resident has the right to file a grievance and to be given assistance in doing so.

▲ The nursing assistant must provide privacy for the resident when giving personal care.

▲ The nursing assistant must cooperate with the activity department in helping residents attend activities of choice.

▲ Showing respect for the resident includes handling the resident's personal possessions carefully.

▲ Any abuse, neglect, or poor care must be reported to the appropriate staff person.

▲ Allowing the resident to make decisions and personal choices is important.

REVIEW QUIZ

1. The purpose of the Resident's Bill of Rights is to:
   a. limit the cost of health care.
   b. list the cost of services provided for residents.
   c. ensure dignity and respect for residents in long-term care facilities.
   d. provide a list of rules and regulations for residents to follow.

2. Which of the following is included in the Resident's Bill of Rights?
   a. to be given privacy when receiving care
   b. to be told the cost of services
   c. to send and receive mail
   d. all of the above

3. When the resident is admitted to the long-term care facility, he should be:
   a. given a copy of the Resident's Bill of Rights.
   b. referred to by his room number.
   c. kept in his room alone until he has time to adjust.
   d. all of the above.

4. An example of a violation of the resident's right to confidentiality would be:
   a. discussing the resident's condition during a staff conference.
   b. reporting an observation to the nurse.
   c. discussing the resident's condition on a crowded elevator.
   d. writing the resident's temperature on a scrap of paper.

5. What is your best response when a resident complains about the long-term care facility?
   a. Call the family and ask them to transfer the resident.
   b. Listen to the resident carefully and report the complaint to the nurse.
   c. Help the resident write a letter of complaint to the state.
   d. Listen to the resident and then explain that some things cannot be changed.

6. When a resident feels that his rights have been violated, the resident has the right to:
   a. leave the facility without paying for the care.
   b. remain in the facility without paying any additional cost.
   c. call the police or sheriff.
   d. file a grievance.

7. When preparing the resident to take part in activities, it is important to:
   a. ask the resident which activity he would like to attend.
   b. take the resident to activities only after you have finished your other work.
   c. take the resident to the activity of your choice so that you may also attend.
   d. wait for the family to come and take the resident to the activity.

8. You see another nursing assistant abusing a confused resident. What is your best response?
   a. Call the resident's family immediately.
   b. Report this to your supervisor.
   c. Tell the other nursing assistant that you will not turn him in if he promises not to do this again.
   d. Do nothing, because it is not your responsibility to watch other employees.

9. You hear a housekeeper cursing at a resident because of a mess on the floor. You should:
   a. pretend that you did not hear.
   b. tell the other nursing assistants what happened and ask their advice.
   c. report this information to your supervisor.
   d. report this information to the housekeeper's supervisor.

10. You can assist the residents in maintaining dignity and self-worth by:
    a. doing everything for each resident exactly the same.
    b. always calling residents endearing names, such as "honey" and "dear."
    c. doing things for the residents yourself so that you can get your work done quickly.
    d. allowing residents to make choices whenever possible.

11. Residents' possessions, such as photos and letters, should be:
    a. placed in the facility's safe.
    b. sent home with family members.
    c. handled with respect and care.
    d. put away where no one can see them.

12. The Resident's Bill of Rights:
    a. is a law for doctors to follow.
    b. must be respected by all employees of the health care facility.
    c. is a guideline for states to follow in providing services to residents.
    d. all of the above.

13. What should you do when tidying a resident's room?
    a. Ask the resident before throwing anything away.
    b. Remove all plants and flowers from the room.

c. Throw out any newspapers or old magazines.

d. Clean the room without telling the resident.

14. When the resident exercises the right to refuse treatment,
    a. the resident must move out of the facility as soon as possible.
    b. the doctor and the family must be called immediately in all cases.
    c. the resident must inform the facility in writing before refusing treatment.
    d. an explanation of the likely results of the refusal must be given to the resident.

15. The resident's right to privacy would be violated if you:
    a. opened the resident's mail without permission.
    b. closed the door after taking the resident into the bathroom.
    c. pulled privacy curtains when the resident wanted to be alone.
    d. exposed only necessary body parts when bathing the resident.

16. A resident asks for help to go to the facility gift shop to buy a teddy bear for a new grandchild. Your best response is:
    a. "That teddy bear is expensive. How will you pay for it?"
    b. "It would be a waste of time. You don't have any money."
    c. "I'll try to take you after lunch or find someone who can."
    d. "Does your doctor know about this?"

17. Adaptive equipment is that which is:
    a. surgically attached to the resident's body to replace a missing part.
    b. designed to help the resident be more independent.
    c. always used by the physician during an examination.
    d. used in emergencies only.

18. Restraints should:
    a. always be used to prevent wanderers from leaving the facility.
    b. be used to punish the resident for misbehaving.
    c. not be used if other measures will keep the resident safe.
    d. never be used.

19. Restraints:
    a. restrict access to the resident's body.
    b. may be used for a brief time to allow the nurse to perform a medical procedure.
    c. restrict freedom of movement.
    d. all of the above.

20. Mr. and Mrs. Schneider have been married for 52 years. They reside in room 308 of your long-term care facility. You are about to enter the room to give bedtime care. You knock on the door and wait. No one answers, so you open the door. You find that Mr. and Mrs. Schneider are in the same bed. You should:
    a. apologize to the residents and leave the room at once.
    b. scold the residents for their childish behavior and assist them into their own beds.
    c. tell the other nursing assistants that you caught Mr. and Mrs. Schneider having sex.
    d. go about your duties in the room as if nothing is wrong.

21. You are assigned to care for Mrs. Sanchez, a 73-year-old resident who has heart problems. When you are bathing her, you notice that she has bruises on her upper arms. She tells you that Mary Atkins, another nursing assistant, held her down and forced her to eat. Mrs. Sanchez asks you not to tell anyone about the bruises. You should:
    a. say nothing, as this is what the resident wants.
    b. call the doctor and advise him of the bruises.
    c. ask Mary Atkins what happened.
    d. inform the charge nurse of the bruises.

22. You are assigned to care for Dr. Palmer, a retired physician who has had a stroke. Normally this resident is alert and able to visit with you when you help her with morning care. Today the resident seems confused and her speech is slurred. You should:
    a. inform the nurse of Dr. Palmer's condition right away.
    b. ask another nursing assistant what to do.
    c. do nothing, as mental confusion is a normal part of aging.
    d. assume that Dr. Palmer did not get enough sleep last night and allow her to rest.

23. You are working the 6:00 AM to 2:00 PM shift on C wing. Your unit is very busy this morning and Susan Birch, CNA, did not come to work. The nurse divides the residents in Susan's assignment and assigns a few of them to each of the other nursing assistants. You have three additional residents to care for from Susan's assignment. At 9:30 AM, you enter Mrs. Mosier's room and find her sleeping with her side rails up. Her breakfast tray is uneaten on the overbed table. You should:
    a. remove the tray so that no one knows that you forgot to feed the resident.
    b. find the nursing assistant who passed the trays and advise her to feed Mrs. Mosier immediately.

c. get another tray from dietary or warm the food in the microwave and feed Mrs. Mosier.

d. tell the nurse that someone neglected the resident.

24. Mr. Springer likes to attend an activity called Current Events. You notice that this activity is scheduled for 9:00 AM. Mr. Springer is scheduled to have a shower on the day shift. If the resident attends the activity, he will miss his shower time. What is the best way of handling the situation?

a. Do not tell Mr. Springer about the activity.

b. Ask Mr. Springer if he would like his shower at another time during the shift.

c. Tell Mr. Springer that the activity is scheduled, but that he must take a shower before he can attend.

d. Tell the activities director to schedule Current Events at a different time of day.

25. State surveyors are in the facility for their annual review. Mr. Connolly asks you to tell the surveyors that he wants to speak with them. You should:

a. inform the nurse of Mr. Connolly's request so that he can tell the surveyors.

b. tell the social worker to visit with Mr. Connolly immediately before he complains to the state.

c. pretend that you did not hear Mr. Connolly and leave the room quickly.

d. tell the resident that the surveyors are too busy reviewing care to speak with him.

26. Mr. James keeps the volume on his television loud. He likes to watch television late at night. The other residents complain that the noise from the television keeps them awake. Your best response would be to:

a. tell the other residents that it is Mr. James's right to watch television if he wants to.

b. go to Mr. James's room and turn the television off.

c. close the doors of the residents who are still awake.

d. tell Mr. James that the television is bothering others and ask him to turn the volume down.

CHAPTER 3
CROSSWORD PUZZLE

Directions: Complete the puzzle using these words found in Chapter 3.

abuse	exercise	protect
activities	explain	refuse
adaptive	grievance	reprisal
choices	law	restraints
communication	name	rights
confidentiality	neglect	self
councils	ombudsman	survey
dignity	privacy	vote

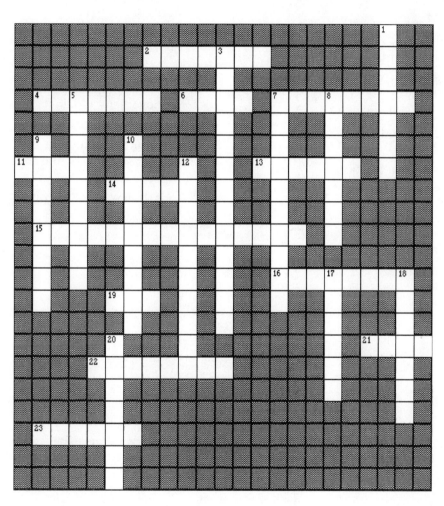

CHAPTER 3
PUZZLE CLUES

ACROSS

2. Offer the resident _____ whenever possible.
4. Treating residents with respect, honor, or esteem is treating them with _____ .
6. Call the resident by her preferred _____ .
7. A device that makes it easier for a resident to do something is called _____ equipment.
11. Residents have the right to _____ in elections.
13. Resident's Bill of _____
14. Intentional harm
15. Keeping facts or information private
16. The nursing assistant must help residents to _____ their rights.
19. The Resident's Bill of Rights is a _____ .
21. Making choices is good for the resident's _____ -esteem.
22. An act of revenge or retaliation
23. Residents may review state _____ findings.

DOWN

1. The resident has a right to _____ during procedures in which her body is exposed.
3. Writing letters and talking on the phone are forms of confidential _____ .
5. A complaint
7. Recreational and social programs
8. The nursing assistant must _____ the resident's rights.
9. Residents may organize and participate in resident and family _____ .
10. A resident advocate
12. Any equipment or device that restricts freedom of movement and limits access to one's body
17. A resident has the right to _____ treatment.
18. If a resident refuses a procedure, health care workers must _____ the consequences of the refusal.
20. Deliberately or carelessly not taking care of a resident

4

Mental Health and Social Needs

OBJECTIVES

In this chapter you will learn how you can help residents meet their mental health and social needs. After reading this chapter, you will be able to:

- Spell and define key terms.
- Identify characteristics of residents with mental health needs.
- Describe considerations to be given to the resident with mental impairment.
- Describe the purpose of validation therapy.
- Describe techniques of behavior management.
- List guidelines for interacting with residents with mental impairments.
- Describe ways to modify your behavior in response to resident behavior.

KEY TERMS

Alzheimer's disease: a disease of unknown cause resulting in gradual loss of mental abilities. This irreversible disease may take from a few months to years to progress to the stage of complete helplessness

catastrophic reaction: unpredictable behavior that may become violent

confusion: behavior that is different from the usual and accepted; mixed up

dementia: impairment of mental abilities involving thinking, memory, and judgment

disorientation: loss of or confusion about one's identity, the place, or time

empathy: compassionately understanding how a resident feels without feeling sorry for her

lethargy: abnormal drowsiness

mental illness: a disorder of the mind

mental retardation: lower than average intellectual development; can range from mild to severe

validation therapy: a program that helps confused residents feel good about themselves by helping them explore their thoughts and feelings

CHARACTERISTICS OF RESIDENTS WITH MENTAL HEALTH NEEDS

Many residents in long-term care facilities need some help in meeting their psychosocial needs. Individuals with some illnesses and conditions have special mental health needs. You will be caring for some residents who have mental disease. These residents may need physical care, but they will also need extra help related to their mental health problems. Knowing about mental impairments will help you care for these residents. Residents with **mental illness, mental retardation, Alzheimer's disease,** and other mental disorders will need special help from you. Individuals with mental problems also have accompanying physical problems.

Mental Orientation

Residents with mental impairments often experience **disorientation.** That is, they feel **confusion** about where they are and the current situation. It is a frightening experience to feel disoriented. Understanding this feeling in yourself will help you relate to the disoriented resident. Orientation is knowing:

- who you are.
- where you are.

- who other persons around you are.
- the time (year, month, date, day of week, and time of day).

POPULATION OF THE LONG-TERM CARE FACILITY

There are many residents in the long-term care facility who fit into broad categories of mental health needs. Residents with different health needs have different characteristics.

Residents with Mental Retardation

Residents with mental retardation often have the following characteristics:

- varying levels of ability
- difficulty adjusting to new situations
- poor judgment and inability to see the consequences of behavior
- socially inappropriate sexual behavior
- ability to learn appropriate and necessary ADL skills with proper training, support, and guidance from a knowledgeable, patient, and caring staff

Residents with Mental Illness

Residents with mental illness often reflect the following characteristics:

- changes in personality that vary between residents and type of mental illness
- tendency to benefit from medication, psychotherapy, and a supportive staff who have knowledge and understanding of behavior techniques

Residents with mental illness often display the following common behaviors:

- Inappropriate social behavior
  - varies from not sleeping to talking excessively
  - poor hygiene and grooming
  - alcoholism
  - sexual addiction
  - eating disorders
- Unusual level of activity
  - overactivity (pacing)
  - underactivity (refusing to move)
- Sleep disturbances
  - excessive sleeping
  - difficulty getting to sleep or awakening extremely early

- Delusions
  - having false beliefs
- Hallucinations
  - seeing, hearing, or smelling things that are not present
- Compulsive behaviors
  - performing a behavior repeatedly
- Other behavior
  - anxiety
  - confusion
  - angry outbursts (Figure 4-1)
  - weeping for no reason
  - laughing without cause
  - fear
  - withdrawal
  - suicidal thoughts and behavior
  - mood swings
  - depression
  - restless, agitated behavior
  - wandering and pacing

Residents with Alzheimer's Disease and Other Related Disorders

Alzheimer's disease is a form of dementia or mental illness of unknown cause. It creates changes in the brain tissue that cause a gradual loss of mental abilities. **Dementia** is a deterioration or decline of the brain that impairs mental capabilities. Dementia can be caused by acute (short-term) or chronic (long-term) disease. Characteristics of Alzheimer's and other dementias include:

- Sleep disturbances
  - difficulty sleeping
  - **lethargy,** depression, or restlessness
- Problems with wandering
  - wandering and confusion that worsens in the evening
- Memory and orientation
  - poor memory of recent events (short-term memory loss)
  - good long-term memory
  - lack of orientation to time and place
  - misidentification of people and common objects
  - lack of safety awareness

Figure 4-1 Residents with mental illness may have angry outbursts.

- Behavior problems

    — easily agitated and cannot be calmed readily

    — careless behavior

    — repetitious speech or behavior

- Neurological problems

    — problems with movement and coordination

    — incontinence of bowel or bladder

    — short attention span

    — poor judgment

- Other problems

    — creating new words

    — repetitious speech or verbally unresponsive

    — messy appearance

These symptoms may increase in severity over time until the resident needs help with all activities of daily living.

Catastrophic Reactions

Catastrophic reactions occur when a resident with Alzheimer's disease becomes overwhelmed by stimuli or when startled. Be careful when approaching the resident with Alzheimer's from behind. Speak quietly and gently so that you do not surprise the resident. Catastrophic reactions may be recognized by an increase in activity or talking. In a severe reaction, the resident becomes violent. You should avoid catastrophic reactions by making sure that the resident is not stimulated by too much noise and activity. Make sure that the resident's basic physical needs, such as hunger, thirst, and need to use the bathroom, are met. If a catastrophic reaction occurs, do not try to reason with the resident. Be calm and gentle in your approach. Touch may cause the resident to become more violent. Avoid restraining the resident, if possible.

If a resident has a catastrophic reaction or other behavior problem, do not take it personally. Understand that the problem is caused by the resident's disease.

CONSIDERATIONS FOR RESIDENTS WITH MENTAL IMPAIRMENTS

The resident with mental impairment needs the same physical care as any other resident. Remember, all people have the same basic physical and psychosocial needs. Be aware of these basic human needs as you care for the resident with Alzheimer's disease, dementia, or another mental impairment. Consider the following in caring for residents with mental impairments:

- Environment

    — Provide a structured, safe environment.

    — Avoid change in routines.

    — Avoid excessive stimulation. Too much activity and noise often add to confusion and anxiety.

    — Avoid isolating the resident. Isolation leads to further confusion.

    — Supervise wandering residents adequately.

- Verbal communication

    — Call residents by their preferred names. All staff members should be consistent.

    — Maintain eye contact with the resident.

    — Use a calm voice and speak softly.

    — Keep communication simple. Give short, simple instructions.

    — Avoid arguing with the resident. A resident with dementia may have many false beliefs that you cannot change. Arguing will cause the resident to become very agitated. The resident has lost the ability to reason.

    — Allow time for the resident to respond.

    — Mention the resident's emotions that are evident, such as fear or sadness.

- Body language

    — Approach residents from the front. Some residents with Alzheimer's disease have decreased ability to see side views.

    — Face the resident and make eye contact.

— Bend down to the same level as the resident instead of standing over the resident when talking.

— Use slow, deliberate hand movements to enhance understanding.

— Remain calm and reassuring.

— Use calm body language. Avoid jerky, rapid movements.

— Use touch to reassure the resident, if he or she is not combative.

• Knowledge of residents' past

— Listen to the resident's family. They can probably give suggestions or ideas to help you in the resident's care. Many families cared for residents for a long time at home.

— Ask the nurse or social worker for information.

— Remember that information about the resident is to be held in confidence.

VALIDATION THERAPY

Validation therapy is a behavior management technique that helps to maintain the resident's dignity and self-esteem by acknowledging how the resident feels. Validation therapy also acknowledges the resident's memories. It recognizes that all behavior has a purpose, even if we do not understand the reasons for the behavior. Sometimes the purpose of the behavior is a memory that the resident has. The nursing assistant should recognize that even confused residents are human beings and that they can feel pleasure by expressing their feelings and memories.

BEHAVIOR MANAGEMENT

All behavior has a purpose. It may mean one thing to the resident and something completely different to the staff. Understanding the resident's behavior may be very difficult. The behavior has meaning to the resident, however. Many behaviors that we consider problems are actually caused by fears, unmet needs, and lack of coping mechanisms. If an alert resident displays a behavior problem, it is usually because of an unmet psychosocial need.

Many residents have lost some control over their lives due to their disabilities. When they come to the long-term care facility, they feel that they have also lost control over their environment. They have given up many things that are important to them, includ-

ing homes, possessions, and pets. This combination of losses often causes inappropriate behavior. Giving the resident control over routines and the environment will often reduce frustration and eliminate behavior problems. **Empathy** is compassionate understanding. Be empathetic. Understand how frustrated the resident is feeling.

If a resident who is mentally confused exhibits a behavior problem, it is often the result of an unmet physical need, such as hunger, thirst, pain, need to use the bathroom, or need to change position. Sometimes the behavior is caused by too much noise and stimulation in the environment. Often the resident is unable to express the need in other ways. What we think is a behavior problem really is a method for the resident to tell us something. If the cause of the behavior can be discovered and eliminated, the behavior will stop.

Remembering that all behavior has meaning is important for the nursing assistant. Do not take the behavior personally (Figure 4-2). Treat each resident with patience, respect, and dignity.

Techniques to Reinforce Appropriate Behavior

Assist residents by reinforcing appropriate behavior in the following ways:

• Refer to the care plan regarding special methods, techniques, or strategies.

• Respond to appropriate behavior with genuine compliments and praise.

Figure 4-2 Don't take the resident's anger personally.

- Show pleasant responses to appropriate behavior by nonverbal communication such as a smile or soft touch.
- Never laugh at or ridicule a resident's behavior.
- Remember that all behavior has a meaning, even if you do not understand what the meaning is.

INTERACTING WITH RESIDENTS WITH MENTAL IMPAIRMENTS

This section lists some general techniques to follow when interacting with residents who have a mental impairment. Because each resident is an individual, certain residents may have special instructions or restrictions. Being empathetic is important for the nursing assistant. Try to understand how the resident feels.

The need for individualized care is essential. Be sure to follow special instructions listed on the care plan for the resident. Consistency is important when caring for mentally impaired residents.

How to Respond to the Resident's Behavior

Become aware of your own responses and reactions to the resident's behavior, and modify your own behavior if necessary. Monitor your body language for hidden messages. Even mentally confused residents are sensitive to the nursing assistant's body language. Develop caring attitudes by demonstrating:

- patience
- kindness
- pleasantness
- gentleness
- caring
- understanding
- empathy

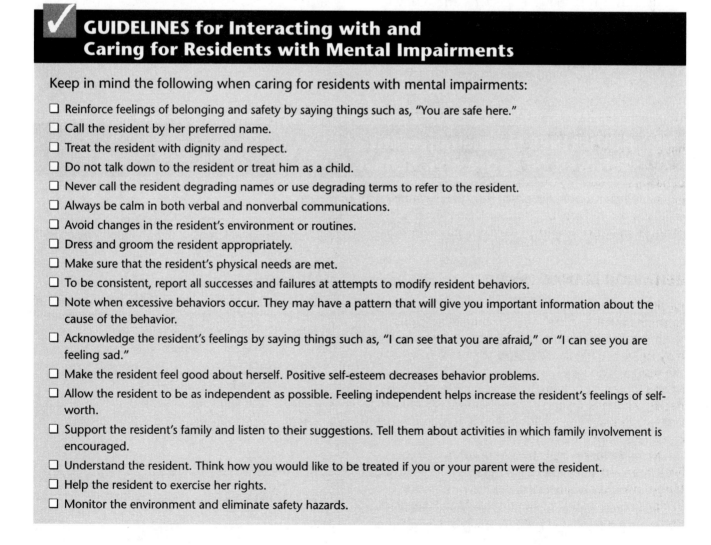

✔ GUIDELINES for Interacting with and Caring for Residents with Mental Impairments

Keep in mind the following when caring for residents with mental impairments:

❑ Reinforce feelings of belonging and safety by saying things such as, "You are safe here."

❑ Call the resident by her preferred name.

❑ Treat the resident with dignity and respect.

❑ Do not talk down to the resident or treat him as a child.

❑ Never call the resident degrading names or use degrading terms to refer to the resident.

❑ Always be calm in both verbal and nonverbal communications.

❑ Avoid changes in the resident's environment or routines.

❑ Dress and groom the resident appropriately.

❑ Make sure that the resident's physical needs are met.

❑ To be consistent, report all successes and failures at attempts to modify resident behaviors.

❑ Note when excessive behaviors occur. They may have a pattern that will give you important information about the cause of the behavior.

❑ Acknowledge the resident's feelings by saying things such as, "I can see that you are afraid," or "I can see you are feeling sad."

❑ Make the resident feel good about herself. Positive self-esteem decreases behavior problems.

❑ Allow the resident to be as independent as possible. Feeling independent helps increase the resident's feelings of self-worth.

❑ Support the resident's family and listen to their suggestions. Tell them about activities in which family involvement is encouraged.

❑ Understand the resident. Think how you would like to be treated if you or your parent were the resident.

❑ Help the resident to exercise her rights.

❑ Monitor the environment and eliminate safety hazards.

BEHAVIOR MODIFICATIONS FOR NURSING ASSISTANTS

This section describes specific ways that you can change your behavior in response to the resident. These techniques can help you when working with residents who have mental impairments. With all techniques, remember to treat the resident with respect and dignity. Never assume that a particular behavior is "normal for the resident." If you can change a resident's behavior by eliminating the cause, be sure to share this information with the nurse and other members of the health care team.

Use of Body Language

Body language is an important tool for helping residents.

- Use body language that expresses a listening approach toward the resident (Figure 4-3).
- Place yourself near the resident, but do not get too close. This shows respect for the resident's personal space.
- Position yourself at the resident's level. Sit if the resident is sitting. Stand if the resident is standing.
- Face the resident and maintain eye contact.

- Assume an open posture by avoiding crossed arms and legs.
- Lean toward the resident.
- Appear relaxed and focus on the resident. Avoid looking around.
- Use nonverbal behavior to show that you are interested in what the resident is saying by smiling, nodding your head, etc.
- Report or record the resident's behavior and responses to your behavior.

Figure 4-3 Use your body language to show the resident that you care.

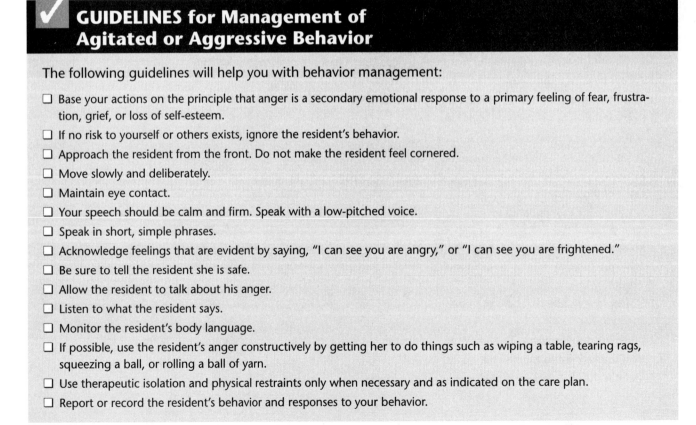

✓ GUIDELINES for Management of Agitated or Aggressive Behavior

The following guidelines will help you with behavior management:

- ☐ Base your actions on the principle that anger is a secondary emotional response to a primary feeling of fear, frustration, grief, or loss of self-esteem.
- ☐ If no risk to yourself or others exists, ignore the resident's behavior.
- ☐ Approach the resident from the front. Do not make the resident feel cornered.
- ☐ Move slowly and deliberately.
- ☐ Maintain eye contact.
- ☐ Your speech should be calm and firm. Speak with a low-pitched voice.
- ☐ Speak in short, simple phrases.
- ☐ Acknowledge feelings that are evident by saying, "I can see you are angry," or "I can see you are frightened."
- ☐ Be sure to tell the resident she is safe.
- ☐ Allow the resident to talk about his anger.
- ☐ Listen to what the resident says.
- ☐ Monitor the resident's body language.
- ☐ If possible, use the resident's anger constructively by getting her to do things such as wiping a table, tearing rags, squeezing a ball, or rolling a ball of yarn.
- ☐ Use therapeutic isolation and physical restraints only when necessary and as indicated on the care plan.
- ☐ Report or record the resident's behavior and responses to your behavior.

KEY POINTS IN THIS CHAPTER

▲ Residents with mental impairments need special assistance in meeting their psychosocial needs.

▲ The symptoms of mental impairment vary according to the disease.

▲ Special consideration must be given to the resident with a mental impairment.

▲ Alzheimer's disease is a form of dementia resulting in gradual loss of mental and physical abilities.

▲ All behavior has meaning, even if the meaning is not clear to others.

▲ Attempt to determine the cause of the behavior and eliminate the cause.

▲ Report successes and failures in modifying resident behavior to the charge nurse.

▲ Inappropriate behavior often is caused by feelings of loss of control over life or by other unmet needs.

▲ Offering choices and allowing residents to do as much as possible gives them some sense of control and promotes feelings of self-esteem.

▲ Consistency in care is extremely important for the resident with mental impairment.

▲ The nursing assistant should modify his behavior in response to the resident's behavior.

▲ Do not take resident behavior outbursts personally.

REVIEW QUIZ

1. A resident who is disoriented is:
   a. usually retarded.
   b. confused as to time and place.
   c. not allowed to eat.
   d. also destructive.

2. Changes in a resident's personality may be a sign of:
   a. mental illness.
   b. too much socializing.
   c. lack of exercise.
   d. all of the above.

3. Alzheimer's disease creates changes in the:
   a. brain.
   b. heart.
   c. lungs.
   d. all of the above.

4. A resident with dementia needs:
   a. increased activity to stay alert.
   b. to be isolated from others.
   c. a structured, safe environment.
   d. freedom from rules.

5. All behavior has meaning to the:
   a. facility psychologist.
   b. person doing the behavior.
   c. person observing the behavior.
   d. person who is talking.

6. Inappropriate behavior may be caused by:
   a. frustration.
   b. loss of control.
   c. unmet needs.
   d. all of the above.

7. When speaking with residents, the nursing assistant should call them:
   a. granny or gramps.
   b. the name preferred by the resident.
   c. "honey" or "dear."
   d. a friendly nickname.

8. When residents have feelings of positive self-esteem, behavior problems:
   a. decrease.
   b. increase.
   c. stay the same.
   d. get started.

9. When caring for residents with a mental impairment, you should keep the daily routine:
   a. full of recreational activities.
   b. varied to maintain interest.
   c. structured.
   d. free from any exercise.

10. To build feelings of self-esteem in residents with mental illness,
    a. do things for them quickly so they do not have to wait.
    b. always feed them so they don't spill food.
    c. tell them what clothing to wear.
    d. allow them to do as much as possible for themselves.

11. When you empathize with residents, you are feeling:
    a. like you think the resident feels.
    b. very sorry for them.
    c. very happy for them.
    d. all of the above.

12. A good listening approach to use when communicating with residents who have mental impairment is to:
    a. tell the resident to stop talking.
    b. stay at least six feet away from the resident.
    c. sit by a resident who is in a chair.
    d. avoid making eye contact.

13. When a resident is angry or agitated, the underlying feeling may be:
    a. fear.
    b. depression.
    c. hate.
    d. happiness.

14. A resident seems very angry and announces, "No one is going to tell me what to do." Your best response is to:
    a. apply a restraint.
    b. tell the resident to settle down.
    c. allow the resident to talk about the anger.
    d. none of the above.

15. A good example of providing choices to a resident would be to:
    a. tell the resident to go for a walk outside.
    b. allow the resident to choose a dessert if all of the dinner is eaten first.
    c. explain that if the resident chooses to be angry there will be no bingo games.
    d. allow the resident to pick out clothes to wear today.

16. Mr. Rimer is a 67-year-old resident with dementia. He is not able to express his needs verbally. He sits quietly much of the time, but you notice that he wanders quickly around the nursing facility about four times on your shift. Mr. Rimer usually urinates in his clothing when he wanders. What might be the purpose of Mr. Rimer's wandering behavior?
    a. The resident is bored.
    b. He is looking for the bathroom.
    c. He is trying to escape the noise in the environment.
    d. The resident is upset with you.

17. Mrs. Lee is an alert, demanding resident who uses the call signal frequently. If you do not answer it immediately, she yells, "Help! Help!" When you answer the call signal, her requests are never urgent. She speaks sharply to you when you are in the room. What would be your best response?
    a. Tell the nurse that Mrs. Lee doesn't like you and ask not to be assigned to her again.
    b. Take Mrs. Lee's call signal away.
    c. Tell Mrs. Lee that you have sick people to take care of and not to use the call signal unless it is an emergency.

    d. Give Mrs. Lee choices and control over her routines and environment.

18. Mr. Green is a 75-year-old resident who has a long history of mental illness. Mr. Green often smiles and talks when no one else is around. You are assigned to care for Mr. Green. He does not want to bathe and change his clothes. He says that God commanded him to wear the same clothes every day. Your best response would be to:
    a. check with the charge nurse or care plan for further directions.
    b. tell the resident that you are God and that he should change his clothes.
    c. attempt to remove Mr. Green's clothing anyway.
    d. leave and care for the next resident on your assignment and do not return to Mr. Green's room.

19. You are caring for Mrs. Clark, a 69-year-old resident with Alzheimer's disease. It is time for lunch and you go to find the resident to take her to the dining room. Mrs. Clark is very upset when you enter her room. She is throwing things on the floor and yelling. You ask her what is wrong, but her response makes no sense. Your best response would be to:
    a. apply a restraint so that Mrs. Clark does not injure herself.
    b. acknowledge Mrs. Clark's feelings by saying, "I see that you are angry."
    c. tell Mrs. Clark to stop acting childishly.
    d. advise the resident that she will not be given lunch because of her temper tantrum.

20. Mr. Hassan is a confused resident who seems to get more confused late in the day. You are working the 2:00 PM to 10:00 PM shift on C station. There is quite a bit of activity on the unit after supper. Visitors are coming in and out, and staff is busily trying to get residents ready for bed. Mr. Hassan is sitting in the chair by the nurse's station. You notice that he is becoming restless and agitated. You take him to the lounge, which is quiet, and put some music on the radio. You sit next to Mr. Hassan and talk to him. The resident calms down right away. Based on Mr. Hassan's response to your intervention, you should:
    a. always isolate the resident from others.
    b. put Mr. Hassan to bed immediately after he eats supper.
    c. inform the nurse and other members of the health care team of Mr. Hassan's response.
    d. say nothing about Mr. Hassan's behavior because it is just a coincidence.

CHAPTER 4
CROSSWORD PUZZLE

Directions: Complete the puzzle using these words found in Chapter 4.

Alzheimer's   disorientation   psychosocial
catastrophic   empathy   reality
confusion   lethargy   retardation
dementia   mental   validation

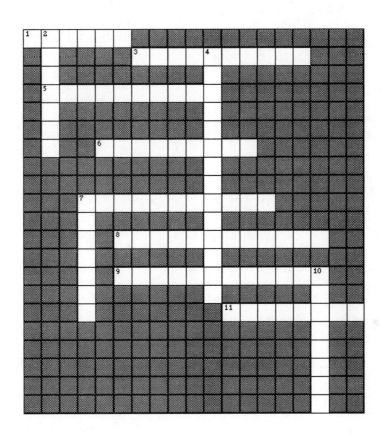

CHAPTER 4
PUZZLE CLUES

ACROSS

1. _____ illness is a disorder of the mind.
3. A program that helps confused residents explore their feelings and makes them feel good about themselves is _____ therapy.
5. _____ disease results in gradual loss of mental ability.
6. Behavior that is different from the usual; mixed up.
7. Lower than average intellectual development is mental _____ .
8. Unpredictable behavior that may become violent is a _____ reaction.
9. _____ needs relate to mental and emotional activity.
11. Impaired thinking, memory, or judgment.

DOWN

2. Understanding how a resident feels.
4. Confusion about identity, place, and time.
7. A program to help the resident relearn dates, time, place, and identity is called _____ orientation.
10. Abnormal drowsiness or sleepiness.

Communication

OBJECTIVES

In this chapter you will learn the importance of good communication with residents and other members of the health care team. After reading this chapter, you will be able to:

- Spell and define key terms.
- Explain why observation is an important part of effective communication.
- Demonstrate effective communication.
- Identify types of communication.
- List characteristics of therapeutic communication.
- Describe barriers to communication.
- Describe how to communicate with residents who have physical disabilities, vision loss, or hearing impairments, residents who are mentally confused, and residents who are unable to speak.
- Describe the importance of communication with staff.
- Give examples of observations to be reported.
- Describe the nursing assistant's role in recordkeeping.
- Identify common medical abbreviations and state their meaning.
- Describe methods of communicating with residents who have vision and hearing impairments.
- Identify common medical abbreviations.
- Answer the resident's call signal correctly.

KEY TERMS

abnormal: unusual, not normal

aphasia: the inability to speak or understand communication because of an injury, illness, or other medical condition

barrier: a barricade; something that hinders or separates

communication: the exchange of thoughts, feelings, and information by verbal or nonverbal messages

legible: plain, clear, easily read

medical record: the resident's chart. The medical record is a written legal record of the history, progress, and care plan of the resident.

nonverbal: sending a message without the use of words. Silence, attire, room decor, and body language are methods of nonverbal communication.

objective: observations made by the senses of the observer; things you can see, feel, hear, and smell

observation: noticing a fact or occurrence

prioritize: organizing your assignment so that the most important tasks are done first

sign: indications of illness, injury, or disease that can be seen by others

subjective: problems experienced by the resident that are not seen by others

symptom: indication of illness, injury, or disease felt by the resident, but not seen by others

verbal: sending a message by using words, tone of voice, and pitch of voice

EFFECTIVE COMMUNICATION

Effective **communication** is essential in your role as a nursing assistant. To do your job well in the long-term care facility, you must develop good communication skills for relating to the residents, family members, visitors, and other staff (Figure 5-1). Communication includes three things:

- a sender
- a message
- a receiver

Effective communication occurs when the receiver understands the message in the same way that the sender meant the message. To communicate well takes time, practice, and skill. Since you will be spending much of your working day with individual residents, you have a responsibility to encourage the resident to talk about her needs. Using the techniques listed will help encourage residents to talk about their needs.

TYPES OF COMMUNICATION

Communication occurs in two ways: **verbal** and **nonverbal.** You will use both forms of communica-

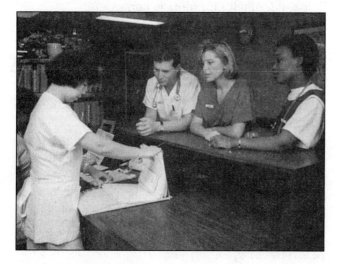

Figure 5-1 Good communication with other team members is an important nursing assistant responsibility.

tion as you work with residents. Verbal communication consists of:

- choice of words
- tone of voice
- speed of voice
- volume and pitch of voice

Monitor the resident's ability to understand the words you use. To achieve effective verbal communication, do the following:

- Get the message across by voice or words that the resident understands.
- Use verbal communication to give and receive information, report facts, and share experiences.

Nonverbal communication conveys a message without using words. Examples of nonverbal communication include:

- facial expression
- posture
- hand gestures
- touch
- dress
- movement
- raising of eyebrows
- smiles
- frowns
- silence
- resident's room decor

Remember that actions speak louder than words. Be aware of your nonverbal behavior when relating to residents, family members, and coworkers.

THERAPEUTIC COMMUNICATION

The words *therapy* and *therapeutic* refer to healing or improving a resident's condition. Therapeutic communication can be either verbal or nonverbal. You have probably used therapeutic communication quite often. You have done this if you have discussed a problem with a friend, or helped someone through a sad situation by just being there. As a nursing assistant, you can provide therapeutic communication for the resident (Figure 5-2). Successful therapeutic communication is possible only if you understand what the resident is really trying to tell you. Important points to remember in therapeutic communication are:

- Listen carefully to what the resident says.
- Observe the resident's body language, facial expression, movements, and actions.

✓ GUIDELINES for Effective Communication

To communicate effectively you must:

☐ Reduce background noise, such as music or television.

☐ Make sure your body language says you are listening.

☐ Speak at a pace that the resident understands.

☐ Give the resident time to talk.

☐ Express an interest in what the resident says.

☐ Make eye contact.

☐ Match body language with what is said.

☐ Speak clearly and at an appropriate loudness level so the resident can hear you.

☐ Do not chew gum when talking.

☐ Do not cover your mouth with your hands.

☐ Refer to the resident by the name she prefers.

- Be sensitive to the resident's feelings. Notice any difference between her words and actions.
- Focus on what the resident is saying.
- Comment on the resident's feelings by giving appropriate responses.
- Respond to what is being said so both you and the resident understand what was communicated.
- Report the resident's responses, actions, and behaviors to the nurse.
- Understand that people sometimes say what they think you want to hear.

COMMUNICATION BARRIERS

Anything that interferes with the communication process can be considered a **barrier,** something that makes communication difficult. The barrier can be from either the sender or receiver and can interfere during any part of communication. Also, both verbal and nonverbal barriers can occur.

Barriers to Effective Communication

The following behaviors and conditions can pose barriers to communication:

- your physical position if you are standing above the resident
- not listening
- background noise
- belittling a person
- talking to a resident as you would a child
- your body language
- your attitude or the resident's attitude, such as when you feel angry, anxious, or pressured
- a resident who is mentally confused
- when the resident's primary language is different from that of the nursing assistant
- taking over the conversation
- avoiding eye contact
- appearing too busy or in a hurry
- making judgments
- not acknowledging what the resident has said
- giving false or inappropriate answers
- using words the resident does not understand
- sensory impairments, such as impaired vision and hearing
- residents with glasses not wearing them, or glasses dirty
- residents with hearing aids not using them; hearing aid batteries dead, or aid in poor repair

Figure 5-2 Whenever possible, take the time to sit and talk with residents.

- physical disability related to injury or disease, such as **aphasia,** which is the inability to speak or understand
- being insensitive to the needs of a resident from a different culture
- preconceived ideas or beliefs

Communicating with the Resident with Vision Impairment

Because some vision loss is part of the normal aging process, you will be working with vision-impaired residents. Vision impairment often is a barrier to communication. The resident's care plan identifies specific methods for helping residents with visual impairments. Helpful techniques for communicating with residents who have visual impairments are:

- Identify yourself when approaching the resident.
- Knock before entering the room.
- Call the resident by the name the resident wants to be called.
- Remember that glare from a window behind you can interfere with the resident's ability to see clearly.
- Encourage the use of eyeglasses and help the resident as needed. The nursing assistant is responsible for keeping the glasses clean.
- Tell the resident where items are. Keep them in the same place so that the environment is familiar.
- Offer your arm to guide the resident. Walk slightly ahead of the resident.
- Speak clearly and slowly, using a moderate tone of voice.
- Do not talk to the resident as if he were a child.
- Provide adequate light in the room. Changes in vision due to aging make seeing in the dark more difficult.

Communicating with the Resident with Hearing Impairment

Some hearing loss occurs in the normal aging process. Hearing loss can be a severe barrier to communication. Specific suggestions will be listed on the resident's care plan. Helpful techniques for communicating with residents with hearing impairments are:

- Identify yourself to the resident.
- Gently touch the resident to get her attention.
- Make sure that the light source is behind the resident, not you, so that the resident can see your mouth clearly.
- Eliminate outside distractions and noise from the radio, television, or other sources.

- Face the resident when speaking. Use hand gestures and facial expressions to help the resident understand you.
- Speak clearly and slowly. Be aware of your own speech patterns and practice so you can speak in a way the resident will understand.
- Keep sentences short.
- Keep your hands away from your face when speaking.
- Stand or sit near the resident.
- Do not eat or chew gum when talking to the resident.
- If the resident does not understand you, choose new words to say the same thing. Do not repeat what you said in a louder tone of voice.
- Write and use other assistive devices to communicate with the resident.
- If the resident uses a hearing aid, help insert it.

Care of the Hearing Aid. Caring for the resident's hearing aid is the responsibility of the nursing assistant. Hearing aids are expensive and difficult to replace. Take care to be sure that it is not accidentally dropped in the linen when changing the bed. Check the resident's ears daily for buildup of wax or other **abnormal** conditions. Follow the manufacturer's instructions or the care plan for cleaning and inserting the hearing aid.

Several different types of hearing aids are available. Some are very small and are worn completely within the ear. Others are larger and have an ear mold. Some are contained within the arm of the resident's eyeglasses. Rules for hearing aid care are as follows:

- Handle the hearing aid with care. Be sure that it is not dropped.
- Do not allow the hearing aid to get wet. If the aid has an outside ear mold, the ear piece can be washed only with mild soap and water. The part of the hearing aid containing the batteries should never get wet. Always remove the hearing aid when bathing the resident or washing the resident's hair.
- Turn the hearing aid off when the resident is not using it.
- If the hearing aid has a cord, check it daily for cracks or breaks.
- Be sure that the ear mold is clean. If the hearing aid is the cannula type, it may be cleaned with a small pipe cleaner or special appliance cleaner. If excess wax is present, notify the nurse.
- Allow the resident to assist as much as possible.

GUIDELINES for Troubleshooting Hearing Aid Problems

Never try to repair a hearing aid yourself. If the resident has problems with the aid, you can perform a few simple activities that may resolve the problem:

☐ Make sure the aid is turned on. Some aids have settings marked on them. These are "M" for microphone, "T" for telephone, and "O" for off. Set the switch to the "M" setting.

☐ Check the volume of the aid; make sure it is turned up loud enough.

☐ Hold the aid in the palm of your hand. Turn the volume up all the way. Cup the aid between your hands. You should hear a loud whistle. If the sound is weak or absent, the battery is low.

☐ Before changing the battery, check the position of the old battery. Put the new one in the same way. Insert a new battery gently. Avoid forcing it.

☐ Check the ear mold and remove wax buildup.

☐ Ask the charge nurse to check the resident's ears with an otoscope.

☐ If the hearing aid makes a whistling sound when it is in the resident's ear, check the position. Make sure it is securely in the ear. Hair, ear wax, and clothing should not interfere with the position. Check the tubing for cracks. Whistling may indicate an air leak.

☐ Check for dirt under and around the battery if the aid works intermittently or makes a scratchy sound. Check the volume control and connections. Make sure the connecting wire is plugged in tightly and is not cracked or bent.

☐ Notify the nurse if the hearing aid does not work properly.

- Insert the hearing aid properly. If the resident complains that it hurts, advise the nurse. Sometimes the shape of the ear changes with aging and the hearing aid may have to be refitted.
- Follow the same guidelines that you use when communicating with a resident with hearing impairment.

COMMUNICATING WITH RESIDENTS WITH DISABILITIES AND OTHER SENSORY IMPAIRMENTS

Many residents in the long-term care facility have disabilities and sensory impairments. Some of these problems interfere with communication. You may be unsure of what to say to residents with other disabilities without being offensive. People with disabilities are like you. They have the same problems, wants, and needs. They can do many of the same things you can. However, they may need to adapt or change the environment to be able to do them. People with disabilities may perform the task differently, but the end result will be the same. Their bodies just work differently! As a rule, people with disabilities do not want to be treated differently from anyone else. Many are self-sufficient. Most have led productive lives. People with disabilities are valuable and equal members of society. You must treat them as such. Al-

though they are physically challenged, most have developed other abilities using nonphysical skills.

You must emphasize the uniqueness and worth of all persons. Treat residents with disabilities the way you like to be treated.

Communicating with Residents Who Have Problems with Language and Understanding

Some residents have illnesses or injuries that affect their ability to speak and understand what is spoken to them. They may understand some things, but not others. Assume that they understand you. Communicate with them as you would other residents. Speak when you are caring for them. If you are silent, the resident may interpret this as a negative message. Some residents may be able to speak, but what they say does not make sense. Certain words or phrases may have meaning to the resident, but not to you. Try to understand what the resident is saying. Avoid frustration. Be empathetic. If you learn what the resident is saying, share this information with others. This will help all team members to meet the resident's needs. Some residents understand what is spoken to them, even if they cannot speak.

Do not assume that residents with speech problems are mentally confused. Test the resident's ability. If she can answer yes-or-no questions, or follow simple directions, she understands you.

GUIDELINES for Communicating with Residents with Disabilities

- ☐ Avoid referring to the resident as a condition, such as "the paraplegic in 525." Say instead, "Mrs. Smith in 525." Avoid identifying the resident by condition. Always emphasize the person over the condition.
- ☐ Use common sense when speaking. Talk to the person the same way you would anyone else. People with disabilities don't want to be treated differently.
- ☐ Do not assume that someone is *not* disabled because you cannot see the disability. Some conditions are severely disabling, but not visible.
- ☐ You may shake hands gently with residents who have upper extremity disabilities or prostheses.
- ☐ Before helping someone with a disability, ask if you can help. Do not assume that the person needs help without asking.
- ☐ It is all right to ask residents about their disabilities. Many residents are comfortable and will talk about them. However, it is also all right if they do not want to talk about it. Residents who are newly disabled may not have accepted the disability, and may be uncomfortable talking about it.
- ☐ Don't assume that the resident can or cannot do something. Assuming is offensive. Always ask.
- ☐ Stress the resident's ability and not the disability.
- ☐ Avoid assuming that residents who use wheelchairs, canes, walkers, and crutches are sick. Avoid making assumptions.
- ☐ Do not treat residents in wheelchairs as if they are mentally impaired! Most have no mental problem. Speak with the person in the wheelchair, not a companion.
- ☐ Position yourself at the resident's eye level when speaking with a resident in a wheelchair.
- ☐ Be polite. Use good manners.
- ☐ Excuse yourself if you walk in front of a resident in a wheelchair.
- ☐ If you are in a crowded area, avoid standing in front of a person in a wheelchair. Standing in front of the resident blocks her view.
- ☐ The wheelchair is an extension of the resident's body. Leaning or hanging on the chair is an invasion of the resident's personal space.
- ☐ It is all right to use words such as "see," "hear," "run," and "walk" when speaking with residents with disabilities.
- ☐ Select words that are positive and nonjudgmental. Avoid using demeaning words like "cripple," "gimp," "spastic," and "retard." Using words like this promotes negative perceptions of people who are physically challenged. Table 5-1 and 5-2 gives examples of acceptable and unacceptable words to use. Always emphasize the person first. Emphasizing the disease is demeaning. Table 5-2 lists phrases to use when speaking about persons with disabilities.
- ☐ People with disabilities like to laugh and have fun. Do not leave them out!
- ☐ Seeing-eye dogs, hearing-ear dogs, and other canine companions are on duty. Do not feed or pet them without permission. This prevents them from doing their job.
- ☐ Do not park in spaces reserved for persons who are disabled. They need them more than you do. Often someone will pull into a disabled parking spot while a companion runs into a store. The driver remains in the car so it can be moved if the police come. When a driver with a disability pulls in, she has no place to park!

TABLE 5-1

Words to Avoid When Speaking with or About Persons with Disabilities

abnormal	cripple	deformity	maimed	stricken with
afflicted	crippled	diseased	moron	sufferer
burden	deaf and dumb	epileptic	normal	suffers with
cerebral palsied	deaf mute	gimp	palsied	suffering
confined to a wheelchair	defect	invalid	poor	unfortunate
courageous	defective	imbecile	spastic	victim

TABLE 5-2

Offensive and Unacceptable— Do Not Use in Conversation	Acceptable— Use This Instead
Disabled person	A person with a disability
Blind person	A person who is vision-impaired
Deaf person	A person who is hearing-impaired
A hunchback	A person who has curvature of the spine
The disabled	People who are disabled; the disabled community
He is a ripple	He has a disability
Dumb (or deaf and dumb)	A person who has a speech or hearing impairment
She is nuts, crazy	She has an emotional disability or mental illness
Retard	A person who is mentally retarded
Birth defect	A person who is disabled from birth
Fit	Seizure
Normal person as compared with a person who has a disability.	A person who is not disabled as compared with a person who is
Confined to a wheelchair	A person who uses a wheelchair

 GUIDELINES for Communicating with Residents who Have Problems with Language and Understanding

- ☐ Knock on the door and identify yourself by name and title before entering the room. Call the resident by the preferred name.
- ☐ Be courteous and friendly when approaching the resident.
- ☐ Assist the resident with glasses and hearing aids, if used.
- ☐ Explain what will be done.
- ☐ Use short, simple words. Speak clearly and slowly.
- ☐ Focus on one topic.
- ☐ Use short sentences.
- ☐ Show that you care with gentle touch.
- ☐ Keep conversations short but frequent.
- ☐ Use gestures and facial expressions to communicate.
- ☐ Allow time for the resident to respond.
- ☐ Do not finish a sentence for the resident.
- ☐ Listen carefully. Pay attention.
- ☐ If you think you understand what the resident is saying, paraphrase the words to give the resident feedback.
- ☐ Do not cut the resident off when he is speaking.
- ☐ Avoid communicating frustration through your body language.
- ☐ If you cannot get a response, assume that the resident understands.
- ☐ Help the resident point to things and use gestures.
- ☐ Use adaptive devices, such as picture boards, if available. The speech-language pathologist will often provide these devices and teach the resident to use them.
- ☐ Tell the resident when you leave the room. Make sure that she is comfortable and safe, with the call signal and needed personal items within reach.

GUIDELINES for Communicating with Residents Who Have Problems Speaking

❑ Knock on the door and identify yourself by name and title before entering the room. Call the resident by the preferred name.

❑ Be courteous and friendly when approaching the resident.

❑ Assist the resident with glasses and hearing aids, if used.

❑ Explain what will be done.

❑ Keep conversations short but frequent.

❑ Ask the resident questions that can be answered yes or no. Instruct the resident to nod her head in response. If the resident cannot nod the head, tell her to blink the eyes once for yes and twice for no.

❑ Allow time for the resident to respond.

❑ See if the resident can write, or use assistive communication devices, such as picture or word boards.

❑ Listen carefully to the response.

❑ If you think you understand what the resident is saying, repeat it.

❑ Do not pretend to understand if you do not.

❑ Emphasize words and gestures that you do understand.

❑ Allow time to complete the conversation.

❑ Avoid showing impatience.

❑ Avoid communicating frustration through your body language.

❑ If you cannot get a response, assume that the resident understands.

❑ Help the resident point to things and use gestures.

❑ Tell the resident when you leave the room. Make sure the resident is comfortable and safe, with the call signal and needed personal items within reach.

Communicating with Residents Who Have Problems Speaking

Residents with some diseases and injuries are unable to speak. Although they can make sounds, they cannot form words. Residents with this problem usually understand what you are saying. Do not make the mistake of thinking that the resident is mentally confused. Some residents will regain their speech with speech therapy. Some develop other methods of communication. They often make their needs known by using gestures, writing, or other adaptive communication devices.

Communicating with People Who Are Mentally Retarded

Three percent of the population in the United States has mental retardation. A person who is mentally retarded has learning problems. The condition was caused by conditions before birth or in early childhood. The resident did not cause the problem. There are many levels of retardation, ranging from profound to mild. Residents with profound retardation function at the level of a newborn. People with mild

retardation function at about the fourth-grade level. Most people with mental retardation are mildly retarded. People who are mentally retarded have the same needs as you do. They learn more slowly. Their learning may be limited. Most live productive lives. Mental retardation is like any other disability.

Residents who are mentally retarded need acceptance and attention. Treat them with dignity and respect. Allow them to express themselves and relieve stress. They may become overwhelmed if they are frustrated. They can make simple choices. Limit the options to avoid frustrating the resident. Consistency is important in their routines. Use the care plan to ensure consistent care. Most are happy and loving. They like to help and feel like they are contributing. Make the resident feel worthwhile.

Avoid pressuring residents with mental retardation to learn or perform new tasks. They can learn new things, but you must be patient and teach them gradually. They may not function well in high-pressure situations, or large, loud, confusing groups. Support a resident who is in this situation. Residents with mental retardation know if others are making fun of them, and feel hurt and rejection.

✔ GUIDELINES for Communicating with People Who Are Mentally Retarded

- ☐ Use short, simple words and sentences.
- ☐ Give simple, clear, concise instructions.
- ☐ Avoid talking down to the resident.
- ☐ Avoid treating the residents like children. They are adults. Avoid dressing them in childish clothing.
- ☐ Listen carefully when the resident speaks. She may know more than you think.
- ☐ People who are mentally retarded are sensitive to the moods of others. If you are upset, the resident will be too. Happiness is contagious.
- ☐ Limit choices to two if making decisions upsets the resident.
- ☐ If the resident becomes frustrated, slow down. Do not push.
- ☐ Praise and compliment the resident frequently.
- ☐ Treat the resident with respect.

COMMUNICATING WITH THE RESIDENT'S FAMILY, FRIENDS, AND VISITORS

You represent the long-term care facility to visitors. Speak and smile when you see visitors in the hallway. Ask if you can be of assistance. Be friendly and supportive. Show them where the lounges, vending machines, cafeteria, restrooms, and smoking areas are. Answer questions about policies and procedures. You must protect resident confidentiality, even with family members. If they ask you questions about the resident's condition, refer them to the charge nurse. You may tell them something about the resident's activities, such as, "He ate a good lunch." Avoid giving them information about other residents.

Families may show anxiety or anger in reaction to a resident's problems. Be patient and understanding. Avoid arguing. Listen carefully and be empathetic. If you believe that family members are upsetting the resident, report to the charge nurse. Relay all complaints to the charge nurse.

If visitors are in the room and you must perform a procedure, ask them to step out. Show them where they can wait. When you are done with the procedure, inform them that they can return to the room. If the procedure is not urgent, wait until the visitors are gone.

ANSWERING THE TELEPHONE

If answering the telephone is your responsibility, answer the phone by stating the name of your facility or unit. State your name and title. Be courteous and polite. A nurse must take the call if a physician is on the line to give orders. If the caller is not a physician, obtain the information, or transfer the caller to the proper person. You may answer the caller's questions. However, avoid giving out personal information about residents. Take a clear message if the person being called cannot come to the telephone. Write down the date, time of the call, name of the caller, and a brief message. Sign your name and title to the message. Inform the caller that you will deliver the message. Thank the person for calling.

COMMUNICATION WITH STAFF

Nursing assistants have frequent and close contact with residents and therefore have the opportunity to observe the resident more closely than the supervising nurse. Communicating with the nurse about the resident is absolutely necessary for continuity of care.

The care plan is an essential tool for staff communication regarding the resident's care. The care plan is a written plan that clearly identifies a resident's needs. Your responsibilities for the resident's care are listed on the care plan. Your supervising nurse will help you develop your assignment based on information in the care plan. Ask the nurse any questions you have when you receive your assignment. Your supervising nurse will help you decide how to **prioritize,** or arrange, your assignment. Setting priorities means that the most important tasks are completed first, and all essential care is done in a timely manner. Remember, the Resident's Bill of Rights gives the resident the right to have privacy regarding all medical records and information.

Be sure you discuss the resident's condition with the nurse in a private setting.

REPORTING OBSERVATIONS

Because of your close contact with the resident, you must know what should be reported to the nurse. Certain **observations** must be reported immediately. If you have any doubts, err on the side of caution and report the change to the nurse right away (Figure 5-3). Report the following observations:

- changes in the resident's physical or mental status, or general mood
- residents' reactions and behaviors
- what the resident says about her health (e.g., pain, numbness, dizziness)
- what you observe using your senses of hearing, sight, touch, and smell
- care that seems to work best for the resident
- care that does not seem to work well

If you report your observations to the nurse and the resident's condition seems to worsen, report to the nurse again. If you make an observation and report it, and you are not sure whether the nurse has responded, ask the nurse for his opinion on what you observed. This will serve as a gentle reminder to the nurse to check the resident if he has not already done so.

How to Recognize and Report Abnormal Signs and Symptoms

A **sign** is an indication of disease. Signs are **objective** findings that can be detected by others. They

are things you can see, feel, hear, and smell. Examples of signs are bruises or reddened areas on the skin. A **symptom** is a **subjective** finding. Symptoms cannot be seen by others. They are felt by the resident, who usually tells you about them. An example of a symptom is pain.

The following signs and symptoms tell you something is abnormal. They may indicate disease or illness in the resident and must be brought to the nurse's attention.

- Evidence of pain
  - in the chest
  - when moving
  - while urinating
  - while having a bowel movement

- Skin changes
  - redness that does not go away quickly when pressure is relieved
  - unusual color, such as blue or gray, of the skin, lips, nail beds, lining or roof of mouth, or mucous membranes
  - breaks or tears in the skin
  - bruises
  - lumps
  - rashes
  - abnormal sweating
  - swelling of feet, ankles, or hands
  - skin that is very warm or cool to touch

- Respiratory changes
  - coughing
  - slow, rapid, or irregular breathing
  - shortness of breath or difficulty breathing
  - "gasping" for breath
  - noisy breathing

- Digestive changes
  - sores or ulcers inside the mouth or gums
  - nausea
  - vomiting
  - choking
  - frequent belching
  - appetite changes
  - excessive thirst
  - difficulty in chewing or swallowing
  - dark or bloody stool
  - loose, watery stool

Figure 5-3 Reporting observations to your supervisor is an important nursing assistant responsibility.

— hard stool or difficulty passing stool

— unusual color of stool

- Urinary changes

  — difficulty urinating

  — dark color

  — strong odor

  — blood, mucus, or sediment in urine

  — urinating frequently in small amounts

  — burning or pain while urinating

  — suddenly cannot control the passage of urine

- Musculoskeletal changes

  — cannot move arms or legs

  — shaky or jerky motions

  — obvious deformities

  — changes in the ability to sit, stand, walk, or move

  — pain on movement

- Change in mental status

  — drowsiness

  — sleepiness for no apparent reason

  — restlessness

  — suddenly more confused

  — problems with coordination

  — changes mood quickly

- Other changes

  — fever or chills

  — any unusual body discharge, such as pus or mucus

RECORDKEEPING

The resident's **medical record** is often called the resident's chart. This is a legal document that contains the history and progress of the resident's care in the facility. It is a true, accurate, and complete record of the resident's care. Recordkeeping policies, or charting, are not the same at all facilities. In many facilities, the nursing assistant is responsible for some important recordkeeping. Patterns or changes in the resident's behavior are noticed and treated because of the nursing assistant's reporting and recording. Most facilities require nursing assistants to do checklist charting (Figure 5-4). Examples of forms that you would use for checklist charting are:

- activities of daily living (ADL) sheets (Figure 5-5)
- bowel sheets

Figure 5-4 Keeping accurate records is an important nursing assistant responsibility.

- intake and output (I&O) sheets
- meal acceptance sheets
- temperature, pulse, and respiration (TPR) and blood pressure (BP) sheets.

Charting is always done after you have given care. Never document a procedure before you actually do it. Charting must be accurate, clearly stated, **legible,** confidential, dated, and signed. Charting is done in chronological order according to the time. Things that happen or are observed first are charted first.

MEDICAL ABBREVIATIONS

You must know some commonly used medical abbreviations to communicate well with the nursing staff. Become familiar with these abbreviations:

ī, ī̄	_____	one, two, etc.
℥	_____	ounces
℥ī, ℥ī̄	_____	one ounce, two ounces, etc.
↓	_____	down
↑	_____	up
Abd.	_____	abdomen
ā̄c	_____	before meals
ad lib	_____	as desired
ADL	_____	activities of daily living
adm	_____	admission
AIDS	_____	acquired immune deficiency syndrome
Amb.	_____	ambulate; to walk
AROM	_____	active range of motion
ax	_____	under the arm
B & B	_____	bowel and bladder program
b.i.d.	_____	twice a day

NURSE ASSISTANT CARE RECORD—A.M. SHIFT

(Reference tags: F309, F310, F312, F315-F318, F327; Cross reference tags: F221, F222, F241, F246-F247)

INSTRUCTIONS: Identify the appropriate code for each item listed under the correct date column. Unless otherwise indicated refer to the following response key: **Y** = Yes; **N** = No; **I** = Independent; **A** = Assist; **D** = Dependent; **—** = Not Applicable. Initial each day's documentation and identify your initials by signing (one time) on the reverse where indicated. Additional notes and comments should also be documented on the reverse.

Month	Year		1	2	3	4	5	6	7	8	9	10	11	12	13	14	15	16	17	18	19	20	21	22	23	24	25	26	27	28	29	30	31
FEEDING	Breakfast	% Eaten																															
	Lunch	% Eaten																															
	Self / Assisted / Fed	S-A-F																															
	Ate in-Bed / Room / Dining Room / Chair	B-R-D-C																															
	Nourishment-Taken / Refused	T-R																															
BODY CARE	Bath-Bed / Shower / Tub / Partial / Whrpl / Shampoo	B-S-T-P-W-SH																															
	Nail Care-Fingers / Toes	F-T																															
	Skin-Clear / Other (Report "O" to Nurse)	C-O																															
	Positioned qh																																
	Pads-Air / Water / Foam / Synthetic	¼-½-1-2 / I-A-D / A-W-F-S																															
	Continent-Bedpan / Urinal / BRP / Commode	P-U-B-C																															
BLADDER	Incontinent	# Times																															
	Catheter	C-N																															
	Intake	cc's																															
	Output	cc's																															
BOWEL	Continent-Bedpan / BRP / Commode	P-B-C																															
	Incontinent	# Times																															
	Enema-Tap Water / Soap / Fleets	T-S-F																															
	Loose Stool	# Times																															
BEHAVIOR	Cooperative-Accepts Assist	C-N																															
	Resistant-Refuses Assist	R-N																															
	Alert-Oriented to Reality	Y-N																															
	Confused / Noisy / Agitated (if ✓'d note reason on reverse)																																
	Behavior Monitored (specify)	# Times																															
	Feeding Program	Y-N																															
	Oral Hygiene	I-A-D																															
	Hair Care	I-A-D																															
	Shave	I-A-D																															
	Dressing / Undressing with ROM	I-A-D																															
RESTORATIVE CARE	Range of Motion-Passive / Active	P-A																															
	Transfers	I-A-D																															
	Bowel & Bladder Program	Y-N																															
	Up in Chair	I-A-D																															
	Restraints-Bed / Wheelchair	B-W																															
	Ambulation-Walker / Cane / Assist / Self	W-C-A-S																															
	Scheduled Activities-Attended / Refused	A-R																															
SAFETY DEVICES	Side Rails Up / Down / Release	U-D-R																															
	Geri Chair / Vest / Wrist / Waist / Pelvic	G-V-W-WA-P																															
	Safety Device / Restraint-Released qh	2-1-1½																															
OTHER	Checked q 30 minutes	✓																															
	Positioned qh	½-1																															
	CHARGE NURSE NOTIFIED (record reason on back)	Y-N																															
	OUT OF FACILITY	Y-N																															
AIDE INITIALS																																		

NAME—Last   First   Middle   Attending Physician   Chart No.

CFS 6-3AHH © 1992 Briggs Corporation, Des Moines, IA 50306 (800) 247-2343 Printed in U.S.A.

NURSE ASSISTANT CARE RECORD
A.M. SHIFT

Figure 5-5 Most long-term care facilities use flow sheets to record daily care. (Compliments of Briggs Corporation, Des Moines, IA; (800) 247-2343.)

BM	_____	bowel movement	PROM	_____	passive range of motion
B/P	_____	blood pressure	PT	_____	physical therapy
BR	_____	bed rest; bathroom	q̄	_____	every, each
BS	_____	blood sugar	q.d.	_____	every day
BSC	_____	bedside commode	q.i.d.	_____	four times a day
c̄	_____	with	q.o.d.	_____	every other day
Ca	_____	cancer	q̄h	_____	every hour
cc	_____	cubic centimeter	q̄2h,q̄3h,⁻		
CC	_____	chief complaint	q4h, etc.	_____	every two hours, every
CHF	_____	congestive heart failure			three hours, every four
c/o	_____	complains of			hours, etc.
COLD	_____	chronic obstructive lung	q̄s	_____	sufficient quantity
		disease	R	_____	rectal, respirations
COPD	_____	chronic obstructive	reg	_____	regular
		pulmonary disease	rehab	_____	rehabilitation
C & S	_____	culture and sensitivity	res, Res	_____	resident
CVA	_____	cerebrovascular accident,	resp	_____	respirations
		stroke, brain attack	R/O	_____	rule out
d/c	_____	discontinue or discharge	ROM	_____	range of motion
DNR	_____	do not resuscitate	Rx	_____	treatment
DOB	_____	date of birth	s̄	_____	without
dx	_____	diagnosis	S.O.B.	_____	shortness of breath
e	_____	enema	S/S, SS,		
et	_____	and	S & S	_____	signs and symptoms
ext	_____	extremities	Stat	_____	immediately, at once
fx	_____	fracture	STD	_____	sexually transmitted dis-
HS or hs	_____	hour of sleep			ease
I&O	_____	intake and output	Std. prec.	_____	standard precautions
MI	_____	myocardial infarction,	Sx	_____	symptoms
		heart attack	T, temp	_____	temperature
ml	_____	milliliter	t.i.d.	_____	three times a day
mm	_____	millimeter	TPR	_____	temperature, pulse, respi-
MRSA	_____	methicillin resistant			ration
		Staphylococcus aureus	Tx	_____	traction, treatment
Na	_____	sodium	UA, U/A	_____	urinalysis
n/c	_____	no complaints	URI	_____	upper respiratory infec-
NG	_____	nasogastric			tion
NPO	_____	nothing by mouth	UTI	_____	urinary tract infection
NV	_____	nausea and vomiting	VS	_____	vital signs
O, PO	_____	oral	WA, W/A	_____	while awake
O₂	_____	oxygen	w/c	_____	wheelchair
OBS	_____	organic brain syndrome	WNL	_____	within normal limits
p̄c	_____	after meals	wt	_____	weight
PRN, prn	_____	whenever necessary	XR, X/R	_____	X ray

KEY POINTS IN THIS CHAPTER

▲ Effective communication occurs when the message received is the same as the one sent.

▲ Communication can be either verbal or nonverbal.

▲ A barrier to communication is anything that blocks communication.

▲ Common barriers to effective communication with elderly residents are vision, hearing, speech, and mental impairments.

▲ People with disabilities should be treated the way you like to be treated. Some people with disabilities have special communication needs.

▲ Courtesy is important when answering the telephone in the health care facility.

▲ The nursing assistant has the most opportunities in the long-term care facility to observe the resident. Reporting these observations to the nurse is an important role of the nursing assistant.

▲ Recordkeeping must be accurate, legible, and confidential. It must be signed and dated by the person doing the recording.

▲ Medical abbreviations are used in the health care setting to help you communicate well.

REVIEW QUIZ

1. Communication is effective when the message is:
   a. sent correctly.
   b. received as the sender wants it to be received.
   c. received as the receiver wants to receive the message.
   d. sent as the sender intends but is received differently.

2. Which of the following are good communication techniques?
   a. Speak clearly and loudly enough for the resident to hear.
   b. Reduce background noise.
   c. Listen carefully to what the resident is telling you.
   d. All of the above.

3. Verbal communication is:
   a. sending a message using words.
   b. using touch to send a message.
   c. the same as nonverbal communication.
   d. sending a message without the use of words.

4. What is an example of a communication barrier?
   a. listening attentively
   b. observing facial expressions
   c. maintaining eye contact
   d. talking down to a person

5. When communicating with a resident who has a vision impairment, it is important to:
   a. speak louder than usual.
   b. encourage the resident to wear his glasses.
   c. give the resident written instructions.

   d. keep the room as dark as possible to avoid eyestrain.

6. Communication with a resident who has a hearing impairment may be improved by:
   a. facing the resident when talking.
   b. standing or sitting close to the resident when talking.
   c. assisting the resident with the use of the hearing aid.
   d. all of the above.

7. What member of the nursing staff has the most frequent contact with the resident?
   a. the medication nurse
   b. the director of nursing
   c. the nursing assistant
   d. the charge nurse

8. The essential tool in staff communication regarding the resident's care is the:
   a. care plan.
   b. interdisciplinary progress note.
   c. flow sheet.
   d. nurses notes.

9. Which of the following is important for you to report to the nurse?
   a. gifts brought to the resident
   b. the television programs that the resident watches
   c. any change in the resident's health
   d. all of the above

10. When observing skin changes in the resident, you should notice and report:
    a. shortness of breath.
    b. redness or swelling.

c. digestive disturbances.

d. drowsiness or restlessness.

11. The legal document that contains the resident's medical history and progress is the:
    a. care plan.
    b. assignment sheet.
    c. medical chart.
    d. medicare report.

12. All of the following are true about charting in the medical record *except:*
    a. Charting must be accurate.
    b. Charting must be clearly written.
    c. No signature is required on any charting.
    d. The information on the medical record is confidential.

13. Medical terms and abbreviations are used in the health care setting to:
    a. encourage staff to learn new words.
    b. discourage residents from understanding medical findings.
    c. keep information in code in case it is overheard by visitors.
    d. assist in making staff communication clear and concise.

14. What does BP at HS mean?
    a. Take blood pressure at bedtime.
    b. Give the resident the bedpan at his side.
    c. Take blood pressure at the resident's side.
    d. Give the resident the bedpan at hour of sleep.

15. Abnormal changes that you should recognize and report are:
    a. swollen ankles.
    b. shortness of breath.
    c. blue color around lips and nail beds.
    d. all of the above.

16. The abbreviation for three times a day is:
    a. 3xid.
    b. t.i.d.
    c. 3 i.d.
    d. t.o.d.

17. When communicating with a resident in a wheelchair, you should avoid using the word:
    a. see.
    b. run.
    c. walk.
    d. none of the above.

18. When caring for residents with vision or hearing loss, you should:
    a. be as quiet as possible when you are in the room so the resident is not disturbed.
    b. make as much noise as possible when you are in the room so the resident knows what you are doing.
    c. announce yourself by name and title when entering the room.
    d. none of the above.

19. When caring for residents who have problems with speech or understanding, you should:
    a. explain the care you will be giving in medical terms.
    b. choose short, simple words and use short sentences.
    c. use sign language that the resident understands.
    d. all of the above.

20. When caring for a person who is mentally retarded, you should:
    a. treat the resident with courtesy and respect.
    b. not explain procedures.
    c. never smile, because this is upsetting to the resident.
    d. all of the above.

21. You answer the telephone on your unit. The caller identifies herself as Dr. Gonzales and states she wants to give orders for Mrs. Keene. You should:
    a. ask the doctor to hold while you get the nurse.
    b. write down the orders the doctor gives you.
    c. tell the doctor to call back later.
    d. none of the above.

22. An abnormal change in the digestive system that you should report is:
    a. dark, hard stools.
    b. pain while urinating.
    c. shortness of breath.
    d. dry, red skin.

23. Mr. King is an 83-year-old resident with a diagnosis of congestive heart failure. He is alert and able to do most of his care by himself. He is usually up, dressed, and in the dining room before breakfast. He remains up and is active in the facility during the day. When you make your first round on the day shift, you enter Mr. King's room and discover that he is still in bed. His ankles are swollen, his breathing is rapid, and he complains of a headache. You should:
    a. tell Mr. King to get up and get ready for breakfast.
    b. notify the nurse immediately of your observations.
    c. help Mr. King get dressed since he does not feel well.
    d. call the kitchen and order a breakfast tray for the resident.

24. You are assigned to help in the facility dining room at lunchtime. Mrs. Hazeldon is an 84-year-old mentally confused resident who wears thick glasses. You observe that she has eaten everything on her plate. However, the resident

has not eaten any of her fruit or dessert. She has not taken a drink of milk or water. You should:

a. return the resident to her room because she has finished eating.

b. leave the resident alone.

c. make sure that Mrs. Hazeldon can see her fruit, dessert, and beverages.

d. report the resident to the nurse.

25. Mr. Kelly is an 87-year-old resident who is very hard of hearing. He wears a hearing aid when he is up and about in the facility. You are assigned to care for Mr. Kelly on Wednesday. You are assigned to give him a shower, wash his hair, and make his bed. You should:

a. remove the hearing aid before Mr. Kelly goes in the shower.

b. check the bed linen before removing it to make sure that the hearing aid was not accidentally dropped in the bed.

c. help Mr. Kelly insert the hearing aid properly after his shower.

d. all of the above.

26. You are assigned to work the 2 PM to 10 PM shift on third floor. When you come on duty, Mr. Allen, the charge nurse, gives you report and posts the assignment sheet. After you get report, you should:

a. complete your charting for the shift.

b. ask another nursing assistant what you should do first.

c. review the assignment sheet and set your priorities for the shift.

d. all of the above.

27. You have been off work for the past two days. You are scheduled to work the 2 PM to 10 PM shift when you return. You are assigned to care for Mrs. Fulmer, a 71-year-old-resident who is mentally confused and does not speak. You are helping Mrs. Fulmer undress and get ready for bed. She is wearing a cardigan sweater and a short-sleeved blouse. When you remove her sweater, you notice a large bruise on Mrs. Fulmer's arm. Because you did not work yesterday, you do not know if the bruise is new or if an injury occurred on your days off. You should:

a. report the bruise to Mr. Allen, the charge nurse.

b. say nothing about the bruise, as this is not your responsibility.

c. do nothing about the bruise as you know that it did not happen on your shift.

d. apply a hot pack to the bruise.

28. You are assigned to care for Mr. Stine, a 77-year-old resident who is normally mentally alert. Mr. Stine speaks with you normally at the beginning of your shift, but as the shift progresses, the resident becomes more confused. You should:

a. do nothing, as this is normal in the elderly.

b. notify the charge nurse of the resident's confusion.

c. call Mr. Stine's daughter and inform her of the confusion.

d. say nothing, but record your findings in the medical record.

29. You are assigned to care for Miss Williams, a 32-year-old resident who has cerebral palsy. The resident has multiple physical deformities and requires total care. Miss Williams is unable to speak, but she understands what others say to her. She is able to nod her head to answer yes-and-no questions. When Miss Williams is using the toilet you must stay in the bathroom with her because she is not able to balance herself on the toilet seat. You notice that she makes a face when she is urinating. Her urine has a very strong odor. You should:

a. report your observations to the charge nurse.

b. notify Miss Williams's doctor of your observations.

c. call Miss Williams's brother and advise him of the problem.

d. all of the above.

CHAPTER 5
CROSSWORD PUZZLE

Directions: Complete the puzzle using these words found in Chapter 5.

abbreviation   impaired   sign
abnormal   legible   subjective
aphasia   medical   symptom
barrier   nonverbal   therapeutic
communication   objective   verbal
hearing   observation

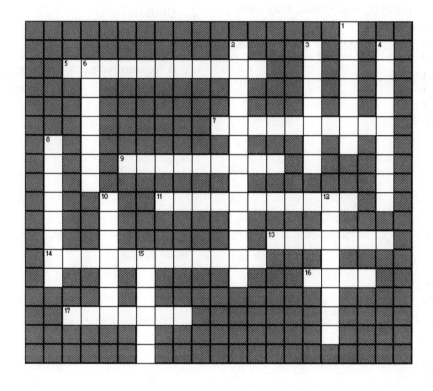

CHAPTER 5
CROSSWORD CLUES

ACROSS

5. Noticing a fact
7. A problem experienced by a resident that cannot be seen by others
9. Indication of illness, disease, or injury that can be detected by using the senses of the observer
11. Care designed to cure, heal, or preserve health
13. A subjective change in the body that may indicate illness, injury, or disease
14. Shortened form of words, used for communication
16. An objective indication of disease, illness, or injury
17. Plain, clear, easily read

DOWN

1. Inability to speak or understand
2. Exchanging thoughts, ideas, and information
3. Document your observations in the _____ record.
4. Sending a message without the use of words
6. A barricade
8. Unusual
10. A device that some residents use so that they can hear what you are saying is a _____ aid.
12. A resident who cannot see well is vision _____ .
15. Speaking is _____ communication.

Infection Control

OBJECTIVES

In this chapter, you will learn the principles of infection control. You must understand these principles to prevent the spread of disease in the health care setting. After reading this chapter, you will be able to:

- Spell and define key terms.
- List principles of medical asepsis.
- Define *infection.*
- Describe the common methods by which infections are spread.
- List the times when you should wash your hands.
- Describe how common infections (HBV, HIV, MRSA, TB, VRE, and scabies) are spread.
- Describe standard precautions.
- Demonstrate proper handwashing.
- Describe when to use gloves, protective eyewear, and surgical masks.
- Perform isolation procedures.
- List the types of isolation and describe personal protective equipment worn in each.

KEY TERMS

airborne precautions: A category of transmission-based precautions that health care workers use to protect themselves from airborne pathogens.

airborne transmission: the spread of disease by very small particles carried or suspended in the air

aseptic: the absence of any disease-causing microbes

bacteria: one-celled microorganisms, some of which cause disease

biohazardous waste: waste products contaminated by contact with blood or body fluid that require special handling

blood and body fluid transmission: a method of transmitting disease that occurs when blood or any body fluid except sweat contacts nonintact skin or mucous membranes

chain of infection: a description of the factors necessary for an infection to spread

communicable: diseases that are easily transmitted to other persons

contact precautions: A category of transmission-based precautions used when caring for patients who have infections that are spread by skin and wound drainage, secretions, excretions, blood, body fluids, or contact with mucous membranes.

contact transmission: the spread of pathogens by direct or indirect contact, such as touching an infectious object or person

contaminated: unclean, soiled articles or equipment

disinfection: the process that destroys or slows the growth of disease-causing microorganisms

droplet precautions: A category of transmission-based precautions used to prevent the spread of infection from patients whose infection is spread by droplets in the air.

droplets: moist secretions produced by sneezing, coughing, laughing, talking, and singing that are spread into the air

droplet transmission: the spread of disease in the air. Droplets usually remain within three feet of the resident. Droplet transmission occurs by inhaling droplets of secretions that contain pathogens.

drug-resistant pathogens: pathogens that cannot be destroyed by most antibiotics

germs: a common name for disease-causing microbes

high-efficiency particulate air (HEPA) filter respirator: this respirator prevents transmission of tuberculosis and other tiny pathogens that are spread by the airborne method of transmission

HBV (hepatitis B virus): the virus that causes hepatitis B, a disease of the liver

HIV (human immunodeficiency virus): the virus that causes HIV disease and AIDS

infection: a disease state caused by germs invading the body

isolation: protective techniques used when caring for a resident with a communicable disease

medical asepsis: the practices and techniques used in the health care setting to prevent the spread of microorganisms from one person or place to another

microbe: a microorganism

microorganisms: living plants and animals that are so small they can only be seen with a microscope

mite: microscopic parasites that live on the skin on animals and humans, causing rashes and irritation

MRSA (methicillin resistant Staphylococcus aureus): a pathogen that is very difficult to eradicate because it is resistant to most antibiotics

N95 respirator: a respirator used when caring for a resident in airborne precautions

pathogen: a microorganism that is harmful and causes disease; disease-causing microbes

personal protective equipment: common medical equipment such as gowns, gloves, masks, and other items that protect the nursing assistant from contact with blood or any other body fluids

PFR95 respirator: a respirator used when caring for a resident in airborne precautions

scabies: a mite that cannot be seen with the eye that causes severe itching and skin rash, and is highly contagious

standard precautions: special protective procedures and practices used in the care of all residents; standard precautions protect both the nursing assistant and the resident

sterile: free from all microorganisms

sterilization: a process that destroys all microorganisms

TB (tuberculosis): a serious disease that is spread by airborne transmission

transmission-based precautions: CDC recommendations for preventing the spread of infection in residents known or suspected to have certain diseases

virus: extremely small microbes that grow in living plants and animals; viruses cause infections that cannot be eliminated by antibiotics

VRE (vancomycin resistant *Enterococcus*): a pathogen found in health care facilities that is resistant to most antibiotics

MEDICAL ASEPSIS

Medical asepsis means practices and techniques used in the health care facility to prevent the spread of disease. **Germs** are also called **microorganisms.** Some of these microorganisms cause disease. **Aseptic** means to be free from disease-causing microorganisms. The staff in a health care facility must use the principles of medical asepsis to prevent the spread of diseases. An understanding of microorganisms will help you to realize the importance of medical asepsis. Practicing medical asepsis protects both the nursing assistant and the resident (Figure 6-1).

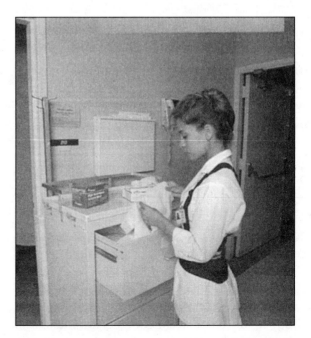

Figure 6-1 Medical asepsis prevents the spread of infection.

Microorganisms

Microorganisms are small, living plants and animals that cannot be seen without a microscope. Microorganisms, also called **microbes,** are found everywhere. They are in the air, in soil, in water, on food, on clothing, and on our bodies. Microbes need food, warmth, and moisture to grow and thrive. They grow best in warm, dark, damp areas. Microorganisms do not grow as well in light and dry areas. Disease-causing microbes are called **pathogens.** Some pathogens can be destroyed by **disinfection.** When something is **sterile,** it is free from all microorganisms. **Sterilization** is required to kill all microorganisms. Sterilization can be done by using heat, gas, or chemicals.

In the long-term care facility, all persons are exposed to many microorganisms. Practicing the principles of medical asepsis is important to protect both the nursing assistant and the resident. Many residents do not have strong resistance to disease because of age and illness. In the health care facility, you must prevent the spread of disease from resident to resident, resident to staff, or staff to resident (Figure 6-2). Sometimes visitors are ill when they come to the long-term care facility. If you believe that a visitor is ill, report this to the charge nurse.

Principles of Medical Asepsis

Principles of medical asepsis include the following:

- Handwashing

  — This is the single most important measure in preventing the spread of infection (Figure 6-3).

- Proper handling of food

- Separation of clean and dirty

  — Follow facility policy for separation of clean and dirty items. For example, the food cart (clean) should be kept at least one room away from the housekeeping cart (dirty) or soiled linen hamper (dirty). Some facilities require that dirty items be completely removed from the hall during food service.

- Disinfection of supplies and equipment

  — As a nursing assistant, you will be responsible for disinfecting reusable resident care items. Take this responsibility very seriously, and disinfect equipment according to facility policy.

- Proper handling of linens

  — Wear gloves when handling linen **contaminated** with blood or any moist body fluid except sweat. The term *contaminated* means the same as dirty.

  — Do not let clean or dirty linens touch your uniform. Carry them away from your body.

  — Do not bring more linen into the room than you need. If linen is stacked in the room, it

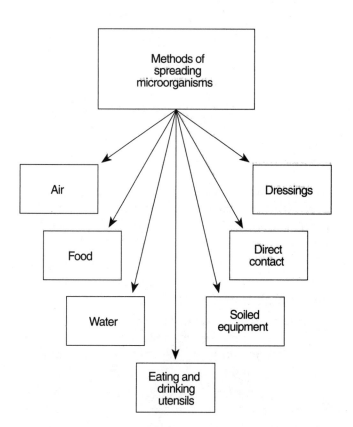

Figure 6-2 Microorganisms can be spread by many different methods.

Figure 6-3 Handwashing is the most important method of preventing the spread of infection.

can only be used there. It is considered contaminated if it is removed.

— Do not place soiled linen on the floor.

— Avoid shaking linens.

— If clean linen falls to floor, place it in the soiled linen hamper.

— Know and follow facility policy for placing clean and soiled linen while you are making a bed and performing resident care in the room.

- Proper disposal of liquids

    — Dispose of soiled liquids directly into sinks, toilets, or according to facility policy.

    — Avoid splashing.

- Facility policy for wearing gloves

    — Wear nonsterile gloves when contact with body fluids and contaminated items is anticipated (Figure 6-4).

    — Some facilities allow one glove to be worn in the hallway to hold a soiled item. The ungloved hand is used to open doors, turn on faucets, etc. Some facilities prohibit the wearing of gloves in the hallway. An alternative is to hold a paper towel in the palm of your hand. Use the paper towel to contact soiled items and the ungloved hand to contact environmental surfaces.

    — Always avoid touching environmental surfaces with used gloves, even if the gloves do not look soiled.

    — Know and follow facility policy for disposing of used gloves.

Figure 6-4 Wear gloves when contact with blood, body fluids (except sweat), secretions, excretions, mucous membranes, or nonintact skin is likely.

- Proper handling of body waste

    — Wear gloves when contact with blood, body fluids (except sweat), secretions, excretions, mucous membranes, or nonintact skin is likely. If you are already wearing gloves, change them immediately before contacting nonintact skin or mucous membranes.

    — Dispose of body waste properly.

    — Follow the infectious waste policy of your facility.

- Maintain good health

    — Eat properly.

    — Get enough sleep.

    — Get adequate exercise.

    — Maintain good mental health.

    — Be sure that your own immunizations of hepatitis B, tetanus, and others are current.

- Personal illness

    — Staff and visitors should avoid coming to the facility when they are ill.

    — Follow your facility policy for notifying your supervisor of illness.

- Personal protective equipment

    — Select the proper type of **personal protective equipment** for the task that you are performing.

- Handwashing

    — Remember that handwashing is the single most effective way to prevent the spread of disease.

INFECTION

An **infection** is a disease state that results from the invasion and growth of pathogens in the body. The infection may be localized, or confined to a certain body part. The infection may also be generalized, involving the whole body.

Development of Infection

The **chain of infection** (Figure 6-5) is a set of factors necessary for an infection to spread. If any of the factors are missing, an infection will not spread. These factors are the:

- source: a carrier of the germ that causes the disease. The source can be human or environmental.

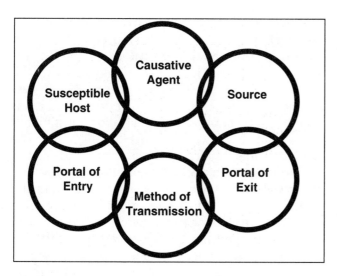

Figure 6-5 The chain of infection.

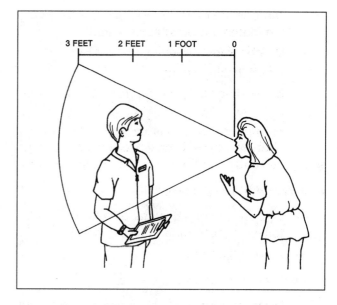

Figure 6-6 Colds can be spread by droplet transmission.

- reservoir or host: a place where the source or germ can grow
- carrier: a reservoir or host, usually a person, who may or may not have the signs of disease; the person may not know that he or she is carrying the disease
- causative agent: the germ that causes the disease
- transmission: the way in which a pathogen is spread from one person to another
- portal of entry: a place where the germ can get into the susceptible host's body
- susceptibility: the ability or inability of the susceptible host's body to resist the disease-causing germ

Spread of Infection

Infections can be spread in many ways. The most common methods are airborne, contact, droplet, and blood and body fluid transmission.

Airborne transmission. In **airborne transmission,** very small pathogens are suspended in the air or in dust particles and may travel for long distances. They are inhaled by the susceptible host.

Contact transmission. In **contact transmission,** pathogens are spread by two different types of contact. Pathogens spread by direct contact are spread when the susceptible host actually touches the source. Touching an infected area or secretions is a form of direct contact. Pathogens that are spread by indirect contact are spread when the susceptible host contacts a contaminated item, such as soiled linen.

Droplet transmission. **Droplets** are moist particles from coughing and sneezing. Pathogens are spread into the air with the droplets. This is called **droplet transmission.** The pathogens usually do not travel beyond three feet from the source (Figure 6-6). The susceptible host usually inhales them.

Blood and body fluid transmission. **Blood and body fluid transmission** of microbes is a form of contact transmission. Diseases can occur when the susceptible host comes into direct or indirect contact with blood, body fluid, mucous membranes, nonintact skin, or any moist body substance except sweat.

COMMON DISEASES

Health care workers must learn to protect themselves from many diseases present in health care facilities. Some diseases are very serious. Practicing medical asepsis, standard precautions, and using **isolation** precautions help protect both the nursing assistant and residents from contracting diseases.

Since the discovery of antibiotics, many lives have been saved. Antibiotics kill **bacteria,** some of which cause disease. Over the years, however, common pathogens have developed resistance to antibiotics so that antibiotics no longer eliminate those pathogens. Sometimes this occurs because people took antibiotics until they felt better but did not finish taking the prescription. The pathogen was still present in the person's body and developed resistance to the antibiotic used. Over time, these pathogens have become quite powerful and now resist most antibiotics. These are called **drug-resistant pathogens.** Although some antibiotics can kill resistant germs, these drugs often are very expensive and may have toxic side effects particularly in the elderly.

Some diseases are caused by a very tiny organism called a **virus.** Antibiotics do not kill viruses.

Several diseases in health care facilities are referred to using abbreviations. Some common diseases are:

- **HBV,** or **hepatitis B virus.** This virus causes permanent damage to the liver and is spread by contact with blood and body fluid.

- **HIV,** or **human immunodeficiency virus.** This virus causes HIV disease and AIDS, a progressively fatal disease that weakens the immune system. It is spread by contact with blood and body fluid. Not everyone who has contact with the virus develops AIDS.

- **MRSA,** or **methicillin resistant *Staphylococcus aureus.*** This pathogen can be spread by either the droplet method of transmission or contact transmission, depending on the location of the germ in the host's body. It usually causes skin infections, but can cause other illnesses in the lungs and urinary tract. This microbe is resistant to most forms of antibiotic therapy. Some people are *colonized* with MRSA. This means that the microbe is in their body, but they do not have an active infection. The pathogen can only be spread to others if the resident has an infection.

- **VRE,** or **vancomycin resistant *Enterococcus.*** This dangerous drug-resistant germ emerged in the 1990s. The pathogen originates in the intestine but can cause infection in any part of the body. It is commonly spread by the contact method of transmission.

Tuberculosis, or **TB,** is a disease spread by airborne transmission. TB is like MRSA in that some people have the TB pathogen in their body but are not infectious. If a tuberculosis skin test is done on these people, it is interpreted as positive. This form of TB is a *latent* infection. Although the microbe is present, the immune system contains it so that it cannot be spread to others. If the individual is treated with drugs, the TB will be eliminated. If the person is not treated, the TB may become active in the future. Some forms of TB also are drug-resistant.

We think of TB as a disease of the lungs, but it can also be found in other parts of the body. All, however, are caused by the susceptible host inhaling the TB microbe. This microbe is very tiny and can spread over long distances in the air on dust and moisture. For this reason, special ventilation systems are used, and all care givers who enter the room wear **high efficiency particulate air (HEPA) filter respirators** (Figure 6-7). Alternatives to the HEPA mask are the **N95 respirator** or **PFR95 respirator.** Any mask worn in an airborne precautions room must be approved by the National Institute of Occupational Safety and Health (NIOSH). The pathogen that causes TB is very small and may fit through the air holes of a regular surgical mask. The respirator mask has extremely tiny pores, and the pathogen cannot fit through them. Not everyone can wear a respirator mask. Before you use one of these masks, you must be fit-tested by a qualified professional. You must also have a medical examination. The physician must state that use of the respirator mask will not harm you. You will learn how to check the fit on the respirator mask yourself. Every time you put a respirator mask on, you must check to be sure that there are no air leaks around your face. The mask must seal tightly to be effective. All respirator masks have two elastic straps that fit around the head. This maintains a tight seal around the face. Men with facial hair cannot wear the respirator mask because the hair prevents a tight seal. Special hoods are available. Some respirator masks are disposable. Disposable masks are used once and thrown away. Other respirator masks are reusable. Many masks are color-coded according to fit size.

Another disease commonly seen in health care facilities is **scabies.** This disease is spread by contact transmission. Scabies is caused by a **mite,** a tiny parasite that can be seen only under a microscope. It lives on the skin and causes severe itching, skin conditions, and rashes. Special lotions and creams are

Figure 6-7 A HEPA respirator (left) and N95 respirator (right).

used to kill the mite. More than one application may be necessary. The environment, furniture, and resident's clothing must also be cleaned to eliminate the mite. Products containing the chemical lindane are not recommended. These can cause toxicity in susceptible individuals. The scabies mite may also be resistant to treatment.

Disease Resistance

It is important to know how infection develops because you will be working with people who can become ill very easily. A person's ability to resist infection and illness is related to:

- age.
- general health and nutritional state.
- medications taken by the person.
- presence of other illnesses and underlying diseases.

STANDARD PRECAUTIONS

Standard precautions are measures that health care workers use to prevent the spread of infection to themselves and others (Figure 6-8). Standard precautions require that all health care workers routinely use appropriate techniques when contact with blood or any other moist body fluid (except sweat), secretions, or excretions is anticipated. They are also used for contact with mucous membranes and nonintact skin. These precautions are used for all residents regardless of their disease or diagnosis. A health care facility may develop specific policies, but most generally include the following:

- Wear gloves when in contact with any body fluids or body discharges (except sweat), secretions, or excretions. Wear gloves for contact with mucous membranes and nonintact skin. If you are already wearing gloves, change them immediately before touching mucous membranes and nonintact skin, even if the gloves do not appear to be soiled. Wearing gloves does not replace the need for handwashing, because the gloves may have small defects that you cannot see, or may get torn during use. Your hands may also accidentally become contaminated when you remove the gloves.
- Wash your hands before applying gloves and after removing gloves.
- Change gloves after contact with each resident.
- Dispose of gloves according to facility policy.
- Always carry gloves with you.
- Wear gloves, gown, mask, cap, face shield, or goggles when indicated to protect you from direct contact with body fluids or accidental splashing of secretions. When you wear goggles or a face shield, you must always wear a face mask as well. A good rule to follow is that you can wear a mask without eye protection, but you cannot wear eye protection without a mask. You must choose the proper protective equipment for the task you are doing. Isolation procedures follow later in this chapter.
- Dispose of trash and linen properly (Figure 6-9). Place in a sturdy plastic bag. Do not allow soiled material to touch the outside of the bag.
- Laundry and trash bags should be labeled as contaminated or as indicated by facility policy. Some facilities require these items to be double-bagged. The Centers for Disease Control state that double-bagging is not necessary unless the outside of the bag becomes contaminated or torn.
- Trash that has contacted blood or body fluid requires special labeling and handling. Follow your facility policy for handling this **biohazardous waste** (Figure 6-10). The biohazard symbol should have a red or orange background with a contrasting color emblem. It means that the contents of the container are potentially contaminated with blood or body fluid. Biohazardous waste requires special storage, handling, and removal. It is not thrown into the regular trash can. Most facilities require staff to dispose of used disposable gloves in a covered trash can. Contaminated disposable gloves and biohazardous waste are discarded in designated covered trash cans. A red bag may be used to line the can, but is not required. The outside of the container should be labeled with the biohazard emblem.
- Know and follow facility policy and procedure regarding special situations.
- Needles, razors, and other sharps must be disposed of in puncture-resistant containers (Figure 6-11). Never recap, cut, or bend needles.
- Clean up broken glass with a broom and dustpan. Never use your hands.

HANDWASHING

As you have learned, handwashing is the single most effective way to prevent the spread of infection. Handwashing should be done:

- when beginning work.
- before and after caring for each resident.
- before and after using gloves.

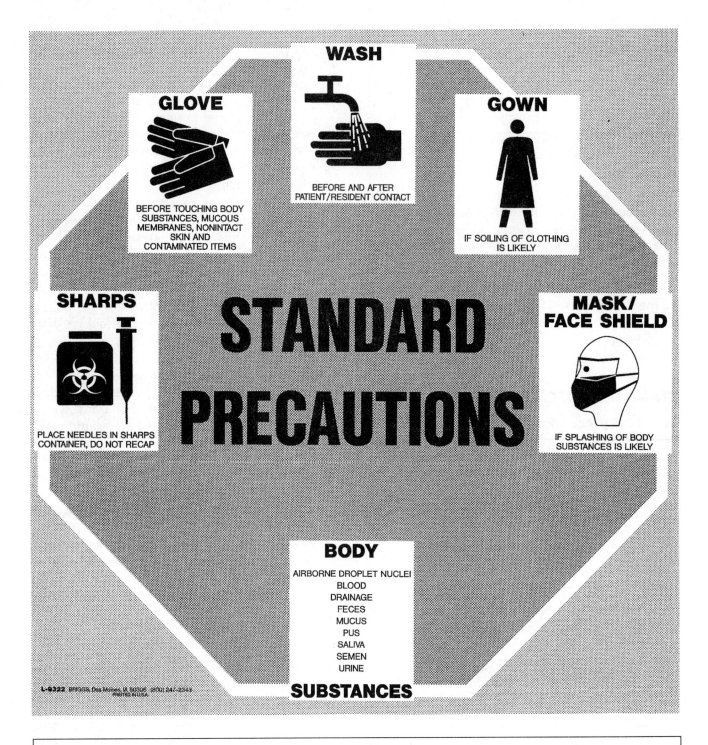

Standard Precautions
1. Wash hands.
2. Gowns are indicated if soiling is likely.
3. Gloves are indicated. When touching body substances, mucous membranes, nonintact skin, and contaminated items, change frequently.
4. Mask/face shield is indicated if splashing of body substances is likely.
5. Place needles in Sharps container. Do not recap.
6. Wash hands.

Figure 6-8 Standard precautions must be used in the care of all residents, regardless of disease or diagnosis. Residents can spread infection even though they do not appear ill. (Courtesy of Briggs Corporation, Des Moines, IA; (800)247-2343.)

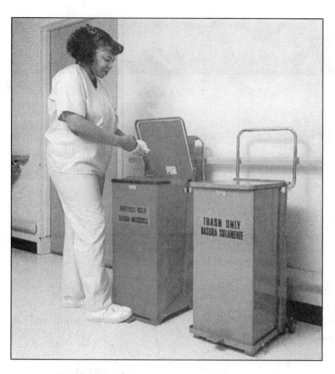

Figure 6-9 Discard trash in the proper container.

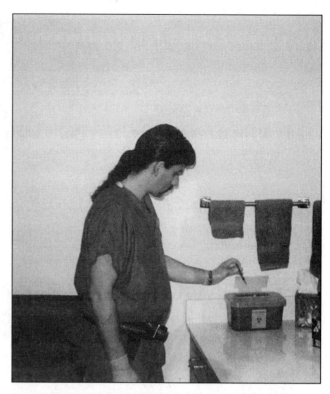

Figure 6-11 Discard needles, razors, and other sharps in a puncture-resistant container.

Figure 6-10 The biohazard emblem is black with a red or orange background. The emblem is used for trash, linen, and other items contaminated with blood, body fluids, secretions, or excretions..

- before handling food.
- after personal use of the bathroom.
- after combing your hair, using a tissue, eating, drinking, or smoking.
- after handling a resident's belongings.
- after working with anything soiled.
- before using lip balm.
- before and after any oral contact.

- before and after manipulating contact lenses.
- before adjusting your eyeglasses.
- after contact with blood, mucous membranes, moist body fluids (except sweat), secretions, excretions, or equipment or articles contaminated by them.
- before leaving work at the end of the day.

WHEN TO USE GLOVES

Residents need to be touched. Avoid wearing gloves for routine contact and care.

Gloves should always be used:

- when touching excretions, secretions, blood, body fluids, mucous membranes, or nonintact skin. If gloves become contaminated with body substances, remove them, wash your hands, and put on a clean pair of gloves before continuing the procedure or care.
- when your hands have cuts, are chapped or scraped, or you have a rash or other skin condition.
- when cleaning spills of any body fluid.
- when cleaning any equipment or environmental surface that may be contaminated.
- when washing or caring for a resident's eyes,

✔ GUIDELINES for Handwashing

Follow these guidelines each time you wash your hands.

☐ Use warm, running water.

☐ Do not lean against the sink when washing. The sink is contaminated.

☐ Always keep your fingertips pointed down when washing your hands.

☐ Wash hands for a minimum of 10 seconds.

☐ Avoid shaking water from your hands. Shaking water may spread the microbes.

☐ *Friction* is required in handwashing. Friction is created by rubbing the hands together briskly. Friction is important to remove germs from the hands.

☐ Dry your hands thoroughly.

☐ Always turn the faucet on and off by using a clean paper towel.

☐ Put lotion on your hands frequently. Frequent washing dries your hands. Dry skin on hands may crack, creating a place for pathogens to enter.

☐ Follow facility policy for use of soap or other hand-cleaning agents. Some facilities use waterless hand-cleaning products as a temporary measure if a sink is not immediately available.

nasal discharges, or discharges from the mouth.

- when providing mouth or oral care, or assisting with a dental procedure.
- when shaving residents.
- any time you perform a procedure in an area where the resident's skin is cut, scraped, torn, or otherwise not intact.
- when changing colostomy or ileostomy bags.
- when collecting specimens.
- when performing perineal care or when cleaning episodes of incontinence.
- during any procedure when you are not sure if an area is contaminated.

Change your gloves:

- before each resident contact.
- after each resident contact.
- *immediately before* touching mucous membranes.
- *immediately before* touching nonintact skin.
- after you touch a resident's secretions or excretions, before moving to care for another part of the body.
- after touching blood or body fluids, before moving to care for another part of the body.
- after touching contaminated environmental surfaces or equipment.
- any time your gloves become visibly soiled.
- if your gloves become torn.
- before caring for another resident.

Avoid:

- double- or triple-gloving, unless you are specifically instructed to do so by the nurse.
- washing your gloved hands.
- touching an environmental surface with used gloves, even if the gloves are not visibly soiled. Gloves are contaminated after resident contact.
- contaminating clean supplies, linen, equipment, or environmental surfaces with gloved hands. Remove one glove and use your ungloved hand, or place a clean paper towel under one glove and contact environmental surfaces with the towel.
- wearing the same gloves to care for more than one resident.

Discarding Used Gloves

Dispose of used gloves according to facility policy. Generally, they are not discarded in an open wastebasket in the resident's room. Some facilities place extra plastic bags in the bottom of the wastebasket. Replace the one currently in use with a new bag from the bottom of the wastebasket. If you must throw soiled gloves and other contaminated items into the wastebasket, remove the bag, tie it, and take it with you when you leave the room. Discard the bag in the biohazardous waste or other designated location.

USE OF PROTECTIVE EYEWEAR

Eye protection should be used any time you anticipate splashes of blood or body fluids. This could occur during a resident care procedure, when cleaning equipment and supplies, or rinsing linen. Protective

2   Handwashing

1 Stand away from the sink. Your uniform and hands must not touch the sink.

2 Turn on warm water with a dry paper towel. Adjust water to a comfortable temperature.

3 Wet hands, keeping your fingertips pointed down.

4 Apply soap over hands and wrists, working it into a lather.

5 Rub your hands together vigorously to create a lather. Rub the hands together in a circular motion for 10 to 15 seconds. Rub all surfaces of the hands. Pay particular attention to the area between your fingers. Wash your thumbs well. Keep your fingertips pointed down (Figure 6-12).

6 Rub the fingernails against the palm of the opposite hand. Clean the nails with a brush or an orange stick if they are soiled.

7 Rinse your hands from the wrist to the fingertips. Make sure that all soap residue is removed. Keep the fingers pointed down.

8 Do not shake water from hands.

9 Dry hands with a clean paper towel. Discard paper towel properly.

10 Use a clean, dry paper towel to turn off the faucet. Do not touch the faucet handle with your hand.

11 Discard the paper towel in the wastebasket.

Figure 6-12 Wash your hands for a minimum of 10 to 15 seconds. Keep your fingertips pointed down.

goggles that fit tightly around the eyes offer protection to the mucous membranes of the eyes. The goggles do not protect the mucous membranes of your nose and mouth. You must wear a surgical mask in addition to the goggles. Face shields are also available. These cover the entire face, from the forehead to the chin. It is possible for secretions to splash under the shield. Additional protection is provided by wearing a surgical mask.

Select eyewear that allows you to see clearly. Protective eyewear that fits over regular eyeglasses is available. Some eyewear is disposable. It is used once and discarded. Other eyewear is reusable. It is disinfected after each use. Become familiar with the eyewear used by your facility before you need it.

GUIDELINES for Wearing a Mask

To ensure full protection, follow these guidelines for wearing a mask:

☐ Wash your hands before putting on the mask.
☐ The mask should cover your nose and mouth. Bend the nose piece of the mask so that it fits securely.
☐ If your face becomes wet, change the mask. It is not effective when moist.
☐ Do not let the mask hang around your neck.
☐ Do not remove the mask when you are performing resident care. Wait until you finish the procedure.
☐ The mask is used only for the care of one resident, then discarded.
☐ Handle the mask only by the ties or elastic straps.
☐ Never touch the front of the mask when you are wearing it.
☐ Wash your hands before removing the mask.

GUIDELINES for Putting on Protective Eyeware and a Mask

☐ Wash your hands.
☐ Apply the surgical mask.
☐ Apply the face shield or goggles.

GUIDELINES for Removing Protective Eyewear and a Mask

☐ Wash your hands.
☐ Remove the face shield or goggles.
☐ Remove the surgical mask.
☐ Wash your hands.

USE OF A SURGICAL MASK

The surgical mask is worn to protect the mucous membranes in your nose and mouth. Some facilities buy masks that have an eye shield attached (Figure 6-13). Masks are disposable. They are worn once, then discarded. They should not be used in more than one resident room. A surgical mask is worn to protect you when a resident is in droplet precautions. It is also worn with goggles or face shield to protect you from splashes of blood and other moist body fluids.

ISOLATION PROCEDURES

Isolation is a method or technique of caring for residents who have **communicable** or contagious diseases. The purpose of isolation is to prevent the spread

Figure 6-13 An alternate type of surgical mask has a face shield attached. This mask proteccts the eyes, as well as the mucous membranes of the nose and mouth.

Figure 6-14 Follow facility policies and procedures for preventing the spread of infection.

of the disease. Knowing isolation procedures will help you stay healthy and prevent the spread of disease.

The procedures for isolation vary with the disease and how it is transmitted from one person to another. Most facilities use a system that lists which procedures to follow. Some isolation procedures include wearing a mask, gown, and gloves (Figure 6-14). *Standard precautions are always used <u>in addition</u> to isolation procedures.*

Transmission-based Precautions

In 1996, the Centers for Disease Control (CDC) issued guidelines that included **transmission-based precautions.** These precautions were designed to replace the isolation categories used previously. The CDC recommends three types of transmission-based precautions. Standard precautions are used with transmission-based precautions. The type of precautions used is selected by the nurse manager and physician according to the mode of transmission of the infection. Transmission-based precautions are used because normal cleanliness and standard precautions are not adequate to prevent the spread of infection with certain pathogens. A private room is used. This confines the pathogen to a single unit. In some situations, residents with the same pathogen will share a unit.

Airborne Precautions. **Airborne precautions**
are used for diseases that are spread a long distance in the air, ventilation system, or by airborne dust and moisture particles (Figure 6-15). An example of a disease requiring use of airborne precautions is tuberculosis. Residents in airborne precautions must have a special ventilation system in their room. Care givers must wear NIOSH-approved respirators when giving care. The HEPA respirator filter N95, and PFR95 respirators are all approved for use in the airborne precautions room. Standard precautions are also used. Figure 6-16 describes how to apply a respirator and check the fit.

Droplet precautions. **Droplet precautions** protect you when a resident has a disease in which the causative agent is spread into the air by large droplets (Figure 6-17). The droplets can be spread by sneezing, coughing, talking, singing, or laughing. An example of a disease requiring use of droplet precautions is influenza. The droplets usually do not travel more than three feet. A surgical mask is worn when caring for a resident in this type of isolation. Standard precautions are also used.

Contact precautions. **Contact precautions** are used for conditions in which a disease is spread by either direct or indirect contact (Figure 6-18). An example of a disease requiring use of contact precautions is scabies. Many skin and urinary tract infections also require the use of contact precautions. Contact occurs by touching the contaminated area on the skin. In the case of a urinary tract infection, contact occurs by touching the urine. Indirect contact can also occur in this type of infection by touching an item, such as linen, that has come in contact with the infectious material. Gloves are put on before you enter the room. Gloves should be changed if they contact highly contaminated matter. After you remove the soiled gloves, wash your hands, then apply clean gloves. Remove the gloves and wash your hands immediately before you leave the room. Use a paper towel to turn the door handle.

A gown is worn when you enter the room if you think that your clothing may contact the resident or items in the room. The gown is removed before you leave the room. After removing the gown, make sure your uniform does not contact the resident or items in the environment. For example, if you are entering the room to leave a food tray on the overbed table, you would wear gloves only. If you will be making the bed or touching the sheets with your uniform, wear both a gown and gloves. Standard precautions are also used.

PERFORMANCE PROCEDURE

3   Isolation Procedures
Putting on disposable gown, gloves, and mask

1   Remove your watch and place it on a clean paper towel. You will carry your watch with you into the isolation room on the paper towel.

2   Wash your hands and dry them thoroughly.

3   Put a mask on, and adjust it over your nose and mouth. Tie the mask securely at the back of your head, or slip the elastic straps over your ears.

4   Put on a gown.

5   Tie the neck ties.

6   Tie the waist ties of the gown, making certain the gown is overlapping and covering your uniform.

7   Put on gloves, covering the cuffs of the gown with the top edge of the gloves.

PERFORMANCE PROCEDURE

4   Removing disposable
gown, gloves, and mask

1   Make sure that all jobs in the isolation unit are complete and that the resident is comfortable and safe. Place needed personal items and the call signal within the resident's reach.

2   Remove gloves by turning them inside out, and dispose of them in the biohazardous waste receptacle.

3   Untie the waist ties of the gown.

4   Using a clean paper towel, turn on the faucet. Wash and dry your hands. Turn off the faucet with a clean paper towel.

5   Remove the mask by grasping only the ties. Untie the bottom tie first, then the top tie, or slip the elastic over your ears.

6   Discard the mask in the covered trash container.

7   Untie the neck ties of the gown and loosen the gown at the shoulders.

8   Slip the fingers of one hand under the cuff of the gown on the opposite arm. Do not touch the outside of the gown. Pull it down over your hand.

9   With your hand inside the gown, pull the gown off the other arm.

10   Fold and roll the gown away from your body, with the contaminated side facing in.

11   Dispose of the gown in the covered biohazardous waste container.

12   Use a clean paper towel to turn on the faucet. Wash and dry your hands. Turn off the faucet with a clean paper towel.

13   Pick up your watch and put it on your wrist.

14   Holding the clean upper side of the paper towel, pick up the towel and discard it in the trash.

15   Obtain a clean paper towel from the dispenser and use it to open the door of the room.

16   Discard the towel inside the room.

17   Repeat handwashing if this is your preference or facility policy.

AIRBORNE PRECAUTIONS
In Addition to Standard Precautions

Visitors - Report to Nurses' Station Before Entering Room

BEFORE CARE	DURING CARE	AFTER CARE

BEFORE CARE

1. Private room and closed door with monitored negative air pressure, frequent air exchanges, and high-efficiency filtration.

2. Wash hands.

3. Wear respiratory protection appropriate for disease.

DURING CARE

1. Limit transport of patient/resident to essential purposes only. Patient resident must wear mask appropriate for disease.

2. Limit use of noncritical care equipment to a single patient/resident.

AFTER CARE

1. Bag linen to prevent contamination of self, environment, or outside of bag.

2. Discard infectious trash to prevent contamination of self, environment, or outside of bag.

3. Wash hands.

Figure 6-15 Airborne precautions. (Courtesy of Briggs Corporation, Des Moines, IA; (800) 247-2343.)

Donning instructions (to be followed each time product is worn):

1 Cup the respirator in your hand with the nosepiece at fingertips, allowing the headbands to hang freely below hands.

2 Position the respirator under your chin with the nosepiece up.

3 Pull the top strap over your head so it rests high on the back of head.

4 Pull the bottom strap over your head and position it around neck below ears.

5 Using two hands, mold the nosepiece to the shape of your nose by pushing inward while moving fingertips down both sides of the nosepiece. Pinching the nosepiece using one hand may result in less effective respirator performance.

6 FACE FIT CHECK
The respirator seal should be checked before each use. To check fit, place both hands completely over the respirator and exhale. If air leaks around your nose, adjust the nosepiece as described in step 5. If air leaks at respirator edges, adjust the straps back along the sides of your head. Recheck.

NOTE: If you cannot achieve proper fit, do not enter the isolation or treatment area. See your supervisor.

Removal instructions:

1 Cup the respirator in your hand to maintain position on face. Pull bottom strap over head.

2 Still holding respirator in position, pull top strap over head.

3 Remove respirator from face and discard or store according to your facility's policy.

Figure 6-16 Check the fit of the respirator each time it is worn. It must fit securely, with no air leaks. (Courtesy of 3M Health Care.)

DROPLET PRECAUTIONS
In Addition to Standard Precautions

Visitors - Report to Nurses' Station Before Entering Room

BEFORE CARE	DURING CARE	AFTER CARE

BEFORE CARE

1. Private room. Maintain 3 feet of spacing between patient/resident and visitors.

2. Mask/face shield for staff and visitors within 3 feet of patient/resident.

DURING CARE

1. Limit transport of patient/resident to essential purposes only. Patient/resident must wear mask appropriate for disease.

2. Limit use of noncritical care equipment to a single patient/resident.

AFTER CARE

1. Bag linen to prevent contamination of self, environment, or outside of bag.

2. Discard infectious trash to prevent contamination of self, environment, or outside of bag.

3. Wash hands.

Figure 6-17 Droplet precautions. (Courtesy of Briggs Corporation, Des Moines, IA; (800) 247-2343.)

CONTACT PRECAUTIONS
In Addition to Standard Precautions

Visitors - Report to Nurses' Station Before Entering Room

BEFORE CARE

1. Private room.

2. Wash hands.

3. Wear gown if soiling is likely.

4. Wear gloves when entering room. Change after contact with infective material.

DURING CARE

1. Limit transport of patient/resident to essential purposes only. Patient/resident must wear mask appropriate for disease.

2. Limit use of noncritical care equipment to a single patient/resident.

AFTER CARE

1. Bag linen to prevent contamination of self, environment, or outside of bag.

2. Discard infectious trash to prevent contamination of self, environment, or outside of bag.

3. Wash hands.

Figure 6-18 Contact precautions. (Courtesy of Briggs Corporation, Des Moines, IA; (800) 247-2343.)

KEY POINTS IN THIS CHAPTER

▲ Medical asepsis refers to practices performed to prevent the spread of disease.

▲ Microorganisms are found everywhere. Many are present on the body.

▲ Microorganisms thrive in warm, dark, damp areas.

▲ Pathogens are microorganisms that cause disease.

▲ Most residents in the long-term care facility have lower resistance to disease, which means that most are susceptible to illness.

▲ Proper handwashing is the single most effective way to prevent the spread of disease.

▲ Friction is required when washing hands.

▲ Infections can be localized or generalized.

▲ The most common routes for infection to spread are airborne, droplet, and contact transmission.

▲ Standard precautions are special procedures used when contacting blood or any moist body fluid (except sweat), secretions, excretions, mucous membranes, or nonintact skin. Standard precautions are used in the care of all residents, regardless of disease or diagnosis.

▲ Isolation procedures may be necessary to prevent the spread of communicable disease.

REVIEW QUIZ

1. Practices used in health care facilities to prevent the spread of disease are called:
   a. sterilization.
   b. disinfection.
   c. medical asepsis.
   d. techniques.

2. Which of the following is *not* true regarding microorganisms?
   a. All microorganisms are harmful to humans.
   b. Microorganisms are small, living plants or animals.
   c. Microorganisms need food, warmth, and moisture to grow.
   d. Microorganisms are present in many places.

3. What is the *most* important measure nursing assistants can take to prevent the spread of infection?
   a. Sterilize all items.
   b. Wear isolation gowns.
   c. Wash hands.
   d. Wear gloves.

4. Proper handling of linens includes:
   a. hold linens away from your uniform.
   b. avoid shaking linen.
   c. wear gloves if linens have moist body fluid, secretions, or excretions on them.
   d. all of the above.

5. Microorganisms can be spread by all of the following *except:*
   a. contaminated dressings.
   b. sterile items.
   c. food and water.
   d. all of the above.

6. Infection is spread:
   a. in the air.
   b. in droplet secretions.
   c. by contact.
   d. all of the above.

7. A germ that causes a disease is the:
   a. source.
   b. host.
   c. carrier.
   d. reservoir.

8. Principles of standard precautions include wearing gloves:
   a. at all times when giving care to residents.
   b. for residents in isolation only.
   c. for contact with all moist body fluids (except sweat), secretions, and excretions.
   d. for contact only with body fluids that contain visible blood.

9. When performing the handwashing procedure, you should:
   a. turn the faucet on and off with a clean paper towel.
   b. wash for a minimum of five seconds.
   c. shake the excess water off your hands.
   d. all of the above.

10. Friction in handwashing is caused by:
    a. lotion applied to hands.
    b. rubbing the hands together.
    c. using a mild soap.
    d. using warm water.

11. A disease state caused by invasion of microorganisms into the body that can be either localized or generalized is:
    a. transmission.
    b. disability.
    c. infection.
    d. contamination.

12. Microorganisms live best in:
    a. cool, dry areas.
    b. warm, sunny areas.
    c. cold, bright, wet areas.
    d. dark, damp, warm areas.

13. Microorganisms that cause disease are called:
    a. toxins.
    b. pathogens.
    c. disinfections.
    d. aseptics.

14. Personal protective equipment includes:
    a. gloves.
    b. gowns.
    c. masks.
    d. all of the above.

15. When working with a resident who has tuberculosis, you should wear a:
    a. surgical mask.
    b. NIOSH-approved respirator.
    c. negative pressure filter.
    d. none of the above.

16. Pathogens that cannot be killed by most antibiotics are:
    a. sterile.
    b. parasites.
    c. drug-resistant.
    d. immune-deficient.

17. A person's ability to resist infection depends on:
    a. general health and nutrition.
    b. medications taken.
    c. underlying diseases and illnesses.
    d. all of the above.

18. Standard precautions are used when caring for:
    a. all residents.
    b. residents with HIV disease only.
    c. residents with MRSA only.
    d. all residents in isolation.

19. Wash your hands:
    a. before applying gloves.
    b. after removing gloves.
    c. after touching blood.
    d. all of the above.

20. An example of indirect contact is:
    a. touching a resident.
    b. touching a tissue used by a resident.
    c. sneezing.
    d. all of the above.

21. Droplet secretions usually do not travel farther than:
    a. one foot.
    b. two feet.
    c. three feet.
    d. twenty feet.

22. When entering an isolation room, you should put on your protective equipment in this order:
    a. mask, gown, gloves.
    b. gown, gloves, mask.
    c. gloves, mask, gown.
    d. gloves, gown, mask.

23. When leaving an isolation room, your protective equipment should be removed in this order:
    a. mask, gloves, gown.
    b. gown, gloves, mask.
    c. gloves, mask, gown.
    d. mask, gown, gloves.

24. Most residents in the long-term care facility have:
    a. low resistance to disease.
    b. strong resistance to disease.
    c. immune deficiency syndrome.
    d. none of the above.

25. You should wear gloves for contact with the resident's:
    a. arms.
    b. perspiration.
    c. hair.
    d. saliva.

26. You are assigned to care for Debra Barber, a 43-year-old resident. Ms. Barber is in a coma and cannot speak to you. She does not have control over her bowels and bladder. You should wear gloves when:
    a. combing her hair.
    b. rubbing her back.
    c. washing her perineum.
    d. all of the above.

27. You are assigned to change the bed for James Tucker, a 77-year-old resident in contact precautions because of an MRSA infection in a wound on his foot. The wound is draining heavily through the bandage. When you go into the room, the resident is sitting in a chair next to the bed. You notice a large amount of drainage from his foot on the top sheet. Select the personal protective equipment that you will need to wear when changing the bed.
    a. gloves only
    b. gloves and gown
    c. gloves, gown, and mask
    d. gloves, gown, mask, and face shield

CHAPTER 6
CROSSWORD PUZZLE

Directions: Complete the puzzle using these words found in Chapter 6.

AIDS	handwashing	reservoir
airborne	HEPA	resistant
aseptic	HIV	scabies
bacteria	indirect	source
biohazardous	infection	standard
carrier	isolation	sterile
communicable	mask	susceptibility
contact	microbe	sweat
contaminated	microorganism	TB
disinfection	mite	transmission
droplet	MRSA	virus
germs	pathogen	VRE
gloves	portal	
gown	protective	

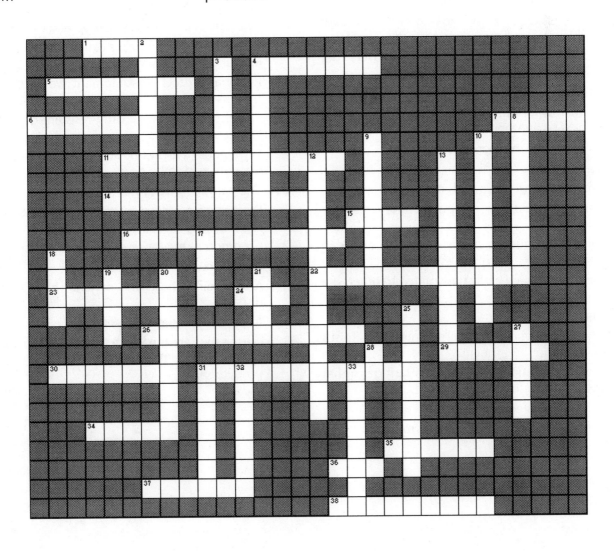

CHAPTER 6
PUZZLE CLUES

ACROSS

1. A special mask worn when working with a resident who is in airborne precautions.
4. A skin condition that is highly infectious and is transmitted by a mite.
5. Touching linen that is contaminated with pathogens is an example of _____ contact.
6. Touching a wound spreads pathogens by direct _____.
7. Extremely small microbe that grows in living plants and animals that cannot be killed by antibiotics
11. A living plant or animal that is so small it can only be seen through a microscope
14. Waste products contaminated with blood or body fluid are disposed of in the _____ waste.
15. Personal protective equipment that covers your uniform
16. Unclean
22. Some way for the germ to get from the reservoir or host to another host
23. Free from all microorganisms
24. The causative organism for AIDS
26. Process that slows growth of microorganisms
29. Personal protective equipment worn on your hands
30. Inhaling pathogens after a resident sneezes is an example of _____ transmission of infection.
31. Diseases that are easily transmitted to others are _____.
34. Perspiration
35. The place where the germ enters the host's body is the _____ of entry.
36. The abbreviation for a drug-resistant germ that is commonly found in the intestine
37. A _____ of infection
38. A place where the source or germ grows

DOWN

2. Absence of disease-causing microbes
3. One-celled microorganisms
4. Routine measures the nursing assistant uses when contacting blood or any moist body fluid (except sweat), secretions, and excretions are _____ precautions.
8. Techniques used when caring for a resident with a communicable disease
9. A microbe that causes disease
10. Personal _____ equipment
12. The ability of the host to resist the disease-causing germ.
13. The single most important measure the nursing assistant uses to prevent the spread of infection
17. Progressively fatal disease caused by the human immunodeficiency virus
18. Personal protective equipment worn to cover the nose and mouth
19. The abbreviation for a drug-resistant germ that causes skin infections
20. Pathogens that cannot be killed by most antibiotics are said to be drug-_____.
21. The parasite that causes scabies
25. Disease state caused by microorganisms invading the body
27. Common name for disease-causing microbes
28. The abbreviation for tuberculosis
31. A reservoir or host who may not have signs of disease
32. A microorganism
33. Germs that are inhaled from the air are spread by the _____ method of transmission.

Safety and Emergency Measures

OBJECTIVES

In this chapter, you will learn the safety and emergency measures you need to know when working in a long-term care facility. After reading this chapter, you will be able to:

- Spell and define key terms.
- Describe common accident hazards in the health care facility.
- List appropriate safety and accident prevention measures for residents.
- List rules to follow when using restraints.
- Apply a vest and belt restraint.
- List beginning procedure actions and procedure completion actions.
- Explain why alternatives to restraints are necessary.
- Describe your role in fire safety measures.
- Identify situations that call for emergency action and perform emergency procedures.

KEY TERMS

cardiopulmonary resuscitation (CPR): an emergency procedure used to establish effective circulation and respiration in a victim whose heart has stopped beating

emergency: an event that calls for immediate action

gait belt: a strong and sturdy belt, usually made of canvas, that is used to move, lift, ambulate, or support residents by placing it securely around the waist

geriatric chair or **geri chair:** a chair with wheels and a tray attached to it

hazard: a potential source of danger

Heimlich maneuver: a procedure done to expel a foreign object from the airway of a person who is choking

immobile: unable to move

impairment: anything that hinders proper function

incident: an unusual occurrence or event

obstructed airway: a blockage of the air passages

oxygen: a tasteless, colorless, odorless gas that is essential for breathing

protective device: a type of restraint that keeps the resident from harm

transfer belt: same as gait belt

RESIDENT SAFETY

As a nursing assistant, you must always make sure the residents are safe. All staff must be concerned for the safety of the resident. Many residents are frail or weak because of disease or old age.

Some residents have **impairments** in vision, hearing, or balance, as well as other disabilities. These, along with decreased strength, may increase the chance of accident or injury. Other residents may have a mental impairment or may be confused. Any of these conditions put the resident at higher risk of injury or accident. Newly admitted residents who may not be familiar with the surroundings also are at high risk for injury. Some residents with mental impairments who are ambulatory or use wheelchairs are at high risk for wandering away from the facility.

Potential Hazards

Some common **hazards** found in many long-term care facilities are:

- hazardous substances that the resident may swallow, such as disinfectants, cleaning supplies, medications, denture cleaning tablets, and nail polish remover. Some of these substances may also harm the resident if they contact the skin or get into the eyes (Figure 7-1).
- lack of proper lighting. Glare is especially hazardous to the elderly person. As we age, our eyes need more light in the room to see properly.
- lack of glasses, hearing aids, and other devices that help the resident stay in touch with her environment. It is the nursing assistant's responsibility to see that the residents who use these devices wear them.
- unsafe equipment.

Figure 7-1 Keep hazardous chemicals locked in a secure location.

- slippery floors (Figure 7-2).
- unlocked wheelchairs, **geriatric chairs (geri chairs),** shower chairs, or beds.
- errors such as giving the resident the wrong tray, treatment, or medication.
- improper use or application of restraints and safety devices.
- improperly placed or nonworking call light (Figure 7-3).
- unsafe or improperly performed procedures.
- unsupervised use of smoking materials.
- cluttered hallways.

PREVENTION OF ACCIDENTS

Preventing accidents is the responsibility of everyone in the health care facility. By being aware of the hazards, an alert staff can prevent many accidents. Ways to prevent injuries or accidents are as follows:

- Respond to emergency calls immediately.
- Follow the care plan at all times.
- Answer call signals as soon as possible.
- Check resident identification before giving care and performing procedures.
- Many injuries occur in the bathroom. Be alert when toileting residents.
- Use wheel locks on beds, lifts, shower chairs, geri chairs, and wheelchairs.
- Fasten safety belts when residents are in shower chairs and whirlpool lift chairs.
- Use side rails as indicated on the care plan.
- Use safety devices and restraints only when indicated on the care plan, and only according to manufacturers' directions.

Figure 7-2 Place a wet floor sign to warn others of a slippery floor.

Figure 7-3 Check the call signal each day to be sure it works properly.

- Clean up spills immediately.
- Be alert for sharp objects and remove them.
- Put all equipment and supplies on the same side of the hallway, leaving the opposite side free of clutter.
- Do not overload electrical outlets or use extension cords.
- Report unsafe equipment, and follow facility policy for removing it from service.
- Know procedures and do them properly. Avoid shortcuts.
  - Ask questions if you are unsure of how to do the task.
  - Do not perform tasks you have not been taught.
- Get help when necessary.
- Know the fire safety policy of the facility. Be alert to fire safety violations. Know smoking rules, oxygen safety, use of electrical equipment, unsafe wires, overuse of extension cords.
- Recognize that some residents cannot stay in the sunlight very long, because of medications or medical conditions. Follow the resident's care plan.
- Maintain your own health. Stay away from the facility if you are ill. Be sure to call the facility when illness prevents you from working.
- Use proper precautions when working with contaminated items.
- Monitor residents who wander. Know what clothing they are wearing and check their whereabouts frequently.
- Be alert for any safety hazard.

Falls

Falls are a serious threat or hazard to the resident. They are a common cause of accidents in the long-term care facility. If a resident starts to fall while you are walking with him, you should do the following:

- Gently guide the resident to the floor while grasping the **transfer (gait) belt,** or wrap your arms around the resident's midsection.
- Lean the resident onto your leg as you go down to the floor.
- Protect the resident's head so it does not hit the floor.

Call for the nurse immediately. Use the call signal or follow your facility policy. Stay with the resident. Do not attempt to move the resident until the nurse has checked him. If you find a resident on the floor, stay with the resident and call for help.

Incidents

When an accident or injury occurs, an incident report must be filled out (Figure 7-4). An **incident** is any event that is not part of the routine care or routine operation of the facility. An incident may involve the resident, the staff, or visitors.

RESTRAINTS AND SAFETY DEVICES

Restraints are **protective devices** that limit a resident's freedom to move about and limit access to his or her own body. These safety devices are an infringement on the resident's rights and may be used only when ordered by a physician. The resident or legal guardian must also consent to the use of a restraint. Restraints must be used only when absolutely necessary and when other means to protect the resident have not been successful. They should be the last choice after other alternatives, such as behavior modification, physical therapy, and changing environmental factors that put the resident at risk of injury have been tried.

Reasons for Using Restraints

Restraints may be used to:

- enable a resident to function at the highest possible level by providing proper positioning and support.
- prevent injury, such as falling.
- prevent the resident from injuring others.
- prevent pulling on tubing or wound coverings.
- prevent residents from accidentally injuring themselves.

Types of Restraints

A variety of protective devices are available. If a resident does not have the physical or mental ability to remove a device, it may be considered a restraint. Common items are not always recognized as restraints. Examples of these items are sheets pulled tightly, trays that attach to the side of a chair with velcro, and seat belts with plastic buckles that are difficult to release. Nursing personnel often cover the resident's lap with a sheet, blanket, or lap robe when the resident is in a wheelchair. If the cover is tied around the back of the chair, it is a restraint. Many other pieces of equipment used in long-term care facilities can restrain residents with impaired physical or mental ability.

Figure 7-4 An incident report must be completed for any unusual occurrence involving a resident, visitor, or staff.

Vest and belt restraints are the most commonly used restraints in long-term care. Some states have discussed eliminating vest restraints completely because they create a high risk of injury, including strangulation and death. Most states, however, still permit facilities to use the vest restraint.

Extremity restraints are used to hold the resident's arms and legs. They are usually used to prevent pulling at tubes or dressings, and to keep the resident still during medical procedures. Many different extremity restraints are available. The most common are mittens and cuffs. Most of these are padded with sheepskin or foam, so additional padding is not necessary. If your facility uses unpadded restraints, wrap a washcloth or other padding around the extremity before applying the restraint, to prevent circulatory problems. Some facilities require the nursing assistant to place handrolls in the resident's hands when wrist restraints are used. Use commercial handrolls. Rolled washcloths as handrolls should be avoided, because they promote squeezing and can cause deformities.

Side rails on beds are restraints. They can also be an enabler. Many residents pull on them to position and turn themselves in bed. Some residents feel more secure if the rails are up. The rails must be up if the resident is restrained in a vest, belt, or extremity restraint.

Studies have shown that serious injuries can occur if residents attempt to climb over side rails and fall. This is a common cause of hip fractures. Leaving the rails down is safer for some residents. Alarms that sound if the resident attempts to get up may be used to alert staff. Facilities and commercial manufacturers have developed many excellent alternatives to the use of side rails. Each resident's care plan will provide instructions regarding use of side rails or alternative devices. Know and follow your facility policy.

Other common restraints are:

- geriatric chairs.
- specially equipped walkers.
- any device that holds the resident in position that the resident does not have the mental or physical ability to remove.

Side Effects of Restraints

Restraints can have many negative side effects. These include:

- swelling of the legs, ankles, and feet.
- decreased appetite and weight loss.
- dehydration.
- confusion, frustration, and anxiety.
- lowered self-esteem.
- change in patterns of bowel and bladder elimination, leading to constipation, urinary tract infection, or incontinence.
- loss of self-care ability.
- weakness.
- decrease in mobility and loss of ability to walk.
- muscle wasting and contractures.
- depression.
- screaming, yelling, calling out, or combative behavior.
- pneumonia, shortness of breath, and accumulation of fluid in the lungs.
- bruising, redness, or cuts.
- pressure sores.
- falls.

 GUIDELINES for the Use of Restraints

Follow these guidelines when using restraints:

☐ Instructions for restraints must be written in the care plan with an order from the physician that specifies the type of restraint, when it is to be applied, the reason for the restraint, and when to release the restraint. The information required to be in the doctor's order varies from state to state.

☐ Information on the care plan also varies according to state. Check the date of the restraint order on the care plan to be sure it has not expired. Sometimes restraints are ordered for limited periods of time.

☐ Restraints are used only when other means of keeping the resident safe have not been effective.

☐ Use the least restrictive restraint that will keep the resident safe.

☐ Restraints must never be used for the convenience of the staff. For example, do not restrain a resident who wanders so that you do not have to watch him.

☐ Always explain to the resident the reason for the restraint.

☐ The restraint must be applied according to manufacturers' directions. Improperly applied restraints put the resident at high risk of injury. For example, vest restraints that cross over in the front should not be put on backwards.

☐ Using the proper size restraint for the resident is very important. If the restraint does not fit the resident, there is a high risk of injury.

☐ When the resident is in a wheelchair, the straps to most belt and vest restraints should be placed across the resident's lap, then threaded *between* the seat and armrest of the chair. This keeps the resident's hips down and prevents standing and tipping the chair. The straps should not be threaded *through* the armrest (Figure 7-5). Follow the manufacturer's directions.

☐ Restraints must always be tied in a slip knot so that they can be removed quickly in case of an emergency (Figure 7-6).

☐ Apply the restraint securely, but do not cut off the resident's circulation. Always check the fit by slipping your fingers under the restraint to be sure that it is not too tight.

Figure 7-5 Always apply the vest restraint so the straps cross in front. The strap placement across the resident's lap keeps the hips down. (Courtesy of the J. T. Posey Co., Arcadia, CA.)

Figure 7-6 Tie the restraint in slip knots at the back of the chair. (Courtesy of the J. T. Posey Co., Arcadia, CA.)

☐ When using restraints in bed, be sure that they are tied to the moveable part of the bed frame and not the stationary part.

☐ Check the skin under the restraint for signs of irritation.

☐ The call signal, water, and needed personal items should be within the resident's reach, even if the resident is mentally confused.

☐ The nursing assistant should visually check the resident who is in restraints every 15 to 30 minutes to be sure that he is safe.

☐ The resident must be completely released from the restraint every two hours or more often. The resident should be repositioned in the bed or chair, allowed to walk, use the bathroom, or be given range-of-motion exercises according to instructions on the care plan. Check pressure areas on the resident's skin for redness or irritation. The resident must be out of the restraint for a minimum of 10 minutes before it is reapplied.

☐ The use and release of the restraint must be recorded on the resident's medical record. Many facilities use a flow sheet for this purpose.

NOTE TO THE STUDENT

The direct care procedures begin in this chapter and continue through the remainder of the text. The beginning and ending steps of all procedures are the same. These steps have been printed inside the covers of your textbook for easy reference. Your text will instruct you to "Perform your beginning procedure actions." Turn to the front cover to refer to these steps. Refer to the back cover when the text instructs you to "Perform your procedure completion actions." Eventually, the steps will be committed to memory. Review them often, because they are very important. Table 7-1 and Table 7-2 summarize these important beginning and ending actions.

ALTERNATIVES TO RESTRAINTS

The OBRA legislation requires nursing facilities to provide alternatives to restraints and to promote a restraint-free environment. Care of residents in restraints is more time-consuming compared with caring for residents who are not restrained. Restraints

TABLE 7-1

Beginning Procedure Action	Rationale
1. Assemble equipment and take to the resident's room.	Improves efficiency of the procedure. Ensures that you do not have to leave the room.
2. Knock on the resident's door and identify yourself by name and title.	Respects the resident's right to privacy. Notifies the resident who is giving care.
3. Identify the resident by checking the identification bracelet.	Ensures that you are caring for the correct resident.
4. Ask visitors to leave the room and advise them where they may wait.	Respects the resident's right to privacy. Shows hospitality to visitors by advising them where to wait.
5. Explain what you are going to do and how the resident can assist. Answer questions about the procedure.	Informs the resident of what is going to be done and what is expected. Gives the resident an opportunity to get information about the procedure and the extent of resident participation.
6. Provide privacy by closing the door, privacy curtain, and window curtain.	Respects the resident's right to privacy. All three should be closed even if the resident is alone in the room.
7. Position the resident for the procedure. Ask an assistant to help, if necessary, or support the resident with pillows and props. Make sure the resident is comfortable and can maintain the position throughout the procedure. Drape the resident for modesty.	Ensures that the resident is in the correct position for the procedure. Ensures the resident is supported and can maintain the position without discomfort. Respects the resident's modesty and dignity.
8. Wash your hands.	Applies the principles of standard precautions. Prevents the spread of microorganisms.
9. Set up the equipment for the procedure at the bedside. Open trays and packages. Position items in a location for convenient reach. Avoid positioning a container for soiled items in a manner that requires crossing over clean items to access it.	Prepares for the procedure. Ensures that the equipment and supplies are conveniently positioned and readily available. Reduces the risk of cross-contamination.
10. Apply gloves if contact with blood, moist body fluids (except sweat), secretions, excretions, or nonintact skin is likely.	Applies the principles of standard precautions. Protects the nursing assistant and the resident from transmission of pathogens.
11. Apply a gown if your uniform will have substantial contact with linen or other articles contaminated with blood, moist body fluid (except sweat), secretions, or excretions.	Applies the principles of standard precautions. Protects your uniform from contamination with bloodborne pathogens.
12. Apply a gown, mask, and eye protection if splashing of blood or moist body fluid is likely.	Applies the principles of standard precautions. Protects the nursing assistant's mucous membranes, uniform, and skin from accidental splashing of bloodborne pathogens.
13. Raise the bed to a comfortable working height.	Prevents back strain and injury caused by bending at the waist.
14. Lower the side rail on the side where you are working.	Provides an obstacle-free area in which to work.

may cause confusion, incontinence, pressure sores, loss of muscle mass, loss of strength, loss of the ability to walk, loss of balance, fecal impaction, and other problems. Sometimes residents who are restrained attempt to remove the restraints and are seriously injured.

Restraints can be psychologically damaging and cause the resident to feel a loss of self-esteem, hu-

miliation, abandonment, anger, and depression. Because of the serious side effects, we must seek other ways to keep residents safe. Examining the reason that the resident is in the restraint in the first place is also important. If we can detect the cause of the behavior that caused the resident to be restrained and eliminate that cause, we can probably eliminate the need for restraints.

TABLE 7-2

Procedure Completion Actions	Rationale
1. Check to make sure the resident is in good alignment.	All body systems function better when the body is correctly aligned. The resident is more comfortable when the body is in good alignment.
2. Remove gloves.	Prevents contamination of environmental surfaces from the gloves.
3. Replace the bed covers, then remove any drapes used.	Provides warmth and security.
4. Elevate the side rails, if used, before leaving the bedside.	Prevents contamination of the side rail from gloves. Promotes the resident's right to a safe environment. Prevents accidents and injuries.
5. Remove other personal protective equipment, if worn, and discard according to facility policy.	Prevents unnecessary environmental contamination from used gloves and protective equipment.
6. Wash your hands.	Applies the principles of standard precautions. Prevents the spread of microorganisms.
7. Return the bed to the lowest horizontal position.	Promotes the resident's right to a safe environment. Prevents accidents and injuries.
8. Open the privacy and window curtains.	Privacy is no longer necessary unless preferred by the resident.
9. Leave the resident in a position of comfort and safety, with the call signal and needed personal items within reach.	Prevents accidents and injuries. Ensures that help is available. Eliminates the need to call or reach for needed personal items.
10. Wash your hands.	Although the hands were washed previously, they have contacted the resident and other items in the room. Wash them again before leaving to prevent potential transfer of microorganisms to areas outside the resident's unit.
11. Inform visitors that they may return to the room.	Courtesy to visitors and resident.
12. Report completion of the procedure and any abnormalities or other observations.	Informs the supervisor that your assigned task has been completed, so that further resident care can be planned and you can be reassigned to other duties. Notifies the charge nurse of abnormalities and changes in the resident's condition for further assessment.
13. Document the procedure and your observations.	Ongoing progress and care given are documented. Provides a legal record. Provides a record of what has been done for other members of the interdisciplinary team.

Most facilities are equipped with the following alternatives to restraints:

- A wheelchair lap tray is a useful restraint alternative (Figure 7-7). Trays fasten to the back of the wheelchair with Velcro straps. They can be used for residents to lean on and as tables during meals and activities. They also are reminders for the resident not to leave the chair. *Trays are heavy. If a mentally confused resident pushes the tray off, it may land on her legs, causing injury. Use these trays only for residents who will not attempt to push them forward. Also note that lap trays are considered to be restraints if they are used for residents who do not have the physical or mental ability to remove them.*

- Lateral body supports improve sitting posture for residents who lean to the side (Figure 7-8). They

Figure 7-7 The wheelchair lap tray provides support and a surface for eating. It is easily removed from the arms of the wheelchair. (Courtesy of Skil-Care Corporation; (800) 431-2972.)

Figure 7-9 The armrest bolsters help keep the resident securely positioned. (Courtesy of Skil-Care Corporation; (800) 431-2972.)

Figure 7-8 The lateral body support helps the resident with paralysis sit without leaning to the side. (Courtesy of Skil-Care Corporation; (800) 431-2972.)

Figure 7-10 The pommel cushion keeps the resident's hips back and prevents sliding forward. (Courtesy of Skil-Care Corporation; (800) 431-2972.)

are commonly used for residents who are paralyzed on one side of the body. The foam support keeps the resident from leaning to the side, and the armrest supports the resident's arm.

- Lateral stabilizer armrest bolsters are also useful for residents who lean to the side (Figure 7-9). These are commonly used for residents who have no paralysis. They provide support for the resident's upper body.

- The slide guard wedge is also called a "pommel cushion." The wedge shifts the resident's weight to the back of the seat (Figure 7-10). The pommel in the center prevents the resident from sliding forward. It is used for residents who slide forward on the seat of the chair.

- A vinyl wedge cushion can be used for residents who slide forward (Figure 7-11). It is also useful to prevent residents from rising in the chair. The cushion

Figure 7-11 The vinyl wedge keeps the hips lower than the knees, making it difficult to stand. The cushion also prevents sliding forward in the chair. When using a wedge cushion, make sure the resident's feet are supported on footrests or the floor. (Courtesy of Skil-Care Corporation; (800) 431-2972.)

PERFORMANCE PROCEDURE

5   Applying a Vest Restraint

1 Obtain a restraint of the proper type and size.

2 Get help if necessary.

3 Perform your beginning procedure actions.

4 Slip the resident's arms through the arm-holes of the vest.

5 Make sure that the clothing under the restraint is not wrinkled and that the vest fits smoothly.

6 Cross the vest in the front and thread the straps through the slots on the sides of the vest. If a vest is used on a female resident, be sure that the breasts are not under the straps.

7 Thread the straps *between* the seat and the armrest if the resident is in a wheelchair. Pull the straps back securely. If the resident is in bed, attach the straps to the moveable part of the bed frame. (This way, if the bed is raised, the resident will not be restricted or strangled by the restraint.) Follow facility policy for the type of beds used. Many different types of beds are used in health care facilities.

8 Finish tying the restraint in a slip knot under the chair or to the bed frame. Refer to the specific manufacturer's directions for the restraint you are using.

9 Insert three fingers under the restraint and check to be sure that it is not too tight.

PERFORMANCE PROCEDURE

6   Applying a Belt Restraint

1 Perform your beginning procedure actions.

2 Get help from another nursing assistant, if necessary.

3 If the resident is in a wheelchair, move the hips as far back as possible, position the footrests to support the feet, and lock the brakes.

4 Place the belt around the waist. Cross the straps through the loops behind the resident.

5 After the straps are threaded through the loops, tighten the belt securely around the waist.

6 Insert the straps between the seat and arm-rest, or between the seat and back rest, according to the manufacturer's recommendations for the type of restraint you are using.

7 Bring the straps down and tie them to the kickspurs of the wheelchair, using a quick-release knot, according to the manufacturer's directions.

8 Insert three fingers under the restraint and check to be sure that it is not too tight.

9 Perform your procedure completion actions.

makes standing difficult because the hips are lower than the knees when the wedge is in place.

- Nonslip matting is sometimes called *gripper* or *dycem* (Figure 7-12). It has many purposes. It can be used as a placemat for residents whose dishes slide away from them when they eat. It can be used alone on the seat of a wheelchair to prevent a resident from sliding. It can also be placed under a wedge cushion for extra security for residents who slide. This product comes on a roll, and a section of the correct size is cut off. The matting may be rinsed with water if it becomes soiled. Hang the matting to dry. The surface of the matting becomes slippery when wet, so do not use it until it is completely dry.

- Support the resident's feet when he is seated in the chair. Dangling freely is painful for the legs, and complications may develop. Sometimes the resident's legs are too short to touch the floor or the footrests of the wheelchair. In this case, a footrest extender pad is used (Figure 7-13). The footrest also provides a firm base of support and makes it more difficult for the resident to tip the chair.

- Side rails can be considered a restraint. If a resident tries to get out of bed by climbing over the rail, he is at high risk for injury. Bed control bolsters may be used (Figure 7-14) alone or in pairs. They keep the resident from rolling off the bed and serve as a reminder not to get up. The bolsters are half the length of the bed. They can also be used as a prop to keep the resident in good body alignment. Residents who are restless benefit from the use of bolsters because they protect the resident from injury caused by striking the side rails.

Other restraint alternatives include:

- sensor bracelets that set off alarms if the resident tries to leave the facility.
- self-releasing seat belts similar to the lap belts used in a car.
- "lap buddies" or foam cushions placed on the resident's lap when she is in the chair.
- special chairs designed to make it more difficult for the resident to get up. Other types of chairs are used for residents with special positioning needs.
- Participation in activity programs that keep residents busy.
- Increased personal attention that the staff gives to the resident.

As a nursing assistant, you spend more time with the residents than the other members of the interdisciplinary team. If you have an idea that could be used

Figure 7-12 Nonslip matting is cut from a roll and has many uses. The matting can be rinsed and reused, but should not be used when wet. (Courtesy of Skil-Care Corporation; (800) 431-2972.)

Figure 7-13 The footrest elevator prevents pain and deformity. (Courtesy of Skil-Care Corporation; (800) 431-2972.)

to eliminate or reduce restraints, share this information with the interdisciplinary team. If you observe a problem, such as too much noise in the environment that causes a behavior problem in a resident, sharing this information is important. If all team members work together, keeping most residents safe and secure without using restraints is possible.

Many excellent alternatives to restraints are available. However, you must remember that any device is a restraint if the resident does not have the physical or mental ability to remove it.

Figure 7-14 Bed control bolsters eliminate the need for side rails, and help prevent injuries. (Courtesy of Skil-Care Corporation; (800) 431-2972.)

FIRE SAFETY

Your facility will have special fire safety procedures. All staff must watch for fire hazards and report them immediately to the proper authority. Because fire safety is extremely important, most states have laws requiring long-term care facilities to have frequent fire drills. Know where the alarms and fire extinguishers are in your facility and how to use them. Know your facility evacuation plan in case of fire (Figure 7-15).

Major Causes of Fire in Long-Term Care Facilities

Fires often are caused by the following:

- improper or unsupervised use of smoking materials
- defects in the heating system
- improper trash disposal
- misuse of electrical equipment
- spontaneous combustion
- lint buildup in dryers

In order for a fire to occur, three things must be present (Figure 7-16):

- material that burns
- flame or spark
- **oxygen** in the air

Fire safety is very important when oxygen is being used. A tiny spark from turning on a hair dryer

Figure 7-15 Know your facility evacuation plan.

or a cigarette ash can cause a fire when oxygen is present in larger amounts than is normally present in the air. Special procedures must be followed when oxygen is used. Follow your facility policy for use of oxygen, oxygen signs, and modifications in procedures you must take when a resident is using oxygen.

Actions to Take When You Discover a Fire

If you discover a fire, take these actions:

- Follow the facility's procedures.
- Alert and assist residents who have vision and hearing impairments.

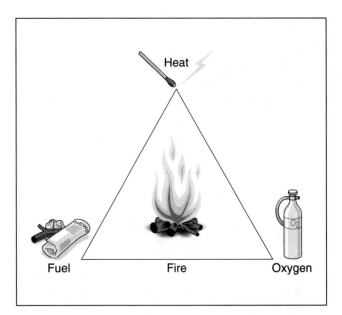

Figure 7-16 Three elements are necessary to start a fire.

Extinguish or

Activate

Evacuate

Contain

Figure 7-17 The RACE system

- Follow facility policy for getting **immobile** residents out of dangerous areas. This may include placing the resident on a blanket on the floor and pulling the resident, or moving the entire bed with the resident in it. Nursing facility doors are required to have fire ratings. Close the doors to place a barrier between the resident and the fire.

The RACE System

Many facilities use the R A C E system (Figure 7-17) as a general guideline in fire safety.

- **R**emove residents in immediate danger.
- **A**ctivate the alarm to alert others (Figure 7-18).
- **C**onfine the fire by closing doors.
- **E**xtinguish the fire, if possible.

EMERGENCY MEASURES

There may be times when **emergency** measures must be performed. Your facility will have a specific policy for emergency procedures. Your responsibility is to tell the nurse immediately and follow the nurse's instructions. Knowing some emergency procedures is important. You might want to take a CPR and first aid course offered by a community organization.

CHOKING

An **obstructed airway** occurs when food or an object becomes lodged in the throat, cutting off the airway. Some residents have difficulty swallowing. The best measure is to prevent choking, but even with the best care, some residents may choke on food or other objects. Facility policies vary, but there are times when you may have to help a resident who is choking (Figure 7-19).

Choking often occurs when residents are eating, drinking, laughing, or talking at the same time. The food or foreign object goes into the throat. It is usually too far down for the fingers to reach. The foreign body obstructs the airway so that the resident is not able to speak or breathe. The resident may put one or both hands on the neck. This is the universal sign for choking.

If you suspect that the resident is choking, ask the resident, "Are you choking?" If the resident signals yes, you must do something right away. The **Heimlich maneuver** is the common name for the procedure done to remove a foreign object from an obstructed airway.

Figure 7-18 Know where the fire alarms are located and how to use them.

Figure 7-19 Proper hand placement for the abdominal thrust

CARDIOPULMONARY RESUSCITATION

Cardiopulmonary resuscitation (CPR) is a basic, lifesaving procedure given to a person whose heart has stopped beating. This is called cardiac arrest. The techniques of CPR must be taught by a certified instructor. The following outline provides an overview of the CPR procedure. It does not replace a CPR course.

1. Gently shake the resident's shoulder and shout, "Are you O.K.?" Call for help.

2. Position the resident on his back.

3. Open the airway by tilting the resident's head backward and lifting the chin. Look, listen, and feel for breath.

4. Pinch the nose, cover the resident's mouth with a barrier device, and give two full breaths into the mouth.

5. Feel the neck for the carotid pulse. Begin chest compression if there is no pulse.

6. Feel for the landmark at the tip of the breastbone by sliding your fingers up the margins of the ribs. The landmark is two fingers up from the tip of the breastbone. Place the heel of your other hand on the breastbone, next to the landmark. Place the "landmark" hand on top. Keep your elbows straight.

7. Compress the breastbone downward one and one-half to two inches at a rate of eighty a minute. Use the heels of your hands. Keep the fingers off the chest.

8. Do fifteen compressions, then two breaths. Repeat.

9. Continue the procedure until the resident recovers, help arrives, or you are exhausted and unable to continue.

7   Clearing an Obstructed Airway (Heimlich Maneuver)

Clearing an Obstructed Airway in a Conscious Resident

1 Call for the nurse immediately.

2 Tell the resident that you will help. If the resident is sitting or standing, stand behind her.

3 Wrap your arms around the resident's waist, above the hips.

4 Make a fist with one hand.

5 Place the thumb side of your fist against the resident's abdomen, just above the navel and below the tip of the breastbone.

6 Grasp the fist with the other hand.

7 Push inward and upward on the abdomen with a quick thrust.

8 Repeat the thrusts until the foreign body comes out or the resident loses consciousness. If the resident begins to cough, wait and see if she can expel the object.

Clearing an Obstructed Airway in an Unconscious Resident

It is important that you know your facility's policy regarding this procedure. This procedure may be the responsibility of the nurse. The procedure is listed here for your general understanding only.

1 Call for help, but do not leave the resident alone.

2 Lower the resident to the floor and position her on her back.

3 Open the airway by doing a tongue-jaw lift. Check for signs of breathing. Look at the chest to see if it is rising and falling. Listen and feel for breaths on your cheek and on your ear.

4 If the resident is not breathing, insert your index finger along the cheek and toward the base of the tongue. If an object is felt, try to remove it. Do not push the object farther down the throat.

5 Attempt to ventilate. If the breath does not go in, reposition the head and attempt to

ventilate again. Use a pocket mask or other barrier, according to facility policy.

Note: Follow your facility policy for mouth-to-mouth ventilation. To prevent the transmission of disease, standard precautions should be used. This means that gloves are worn for the finger sweep. A ventilation barrier mask with a valve that prevents the backflow of secretions, or a resuscitation face shield, should be placed between your mouth and the resident's mouth for ventilations. Familiarize yourself with the devices in your facility. CPR classes are offered to teach you how to use ventilation devices correctly. Attending a CPR class will benefit you personally and professionally.

6 If your breath meets resistance, straddle the resident.

7 Place the heel of one hand above the navel. Place the other hand on top. Keeping your elbows locked and shoulders straight, give five abdominal thrusts.

8 Open the airway by doing a tongue-jaw lift. Check the resident's mouth and use your finger as a hook to remove any objects that you can see.

9 Attempt to ventilate.

10 Repeat steps 3 through 7 until the object is expelled.

11 Assist the charge nurse, code team, or emergency medical services (EMS), as appropriate.

12 Discard gloves and face shield, or disinfect reusable ventilation device according to facility policy.

13 Perform your procedure completion actions.

14 Observe and report to the charge nurse:
- exact time the choking and unconsciousness started and stopped.
- the procedures done and the time that you started and stopped.
- the resident's response.
- factors related to the cause of choking, if known.

KEY POINTS IN THIS CHAPTER

▲ Safety is very important in the long-term care facility because many residents are at high risk for accidents or injuries.

▲ Accident and injury prevention is the responsibility of the entire staff.

▲ Falls are a frequent cause of injury to residents.

▲ Incident reports must be completed when an accident or injury occurs to a resident, staff member, or visitor.

▲ Residents who are restrained require more care and take more time compared with residents who are not in restraints.

▲ Residents should be free from restraints whenever possible.

▲ Restraints may be used only when other means of protecting residents have not been successful.

▲ Restraints require a doctor's order and must be released at least every two hours for ten minutes for exercise and care.

▲ Fire safety is so important that most states require frequent fire drills for long-term care facilities.

▲ In an emergency, you must follow facility policies.

REVIEW QUIZ

1. Which of the following residents are at high risk of injury?
   a. the confused resident who wanders
   b. the newly admitted resident
   c. the resident with vision and hearing impairment
   d. all of the above

2. Which is the safest way to prevent residents from having contact with hazardous substances, such as cleaning supplies and medications?
   a. Label containers with the poison sign.
   b. Tell the resident to stay away from hazardous materials.
   c. Lock cabinets where hazardous materials are stored.
   d. Tell other residents to watch confused residents.

3. Which of the following floor conditions pose a threat to resident safety?
   a. a shiny surface
   b. spilled liquids
   c. beige colored tile
   d. all of the above

4. If the resident begins to fall while you are walking with him, you should:
   a. gently ease the resident to the floor.
   b. ask another resident to help you.
   c. quickly go and get the nurse.
   d. get a pillow for the resident immediately.

5. What must be done when an event that is not part of the normal routine happens?
   a. An incident report must be completed.
   b. The nursing assistant should call the administrator of the facility.
   c. The resident must be restrained.
   d. All of the above.

6. Which is true regarding the use of restraints?
   a. Restraints may be applied when the nursing staff is busy.
   b. Restraints are applied to all confused residents to keep them safe.
   c. Restraints may be applied to any resident who will not stay in bed.
   d. Restraints may be applied only if necessary to protect the resident from harm.

7. Restraints should be released at least:
   a. once every shift.
   b. every two hours.
   c. every three hours.
   d. every four hours.

8. Which of the following rules should you follow when using restraints?
   a. Restraints should be the proper size to fit the resident.
   b. Restraints must always be tied in a slip knot.
   c. The nursing assistant should visually check the restrained resident every 15 to 30 minutes.
   d. All of the above.

9. In order for a fire to occur, what must be present?
   a. oxygen and material
   b. flame, oxygen, and smoke
   c. oxygen, material, and spark
   d. flame and oxygen

10. In case of fire, what should be done first?
    a. Call the fire department.
    b. Remove residents in danger.
    c. Alert other staff.
    d. Announce the location of the fire over the intercom.

11. When an emergency occurs in the long-term care facility, your responsibility as a nursing assistant is to:
    a. follow the directions of your supervisor.
    b. notify the family immediately.
    c. contact the physician for instructions.
    d. all of the above.

12. The universal sign for choking is:
    a. coughing.
    b. clutching the throat.
    c. shouting.
    d. waving arms about.

13. If a resident is coughing and able to breathe, you should:
    a. perform the Heimlich maneuver.
    b. use finger sweeps to remove the object.
    c. stay with the resident and let him continue coughing.
    d. give the resident oxygen.

14. The correct procedure for clearing an obstructed airway in an unconscious adult is to place the heel of your hand:
    a. on the chest.
    b. below the navel.
    c. above the navel.
    d. on the back.

15. One of the most frequent causes of accidents to residents in long-term care facilities is:
    a. falls.
    b. smoking.
    c. choking.
    d. all of the above.

16. Accident prevention is the responsibility of the:
    a. safety committee.
    b. maintenance department.
    c. nursing department.
    d. entire staff.

17. You are assigned to care for Jeffrey Greene, a 54-year-old resident with Alzheimer's disease. Mr. Greene is very confused and restless. The care plan states that he is to use a vest restraint when he is in the wheelchair. You get Mr. Greene up and apply the vest restraint. Before leaving the room you should:
    a. tie the restraint securely in a knot so that the resident cannot untie it.
    b. ask Mr. Greene to behave himself until you come back in two hours.
    c. move Mr. Greene's wheelchair away from the other furniture so that he does not get hurt.
    d. place the signal cord so that Mr. Greene can reach it.

18. You are assigned to work in the dining room during the evening meal. You are passing food trays when you notice that Mrs. Hernandez is sitting at the table with her hands on her throat. You should:
    a. continue passing trays, as you are not assigned to care for Mrs. Hernandez.
    b. go immediately to Mrs. Hernandez and ask her if she is choking.
    c. leave the dining room immediately and get the nurse.
    d. help Mrs. Hernandez to the floor and perform abdominal thrusts.

19. You are working the 10 pm to 6 am shift on C-wing. As you walk down the hallway, you look into Mr. Griffin's room and notice that he is on the floor next to the bed. You should:
    a. call for the nursing assistant who is assigned to care for Mr. Griffin.
    b. go and get the nurse.
    c. continue walking and pretend that you did not see the resident.
    d. go into the room and check the resident.

20. You are assigned to straighten the drawers in Mr. Atkins room. Mr. Atkins is a confused resident with Alzheimer's disease. When you open the drawer to the nightstand you find a comb, a wrapped candy bar, a roll-on deodorant, an electric razor, a toothbrush, a package of denture cleaning tablets, and an emesis basin. Which of these items is most likely to cause harm to Mr. Atkins?
    a. the razor
    b. the denture tablets
    c. the roll-on deodorant
    d. all of the above

CHAPTER 7
CROSSWORD PUZZLE

Directions: Complete the puzzle using these words found in Chapter 7.

airway   immobile   oxygen
CPR   impairment   restraint
emergency   incident   spark
gait   material   transfer
geriatric   protective
hazard   obstructed

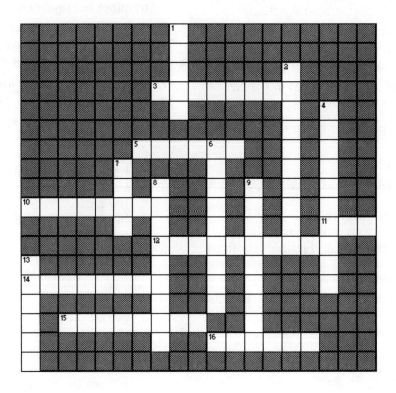

CHAPTER 7
PUZZLE CLUES

ACROSS

3. A device that the nursing assistant uses to assist a resident when moving from the bed to a chair is a _____ belt.
5. A potential source of danger
10. Unable to move
11. Cardiopulmonary resuscitation
12. Something that hinders proper function
14. An unusual occurrence or event
15. In order for a fire to start, you need oxygen, a spark, and _____ that will burn
16. A colorless, odorless, tasteless gas in the air

DOWN

1. A sudden quick light
2. A type of restraint that is used to keep a resident from harm is called a _____ device.
4. The Heimlich maneuver is done if a resident has an _____ airway.
6. A device that is applied to the resident to restrict freedom of movement
7. A _____ belt is used to assist residents in walking.
8. A _____ chair is a chair with wheels and a tray that is a type of restraint.
9. An event that calls for immediate action.
13. The breathing passage in the throat.

The Resident's Unit

OBJECTIVES

In this chapter, you will learn how to care for the resident's unit in a long-term care facility. After reading this chapter, you will be able to:

- Spell and define key terms.
- Care for the resident's unit.
- Discuss the importance of maintaining a homelike environment and respecting the resident's personal items.
- List safety practices to follow in the resident's unit.
- Describe infection control practices to follow in the resident's unit.
- Demonstrate the separation of clean and dirty items in the resident's unit.
- Make the unoccupied bed.

KEY TERMS

bedside stand: a nightstand or table used for personal possessions and equipment used for personal care of the resident

gatch handles: the handles at the end of some beds used to raise the head, foot, or height of the bed

overbed table: a narrow table on wheels; the height of the table is adjustable

resident's unit: the space for one resident in a long-term care facility

THE RESIDENT'S UNIT

When we speak of the **resident's unit,** we are referring to the area that is for a resident's personal use (Figure 8-1). The items in the unit are a bed, chair, an overbed table, bedside stand, dresser, waste basket, closet, and sometimes a television set or radio. Many facilities allow some furniture items from the resident's former home. The nursing assistant must realize that the long-term care facility is now the resident's home. Caring for the resident includes some care of the unit.

The OBRA legislation emphasizes the importance of maintaining a homelike environment. The unit should be comfortable and attractive in appearance. The resident's personal items should be used to decorate the room whenever possible (Figure 8-2). These items are important because they bring back memories of the past. The items brought to the nursing facility are often the most important to the resident and may be the only possessions that she has left in the world. Handling these items with respect and care shows the resident that you care. Showing respect for personal belongings is one way you can help the resident with grief and loss issues.

The resident has a right to expect his or her unit to be treated with respect and dignity. This includes knocking on closed doors and giving the resident and visitors the right to privacy when requested. When giving the resident personal care, you must close the door, pull the privacy curtain, and close the drapes on the window, even if you are alone in the room with the resident.

Unit Safety and Infection Control

Think safety each time you enter and leave the resident's room. Check the resident's unit each day for safety. Some considerations to note are:

Figure 8-1 The resident's unit.

Figure 8-2 Make the room as homelike and comfortable as possible by displaying the resident's belongings.

- Check side rails to be sure they are secure. These are used by the resident to prevent falling and assist with turning in bed.
- Check the call signal. Make sure the signal is working and within the resident's reach at all times, even if the resident is confused.
- If the resident is confined to bed or chair in the room, make sure that water, tissues, and other needed personal items are within reach.
- Keep the unit tidy. Major cleaning is the job of other departments. However, the nursing assistant may be responsible for caring for the resident's personal items.

Figure 8-3 Tuck the gatch handles under the foot of the bed when not in use to prevent injury to residents and staff.

- Keep the top of the **overbed table** clean at all times. The overbed table is used when giving personal care, such as a bed bath. The height of the table can be adjusted to a high or low position. The resident uses the overbed table for drinking water and meal trays. You may need to wipe this table frequently throughout the shift so that it is kept clean at all times.
- You may be responsible for changing the resident's drinking water one or more times during your shift. Most facilities collect the water pitchers and drinking glasses and wash them in the dishwasher at least once a day.
- Always respect the resident's choices. Ask her how and where she wants items, if possible.
- Respect the resident's right to privacy when you straighten closets and drawers.
- Make sure that the **gatch handles** to manually operated beds are kept under the bed when not in use (Figure 8-3). The gatch handles are found at the foot end of the bed. The gatch handle on the left is used to raise the head of the bed. The gatch handle on the right is used to elevate the knee area of the bed. Adjusting the position of the bed assists in maintaining resident position and comfort. Many beds also have a gatch handle in the center of the bed. The center handle is used to raise or lower the height of the bed. When the nursing assistant is providing care or making the bed, the bed should be raised with the center handle until it is at a good working height for you. Raising and lowering the height of the bed will help prevent fatigue and protect your back. If the resident is in the bed, the bed should be placed in the lowest possible position. If the bed is in an elevated position, the side rails should be kept up at all times. The gatch handles of the bed should be tucked under the foot end of the bed when they are not in use, to prevent injury and falls to residents and staff.

- Check for items on the floor that the resident and staff could trip or slip on.
- If you notice personal items in the room that you feel may be unsafe for the resident, check with the nurse regarding what to do with them.
- If an electrical or mechanical safety hazard exists, follow your facility policy for having the equipment removed or repaired.
- Check the unit for sharp items, chemicals, improperly stored food items, medications, and other items, such as aerosol cans, that may not be kept in the room according to your facility policy or state law.

The Bedside Stand

The **bedside stand** is an important piece of equipment for resident care. The bedside stand is used to store personal items and articles used by the nursing assistant to deliver care to the resident. Bedside stands vary in design. Most have at least one drawer at the top. The lower portion of the stand may have a cupboard-type door or several drawers. Follow your facility policy for storage of items in the bedside stand. Clean and dirty items must be kept separate. For example, the drawer in the top of the bedside stand is often used to store the resident's toothbrush, brush, and comb. It is important that these items do not come into contact with each other. The lower part of the bedside stand often contains the washbasin and bedpan or urinal. The washbasin is considered a "clean" item. It should not come into contact with the bedpan and urinal, which are considered "dirty." In the cupboard-type bedside stand, the inside is typically divided by two shelves. Many facilities keep the washbasin on the top shelf and the bedpan on the bottom shelf so that they are separated. In bedside stands with drawers, these items may be stored in separate drawers (Figure 8-4). Follow your facility's infection control policies for separation of clean and dirty personal care articles in the bedside stand.

Making the Resident's Bed

The nursing assistant is responsible for making the resident's bed each day. When the resident is out of bed, you will use the unoccupied bedmaking procedure. Facilities use many different types of linen for bedmaking. Some use flat sheets. Many use a fitted sheet on the bottom. Some facilities use draw sheets. Some use plastic or rubber draw sheets on the bed if the resident is incontinent or uses the bedpan or urinal when in bed. Other facilities use large disposable or reusable underpads in place of rubber sheets. Many types of bedspreads can be used to make the resident's room appear homelike and attractive.

When making the bed, raise it to a comfortable working height for you. Avoid walking around the bed many times. Make one side of the bed first, then go to the other side and complete the bedmaking procedure. By raising the height of the bed and making one side of the bed at a time, you will reduce fatigue and prevent injury to your back.

Knowing your facility policy for placement of clean and dirty linen when making the bed is important. Always wash your hands before handling clean linen. Wash your hands again after discarding soiled linen, even if you were wearing gloves. Carry clean and dirty linen away from your uniform. Most facilities have specific locations where clean linen should be placed. Dirty linen should never be placed on the floor. Know and follow your facility policy for placing soiled linen until it can be placed in the linen hamper (Figure 8-5). When placing soiled linen in the hamper, secure the lid tightly. Linen should not overflow the top of the hamper. Never allow clean and dirty linen to touch each other.

Figure 8-4 Store clean and soiled items in separate drawers of the resident's bedside stand.

Figure 8-5 Always keep the lid to the soiled linen hamper tightly closed.

PERFORMANCE PROCEDURE

8   Making the Unoccupied Bed

1 Wash your hands. Gather supplies needed: two large sheets (or one flat and one fitted sheet), a linen draw sheet (if used), plastic or rubber draw sheet (if used), pillowcase, laundry bag or hamper, and clean bedspread, if needed. Stack the linen in the order in which it will be used. Obtain disposable gloves if the linen is soiled with blood or any moist body fluid.

2 Perform your beginning procedure actions.

3 Carry the clean linen away from your uniform (Figure 8-6).

4 Place the linens on a clean area near the bed in the order of use, from bottom to top.

5 Elevate the bed to a good working height for you.

6 Position the bed so that it is flat.

7 Remove and fold the bedspread if you are reusing it.

8 Apply gloves if linen is soiled.

9 Remove the linen from the bed by rolling it in a ball, without letting it touch your uniform.

10 Place soiled linens in a laundry bag, or dispose of it according to facility policy. If gloves were used, remove them and dispose of them according to facility policy. Check the mattress to be sure it is in good repair. Wash your hands before handling clean linen, even if gloves were worn.

11 Follow your facility policy for wiping the mattress. Some facilities require that the mattress be wiped with disinfectant if the linen is soiled with excretions or secretions. (Wear gloves for this task).)

12 Place the bottom sheet on the bed, centering the lengthwise middle fold of the sheet in the middle of the bed.

13 Open the sheet.

14 Place the sheet with small hem even with the foot edge of the mattress (Figure 8-7).

15 Tuck the top of the sheet under the top of the mattress.

16 Miter the corner of the sheet at the head of the bed on the side where you are working (Figure 8-8).

OR

Secure upper and lower corners of fitted sheet.

17 Tuck in the bottom sheet on the side of the bed, working from head to foot.

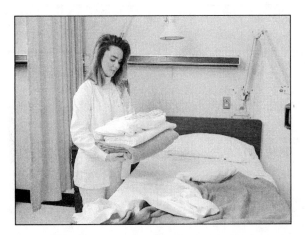

Figure 8-6 Carry clean linen away from your uniform.

Figure 8-7 Align the hem of the bottom sheet even with the end of the mattress.

(continues)

8 *continued*

18 Place the plastic draw sheet, if used, over the middle one-third of the bed.

19 Place the linen draw sheet over the plastic sheet, covering the entire plastic sheet.

20 Tuck the edge of the plastic sheet and draw sheet under the mattress (Figure 8-9).

21 Place the top sheet on the bed, centering the lengthwise middle fold in the center of the bed.

22 Position the sheet with the top edge even with the top of the mattress (Figure 8-10).

23 Tuck the bottom of the sheet under the mattress at the foot of the bed.

24 Place the bedspread on the bed.

25 Position the bedspread about four inches above the top edge of the mattress.

26 Miter linens at the foot of the bed (Figure 8-11).

27 Move to the other side of the bed.

28 Pull and smooth out the bottom sheet.

29 Tuck the bottom sheet under the mattress at the head of the bed, pulling tight.

30 Miter the corner of the sheet at the head of the bed (Figure 8-12),

OR

Figure 8-8 Miter the corner of the sheet by following steps A through D.

Figure 8-10 Position the hem of the top sheet even with the top of the mattress, then fold it down.

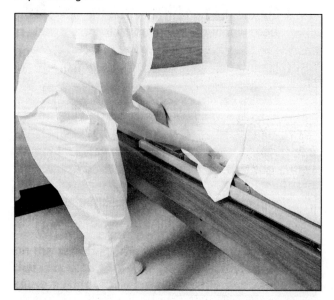

Figure 8-9 The draw sheet is positioned so it is under the resident's shoulders to below the hips.

Figure 8-11 Miter the corners of the top sheet and bedspread together at the foot of the bed.

(continues)

8 *continued*

Secure upper and lower corners of the fitted sheet.

31 Pull and tightly tuck the side of the bottom sheet under the mattress.

32 Pull the plastic sheet tightly.

33 Tuck the plastic sheet under the mattress, pulling and tucking from the middle of the plastic sheet first. Then pull and tuck the edges of the sheet.

34 Pull the linen draw sheet tightly.

35 Tuck the linen draw sheet under the mattress, pulling and tucking from the middle of the draw sheet first. Then pull and tuck the edges of the sheet.

36 Check the foundation of the bed. Make sure the bed is smooth and wrinkle-free.

37 Pull and smooth the top sheet.

38 Pull and smooth the spread.

39 Tuck the sheet and spread under the foot of the mattress.

40 Miter the top linens at the foot of the bed.

41 Fold the spread back about 30 inches.

42 Make a cuff on the top sheet by folding it back about four inches at the top edge of the sheet (Figure 8-13).

43 Place the pillow on the bed.

44 Fold the pillow in half and insert the zippered end of the pillow in the pillowcase toward the closed end (Figure 8-14).

45 Straighten the pillowcase on the pillow.

46 Place the pillow at the head of the bed with the open end facing away from the door.

47 Cover the pillow with the bedspread.

48 Perform your procedure completion actions.

Figure 8-13 Fold the top sheet and spread down, forming a cuff.

Figure 8-12 Make the bed systematically, beginning at the top and working your way down. Make one side at a time, then move to the other.

Figure 8-14 Fold the pillow in half and slip it into the pillowcase.

KEY POINTS IN THIS CHAPTER

▲ The resident's unit is an area for personal use.

▲ The OBRA legislation promotes a homelike environment.

▲ Respect the resident's rights when performing care and handling the resident's possessions.

▲ You show respect for the residents by treating their possessions with care.

▲ *Think safety* each time you enter and leave the resident's room.

▲ Follow your facility infection control policies for linen handling and separation of clean and dirty items in the resident's room.

REVIEW QUIZ

1. The resident's unit includes:
   a. the floor or wing of the facility in which the resident's room is located.
   b. the nurse's station.
   c. the resident's room and furnishings.
   d. all of the above.

2. The nursing assistant's responsibility for daily care of the resident's unit includes:
   a. washing the bed.
   b. mopping the floor.
   c. cleaning the bathroom.
   d. checking for safety and properly working side rails and call lights.

3. The resident's room should appear:
   a. homelike.
   b. institutional.
   c. like a hospital.
   d. none of the above.

4. When entering and leaving the resident's room, you should:
   a. always pull the privacy curtain.
   b. think safety.
   c. always leave the door open so others know where you are.
   d. all of the above.

5. When cleaning the resident's bedside stand, you should:
   a. remove all food items and throw them away.
   b. keep clean and dirty items separated.
   c. remove the bedpan and washbasin, as they do not belong there.
   d. all of the above.

6. If the resident is in a bed that is elevated, you should:
   a. always leave the side rails up.
   b. always leave the side rails down.
   c. leave the gatch handle out at the foot of the bed so that you can adjust the height of the bed quickly.
   d. always elevate the knee rest to make the resident more comfortable.

7. When making the unoccupied bed, you should always:
   a. put the soiled linen on the floor.
   b. put the soiled linen on the chair.
   c. wear gloves if you anticipate contact with blood or moist body fluid.
   d. keep the bed at the lowest possible height.

8. You will prevent fatigue if you:
   a. walk around the bed several times to tuck the sheets in.
   b. make the bed before the resident gets up.
   c. change the resident's linen once a month.
   d. make one side of the bed at a time.

9. You show respect for the resident when you:
   a. provide privacy when performing care.
   b. knock on the door when entering the room.
   c. handle the resident's personal belongings with care.
   d. all of the above.

10. The gatch handles of the bed should be:
    a. tucked under the foot of the bed when not in use.
    b. left out at the foot end of the bed so they can be quickly located.
    c. left out if the resident is in bed all the time.
    d. tucked under the bed only if the resident is ambulatory.

11. You are assigned to straighten Mrs. Hillyer's room. When you enter the room, you introduce yourself and tell Mrs. Hillyer what you are going to do. The resident instructs you to "Leave my things alone." You should:
    a. continue straightening the room as you were instructed to do.
    b. tell the resident that her room is messy and that you were told to clean it.
    c. do as the resident requests and report what she said to the charge nurse.
    d. tell the resident that you will have to report her to the administrator.

12. Mrs. Jaffe is a 93-year-old bedfast resident. She is alert and uses the bedpan independently. You enter her room and find a full bedpan on the overbed table next to her water glass. You should:
    a. remove the bedpan.
    b. wipe the top of the overbed table with disinfectant.
    c. replace the water glass with a clean glass.
    d. all of the above.

CHAPTER 8
CROSSWORD PUZZLE

Directions: Complete the puzzle using these words found in Chapter 8.

bed	home	signal
chair	overbed	stand
clean	respect	unit
dirty	safety	unoccupied
gatch	side	

CHAPTER 8
PUZZLE CLUES

ACROSS

3. Check the call _____ every day to be sure it works properly.
6. The piece of equipment the resident sits on
7. The type of bedmaking procedure used when the resident is not in the bed
9. Check the _____ rails every day to be sure that they work properly.
10. The piece of equipment that the resident sleeps on
11. The resident's room should appear _____ like.
12. Separate clean and _____ items.

DOWN

1. Handling the resident's belongings with care shows _____.
2. Articles used for resident care that are not dirty
3. The table next to the bed that contains personal items and articles used for personal hygiene is the bedside _____.
4. The handles at the foot of the bed are _____ handles.
5. Think _____ when you enter and leave the room.
7. The resident's room is also called the resident's _____.
8. The adjustable table that is used for resident care and for serving food trays on is the _____ table.

Body Alignment and Activity Needs

OBJECTIVES

In this chapter, you will learn the importance of proper positioning, moving, and lifting. After reading this chapter, you will be able to:

- Spell and define key terms.
- Describe the purpose of restorative nursing.
- List the principles of restorative nursing.
- List the effects of immobility.
- Explain how a weakness in one area can affect the resident's state of functioning and well-being.
- Demonstrate the principles of body mechanics.
- Demonstrate good body alignment.
- Move and position the resident.
- Ambulate the resident using a gait belt, cane, and walker.
- Transfer the resident.
- Help the resident do range-of-motion exercises.

KEY TERMS

abduction: moving an extremity *away from* the body

adduction: moving an extremity *toward* the body

ADLs: activities of daily living that include bathing, dressing, grooming, eating, and moving about

alignment: proper position, as in good posture

ambulate: to walk

atrophy: wasting away of muscle

body mechanics: proper use of the body to attain the most strength and reduce injury and fatigue

contracture: abnormal tightening or shortening of muscles from lack of sufficient exercise

contraindicated: not indicated, improper or undesirable

edema: swelling in the tissues often seen in legs, ankles, feet, and hands

extension: straightening out of a joint

flexion: to bend a joint

Fowler's position: sitting with the head of the bed elevated 45 to 60 degrees with the knees bent

friction: rubbing and chafing against the resident's skin so that the skin becomes irritated

hemiplegia: one half (right or left side) of the body is paralyzed

high Fowler's position: same as the Fowler's position but with the head of the bed elevated 90 degrees

immobility: inability to move

lateral position: lying on one side

paralysis: loss of ability to move a part or all of the body

pressure ulcers: red or open areas on the skin caused by prolonged pressure

prone position: lying on the abdomen (stomach)

prosthesis: artificial body part

range-of-motion (ROM) exercises: exercises that move each muscle and joint

rehabilitation: a process designed to restore and maintain a resident's highest level of ability

restorative nursing care: nursing care designed to promote health and restore as much independence as possible

semi-Fowler's position: similar to Fowler's position, but with the head elevated 30 to 45 degrees and the knees lower

semiprone position: a modified prone position in which the body is supported on pillows to relieve pressure from most of the bony prominences

semisupine position: a modified side-lying position in which the body is supported on pillows to relieve pressure from most of the bony prominences

shearing: stretching the skin between the bone inside and the bed or another surface outside the body

Sims' position: lying on the left side with the top knee flexed and supported on a pillow. This position is used for enemas and examinations

supine position: lying on one's back

transfer: moving from one surface to another, as in moving a resident from bed to wheelchair

REHABILITATION AND RESTORATION

Rehabilitation is the process designed to help a resident restore and maintain the highest level of physical and mental ability. As a nursing assistant, you will have a major role in the resident's rehabilitation program. The care plan will describe your responsibilities. Other members of the rehabilitation team include the nurse, physical therapist, occupational therapist, speech therapist, and the activities department (Figure 9-1). Rehabilitation programs are based on the resident's physical condition and ability and desire to cooperate.

Restorative nursing care is given by the nursing team to help the resident to restore health and maintain and improve her level of function and independence. Some people use the terms *rehabilitation* and *restoration* interchangeably. However, they are not the same. Rehabilitation involves skilled care given by therapists and other licensed health care professionals. Restoration, or restorative nursing, involves nursing procedures that are designed to maintain or improve the resident's condition. If a resident does not use her abilities, she may eventually lose them. For example, a resident who sits in a wheelchair all the time may lose the ability to walk. A resident who is spoon-fed by staff may lose the ability to feed herself. Rehabilitation and restorative nursing programs are designed to prevent declines such as these.

The OBRA legislation requires us to assist all residents to achieve their highest level of function. Rehabilitation and restorative care should be part of the care of each resident. We recognize that if the resident is independent, this affects her self-esteem. Residents who are totally dependent on others may feel as if they are not worthwhile. Sometimes we perform care that residents can do themselves because it is faster. Realizing that this goes against the intent of OBRA and is not good for the resident is important. Learn to organize your work so that you can enable residents to do as much for themselves as possible. Perform other duties while the resident is performing self-care. When the resident is unable to complete a procedure, the nursing assistant should step in and assist as appropriate. Before physically assisting the resident, use verbal cues. This means that you tell the resident how to do the task in simple terms. If the resident does not respond to your cues, using hand-over-hand technique may be necessary. This is done by placing your hand on top of the resident's hand and doing the skill. If this is ineffective, you must complete the task for the resident. Sincerely compliment the resident for the part of the task that she was able to complete.

Principles of Rehabilitation and Restorative Nursing

The principles of rehabilitation and restorative nursing care are the same. These are:

- Emphasize the resident's ability, not his disability. For example, stress what the resident can do, not what he can't.
- Use the resident's strengths to help her overcome her weaknesses.

Figure 9-1 Members of the interdisciplinary team meet to plan rehabilitation and restorative nursing care.

- Prevent further disability.
- Begin treatment as early in the illness or injury as possible.
- Treat the whole person. Look at the resident as a whole, not just the condition causing the disability. Look at the resident as a complete individual with many complex needs. A weakness in one area can affect all areas of the resident's life. For example, if the resident becomes depressed, he may refuse therapy. This refusal can affect many other areas of the resident's physical and mental condition.
- Praise the resident's accomplishments.

Considerations for Care.   Some points to remember in any rehabilitation program include:

- Encourage self-care with **ADLs** by using adaptive equipment such as a shoe horn or gripper. By using adaptive equipment, the resident may be able to perform a procedure independently. Enabling the resident to be independent promotes good self-esteem.
- Emphasize the resident's abilities.
- Encourage the resident in active **range-of-motion (ROM) exercises.** During this exercise, the resident moves all limbs freely. If the resident is not able to move all extremities, the nursing assistant should do passive range-of-motion exercises (PROM) on the limbs that the resident is unable to move.
- Encourage the resident to be as independent as possible.
- Follow the care plan for a resident using a **prosthesis** such as an artificial leg or arm.

IMMOBILITY EFFECTS

Immobility affects the resident's physical and psychosocial needs. Try to understand how frustrated residents must feel when they always need help to move. Some residents will not be able to move at all without your help. Besides the mental frustrations, there are medical effects of inactivity on the body.

Physical Effects of Immobility

Some physical problems seen in all body systems because of inactivity:

- Circulatory system

  — Blood in vessels may pool, causing blood clots.

  — Poor blood flow may cause **edema** (swelling) in the tissues.

  — The heart has to work harder.

- Respiratory system

  — The resident has more difficulty expanding the lungs.

  — Fluid accumulates in the lungs and respiratory tract.

  — The risk of lung infection increases.

- Urinary system

  — Without gravity, urine may be retained in the bladder, causing urinary tract infection.

  — Kidney stones may develop.

- Digestive system

  — The resident loses her appetite.

  — Constipation may occur.

- Musculoskeletal system

  — Calcium loss increases when stress is not placed on bones.

  — **Contractures** are deformities. They result from shortening and tightening of muscles and occur in muscles that are not used.

  — **Atrophy,** or wasting of muscle tissue, results in weakness of muscle.

- Integumentary System

  — **Pressure ulcers** that quickly reach deeper tissues, including muscle, tendon, and bone, develop easily.

Mental and Social Effects of Immobility

Inactivity leads to loss of self-esteem, poor body image, sensory deprivation, and increased dependence on others. Inactivity is often a factor leading to depression. Most residents feel better if they have some interaction with others. The resident who cannot move should be helped out of her room and spend time near activity. Inactivity and immobility can lead to withdrawal, isolation, and loneliness. Instructions to help the immobile resident are found on the care plan.

BODY MECHANICS

Body mechanics refers to the correct use of the muscles to help use your strength properly to avoid fatigue and injury to yourself or others (Figure 9-2). Using proper body mechanics is one of the safest

✔ GUIDELINES for Using Proper Body Mechanics

- ☐ Plan what you are going to do.
- ☐ Know what the resident can do to assist.
- ☐ Explain the procedure to the resident.
- ☐ Ask for the resident's help.
- ☐ Get another nursing assistant to help, if necessary.
- ☐ Have a wide base of support. Place your feet 12 to 14 inches apart.
- ☐ Move close to the resident. Do not reach from a distance.
- ☐ Use your "internal girdle." Tighten your abdominal muscles upward and your buttock muscles downward before lifting.
- ☐ Squat to move or lift an object. Bend at the knees and hips. Keep your back straight.
- ☐ Lift by using your thigh muscles.
- ☐ Work smoothly and match your movements when working with a partner.
- ☐ Turn with your feet. Do not twist your body.
- ☐ Do not lift when you can push or pull.
- ☐ Use lifting aids when appropriate, such as mechanical lifts and lift sheets.

Figure 9-2 Make good body mechanics a habit.

things you can to do prevent injury to the resident and to yourself. Nursing assistants move, lift, and turn residents often. Using proper body mechanics can prevent injuries and lessen strain and fatigue. Proper body mechanics involves:

- using good posture and balance. Use the strongest muscles of the body to do the work.
- using a back support belt if this is your preference or the policy of your facility. Good body mechanics should be used along with the belt for maximum effectiveness.
- correctly using your own body and that of the resident.
- enhancing the safety, comfort, and confidence of the resident.
- using pillows, props, and other supports to maintain the resident's body in good alignment.

BODY ALIGNMENT

The correct positioning of the resident's body is called body **alignment.** The resident should be positioned in good posture when sitting or lying. Always follow instructions from the supervising nurse or the resident's care plan. The following points refer to proper body alignment and positioning techniques.

Fowler's Position

The **Fowler's position** is used when the resident is sitting in bed. The headrest of the bed is elevated 45 to 60 degrees, and the knee area of the bed is raised slightly. The **high Fowler's position** is similar, but the head of the bed is elevated 90 degrees. In the **semi-Fowler's position,** the head of the bed is elevated 30 to 45 degrees.

- Have the resident lie on her back with the head of the bed and knees elevated.
- Make sure the resident's hips are at the bend of the bed.
- If necessary, move the resident up in bed at intervals.
- Support the arms with pillows, if necessary.
- Remember that this position increases pressure on the buttocks, increasing the risk of pressure ulcer development. The resident should not be left in this position for prolonged periods. Follow your facility policy or the resident's care plan for the time frame.

Sitting in a Chair

Proper positioning in the chair is important so that the resident can breathe correctly. Good positioning promotes resident comfort and a sense of well-being. Follow these guidelines:

- Place the resident's feet flat on the footrests of the wheelchair, the floor, or a stool. The feet should not dangle.
- Position the hips and knees at right angles.
- Rest the buttocks firmly against the back of the chair. You may wish to pad the seat of the chair for the resident's comfort and to prevent skin breakdown.
- Position the spine straight against the back of the chair.
- Position the resident's head directly over the shoulders.
- Support the forearms and elbows on the armrests of the chair.
- If necessary, prop the resident with pillows or pads to maintain good alignment.

Proper position at mealtime is important to prevent choking. Position the resident upright, using pillows or props for support, if necessary. The elbows should be below wrist level when the resident is eating. Pay attention to table height. If the table is too high for the resident, he will have more difficulty eating. Seating the resident on a cushion may help. Likewise, make sure that the resident is close to the table. Residents who are seated in wheelchairs may be too far away. After meals, residents should remain upright for at least 30 to 60 minutes, if possible.

Supine Position

The **supine position** is used when the resident is lying on the back.

- Place a small pillow under the resident's head. This allows better alignment than a large pillow.

If a large pillow is used, extend it down past the neck so that it supports both the shoulder area and the head.

- Keep the feet in proper alignment and prevent foot drop with a footboard or other device specified on the care plan.
- Use positioning devices such as handrolls, splints, foam, or firm wedges as indicated on the care plan to maintain position.

The **semisupine position** is also called the *tilt position*. Do not confuse it with the lateral position. The resident in the lateral position is lying on the side. This increases pressure on the bony prominences of the ear, shoulder, elbow, hip, and ankle. The resident in the semisupine position is on his or her side, but is tilted at an angle. When used correctly, this position relieves pressure from all bony prominences and keeps the spine straight. The resident is positioned so that he is leaning against a pillow for support. The legs are straight, with the top leg slightly behind the bottom leg. A pillow is placed under the top leg to keep it even with the hip joint. The lower shoulder is pulled forward. This causes pressure to be distributed across the back, not the shoulder joint. The arms can be at the sides or folded across the abdomen.

Lateral Position

The **lateral position** is used when the resident is to lie on the side.

- Support the upper arm and leg with pillows.
- Position the upper leg so that its weight does not rest on the lower leg.
- Place a pillow lengthwise to support the resident's back and maintain the position.

Sims' Position

The **Sims' position** is commonly used when an enema is given or when the physician is doing an examination.

- The resident is positioned on the left side.
- The left arm is positioned behind the back and extended.
- The right arm is flexed and brought forward, supported on a pillow.
- The right knee is flexed and supported on a pillow.
- A small pillow is placed under the resident's head.

Prone Position

The **prone position** is used when the resident is lying on the abdomen. Use this position for residents only if directed to do so by the care plan. Check the resident every 15 to 30 minutes, or according to facility policy, when in the prone position.

- Turn the resident's head to one side when she is lying prone.
- Place a small pillow under the resident's abdomen near the waist.
- Flex (bend) the resident's arms and position them near the head.
- Place the resident's feet in the space between the mattress and the foot of the bed.

The **semiprone position** is the opposite of the semisupine position. It is a very comfortable position for the resident. Like the semisupine position, it eliminates pressure on the bony prominences, reducing the risk of pressure ulcers. To place the resident in this position, begin by turning the resident prone. Lift the shoulder and chest on the side closest to you. Support them with a pillow. Position the opposite arm behind the resident. The legs and spine are straight. Fold a second pillow in half and place it under the top leg. Turn the resident's head to either side. Use a small pillow for comfort.

Moving a Resident with a Draw Sheet

Some residents are too weak, ill, or large for you to move by yourself. Sometimes moving the resident

---

PERFORMANCE PROCEDURE

9 Positioning the Resident in the Supine Position

1 Perform your beginning procedure actions.

2 Position the resident so that she is lying on her back.

3 Place the resident's arms at her sides in a comfortable, functional position, supporting them with pillows if necessary.

4 Check for good body alignment.

5 Pad bony prominences of elbows and heels if indicated.

6 Elevate the knees slightly for comfort, if desired.

7 Perform your procedure completion actions.

PERFORMANCE PROCEDURE

10 Moving the Resident to the Side of the Bed

1 Perform your beginning procedure actions.

2 Stand on the side of the bed opposite from the one on which the resident will lie.

3 Use proper body mechanics to move the resident.

4 Place the resident's arms across his chest. Cross the resident's legs at the ankles.

5 Remove the pillow.

6 Place one of your arms under the resident's shoulder. Place the other arm under the back.

7 Move the upper part of the resident's body toward you.

8 Place one of your arms under the resident's waist and the other arm under the resident's thighs.

9 Move the resident's midsection toward you.

10 Move the resident's legs toward you. Uncross the ankles. Straighten the resident's arms.

11 Replace the pillow.

12 Begin positioning or transferring the resident, or go to the next step of this procedure.

13 If the resident is to be left in this position, straighten the linen and raise the side rails if ordered.

14 Perform your procedure completion actions.

with your arms causes pain for the resident. Using a draw sheet to move and turn the resident prevents **friction** and **shearing** between the resident's skin and the sheets. Another advantage of moving the resident with a draw sheet is that it reduces the risk of a back injury in the nursing assistant. The following procedure assumes that a draw sheet is left on the bed at all times for lifting and moving the resident. In this procedure, you will need a coworker to help you.

Moving the Resident to the Head of the Bed Using a Draw Sheet

Using a draw sheet to move the dependent resident prevents friction and shearing between the resident's skin and the sheets. This procedure assumes that a draw sheet is left on the bed at all times for lifting and moving the resident. In this procedure, you will need a coworker to help you.

TRANSFERRING AND AMBULATING THE RESIDENT

You will be transferring, or moving, residents out of bed and wheelchairs several times a day. It is important that you do this correctly to avoid injury to the resident and yourself. It is always good to practice these skills with another nursing assistant. Practice will reinforce and help you learn the rules of safety. Another task you will be expected to perform is to **ambulate,** or walk with, the resident. Using a transfer belt or gait belt helps assure the resident's and your safety.

Using the Transfer (Gait) Belt

A gait belt and a transfer belt are the same piece of equipment. The belt is called a *transfer belt* when it is used to **transfer** the resident. It is called a *gait belt* when it is used to ambulate the resident. It should be worn around the nursing assistant's waist when it is

PERFORMANCE PROCEDURE

11 Moving the Resident to the Side of the Bed Using a Draw Sheet

1 Perform your beginning procedure actions.

2 Use proper body mechanics to move the resident.

3 Place the resident's arms across her chest. Cross the resident's legs at the ankles.

4 Remove the pillow.

5 Roll the ends of the draw sheet toward the resident until they touch the body.

6 Using an overhand grip, place one hand at the upper end of the draw sheet, by the resident's shoulders. Place the lower hand on the draw sheet in the hip area.

7 The nursing assistant on the side of the bed to which the resident will be moved does most of the work and calls the signals.

8 Move one foot about 12 inches forward to give you a broad base of support. Place your weight on this foot.

9 Flex your knees and keep your back straight.

10 On the count of three, both nursing assistants lift and pull the sheet toward the side of the bed.

11 Uncross the resident's ankles and straighten her arms.

12 Replace the pillow and unroll the draw sheet.

13 Begin positioning or transferring the resident, or go to the next step of this procedure.

14 If the resident is to be left in this position, straighten the linen and raise the side rails if ordered.

15 Perform your procedure completion actions.

PERFORMANCE PROCEDURE

12 Assisting the Resident to Move Up in Bed

1 Perform your beginning procedure actions.

2 Lower the head of the bed.

3 Remove the pillow and lean it against the headboard.

4 Stand next to the bed.

5 Ask the resident to bend her knees and put her feet flat on the mattress.

6 If the resident is able, ask her to bend her arms at her sides, place her hands on the bed, and ask her to push when told to do so.

7 Slide one hand and arm under the resident's upper back and shoulders.

8 Slide the other arm under the resident's hips and buttocks.

9 Instruct the resident to push with her hands and feet on the count of three.

10 On the count of three, move the resident to the head of the bed.

11 Replace the pillow.

12 Check to see if the resident is in good alignment.

13 Perform your procedure completion actions.

PERFORMANCE PROCEDURE

13 Moving the Resident to the Head of the Bed Using a Draw Sheet

1 Perform your beginning procedure actions.

2 Place the resident's arms across his chest.

3 Remove the pillow.

4 Roll the ends of the draw sheet toward the resident until they touch his body.

5 Using an overhand grip, place one hand at the upper end of the draw sheet, by the resident's shoulders. Place the lower hand on the draw sheet in the hip area.

6 Both nursing assistants should stand with feet apart, one foot ahead of the other.

7 Bend your knees and keep your back straight.

8 On the count of three, both nursing assistants should shift their weight from one foot to the other while lifting the draw sheet and moving it toward the head of the bed.

9 Straighten the resident's arms.

10 Replace the pillow and unroll the draw sheet.

11 Straighten the linen and leave the resident comfortable.

12 Perform your procedure completion actions.

not being used on a resident. In some facilities, a belt is left with each resident and the nursing assistant uses only this belt for transferring the resident. Know and follow your facility policy.

A transfer belt is a heavy canvas belt placed closely around the resident's waist (Figure 9-3). You can hold onto it while lifting the resident instead of lifting the resident under the arms. When using the transfer belt, always grasp it with an underhand grasp for good control. While ambulating the resident, a firm underhand grasp on the transfer belt helps you ease the resident to the floor in case of a fall. Never use the resident's own belt in place of the transfer belt.

GUIDELINES for Lifts and Moving Residents

The nursing assistant does a great deal of lifting and moving. Wear uniforms that fit loosely enough to allow you to move comfortably without tearing. Wear nonskid shoes so you do not slip. Use a back support if this is your preference or facility policy. Plan your moves to include the following:

❑ Refer to the care plan for specific instructions.

❑ Explain the procedure to the resident, making certain that she understands what is to be done and how she should help.

❑ Use a transfer belt to prevent injury to yourself and the resident.

❑ Use lifting devices, if indicated.

❑ Position the bed in the lowest possible position.

❑ Get assistance if you are not sure whether the resident can safely move, position, or transfer.

Be alert to safety as follows:

❑ Lock the brakes on beds, wheelchairs, and lifts.

❑ Make sure that lifting and moving devices are in good working condition.

❑ When transferring a resident, move the resident toward her stronger side.

❑ Support the resident's weaker side during transfers, such as when the resident has **hemiplegia.**

❑ Be alert to catheters and other tubing so that tubes are not accidentally pulled or dislodged.

❑ Have the resident wear nonskid shoes or footwear.

❑ Apply artificial limbs and braces properly.

❑ Avoid lifting the resident under the arms. This can cause pain and dislocate the resident's shoulders.

❑ The resident should not use your neck for support.

❑ Support body parts when turning the resident.

❑ When ambulating residents, approach corners slowly and watch for approaching traffic.

❑ Check the rubber tips of canes and walkers before using them, to be sure they are not too worn.

Observe and report changes as follows:

❑ change in color, paleness, sweating

❑ dizziness, unsteadiness, inability

❑ shortness of breath or difficulty breathing

❑ changes in vital signs

❑ signs of skin irritation

❑ resident's comments and concerns

Also be aware of these psychosocial concerns:

❑ Let the resident help as much as possible if consistent with the care plan.

❑ Encourage the resident to be in charge of moving.

❑ Ask the resident to count to three.

❑ Offer the resident choices, such as where and when to be moved.

❑ Realize that the inability to move is a great loss of the resident's independence.

❑ Know the resident's fears, such as falling or being left alone.

Figure 9-3 Using the gait (transfer) belt keeps both the resident and the nursing assistant safe.

Contraindications for Use of the Transfer Belt. The transfer or gait belt is **contraindicated** in residents with these medical conditions:

- colostomy
- a gastrostomy tube
- recent abdominal surgery or a fresh incision
- severe cardiac or respiratory disease
- fractured ribs
- pregnancy

Before using the transfer belt on any resident, check with the charge nurse or care plan.

PERFORMANCE PROCEDURE

14   Using a Transfer (Gait) Belt

1 Perform your beginning procedure actions.

2 Assist the resident to sit on the side of the bed.

3 Assist the resident to put on clothing and shoes or other footwear with nonslip soles.

4 Explain to the resident that the transfer belt is a safety device that will prevent pulling and tugging on the resident. Explain that it will be removed when the resident has been transferred.

5 Always apply the belt over the resident's clothing.

6 Place the belt around the resident's waist and buckle it in the front. Take care with female residents to ensure that the breasts are not under the belt.

7 Thread the belt through the teeth side first. Place the end of the belt through both openings so that it is double locked.

8 The belt should fit snugly, but you should check it by slipping your fingers comfortably underneath to be sure it is not too tight. Monitor female residents to be sure that the breasts are not under the belt.

9 Using an underhand grasp, insert your hands under the belt on each side and assist the resident to stand.

10 Complete the transfer or ambulation procedure.

11 Perform your procedure completion actions.

15   Transferring the Resident from Bed to Wheelchair—One Person

1   Perform your beginning procedure actions.

2   Position the wheelchair so the resident's stronger side will be closest to the wheelchair when the resident is sitting on the edge of the bed. Place the wheelchair within one foot of the bed at a slight angle.

3   Raise or remove the wheelchair footrests.

4   Lock the wheelchair brakes.

5   Raise the head of the bed.

6   Lock the wheels of the bed.

7   Lower the bed to the lowest position. Lower the side rail.

8   Assist the resident to sit on the side of the bed.

9   Assist the resident to put on clothing and shoes or other footwear with nonslip soles.

10   Place the transfer belt around the resident's waist and buckle it in the front.

11   Thread the belt through the teeth side first. Place the end of the belt through both openings so that it is double locked.

12   Check the fit of the belt by inserting your fingers underneath it.

13   Make sure that the resident's feet are flat on the floor. If not, use the transfer belt to move the resident to the side of the bed until his feet touch the floor.

14   Instruct the resident to push off the bed with his hands on the count of three.

15   Using an underhand grasp, insert your hands under the belt on each side, count to three, and assist the resident to stand.

16   Support the resident's weaker side.

17   Pivot and turn the resident with his back to the wheelchair.

18   Continue to hold the transfer belt, and guide the resident backward until he can feel the edge of the wheelchair seat with the back of his legs.

19   Tell the resident to place his hands on the wheelchair arms. Seat the resident in the chair (Figure 9-4).

20   Remove the transfer belt.

21   Adjust the wheelchair footrests.

22   Cover the resident's lap with a lap blanket or other covering. Be sure the blanket does not become caught in the wheels.

23   Perform your procedure completion actions.

Figure 9-4 Maintain a wide base of support and use good body mechanics when transferring residents.

PERFORMANCE PROCEDURE

16 Transferring the Resident from Bed to Wheelchair—Two Persons

1 Perform your beginning procedure actions.

2 Position the wheelchair so the resident's stronger side will be closest to the wheelchair when the resident is sitting on the edge of the bed. Place the wheelchair within one foot of the bed at a slight angle.

3 Raise or remove the wheelchair footrests.

4 Lock the wheelchair brakes.

5 Raise the head of the bed.

6 Lock the wheels of the bed.

7 Lower the bed to the lowest position. Lower the side rail.

8 Assist the resident to sit on the side of the bed.

9 Assist the resident to put on clothing and shoes or other footwear with nonslip soles.

10 Place the transfer belt around the resident's waist and buckle it in the front.

11 Thread the belt through the teeth side first. Place the end of the belt through both openings so that it is double locked.

12 Check the fit of the belt by inserting your fingers underneath it.

13 Use the transfer belt to move the resident to the edge of the bed until his feet are flat on the floor. Each nursing assistant places the hand closest to the resident at the back of the belt and the other hand at the front of the belt and slides the resident forward.

14 On the count of three, both nursing assistants will move the resident at the same time. Coordination of movement is very important.

15 Each nursing assistant places the hand closest to the resident through the belt with an underhand grasp behind the resident.

16 The nursing assistant closest to the chair, on the resident's right side, stands in a position so that she can pivot and move away, allowing the resident access to the chair. This nursing assistant should stand with the left leg further back than the right leg.

17 The other nursing assistant should use her left knee to support the resident's weaker left leg. This nursing assistant's right leg is positioned further back than the left one.

18 Instruct the resident to lean forward and push off the bed, using the palms of his hands, on the count of three.

19 The resident's knees should be spread apart. Tell the resident to put both feet back with the stronger foot behind the weaker foot.

20 Both nursing assistants should bend their knees, squat slightly, and spread their feet to provide a broad base of support.

21 On the count of three, the resident stands. The nursing assistants pivot the resident slowly and smoothly by pivoting their feet, legs, and hips toward the left until the resident can feel the wheelchair with the back of his legs (Figure 9-5).

Figure 9-5 On the count of three, both nursing assistants lift and pivot the resident.

(continues)

16 *continued*

22 Tell the resident to place both hands on the armrests of the chair and lean forward slightly.

23 Both nursing assistants should bend their knees and lower the resident into the chair (Figure 9-6).

24 Remove the transfer belt.

25 Adjust the wheelchair footrests.

26 Cover the resident's lap with a lap blanket or other covering. Be sure that the blanket does not become caught in the wheels.

27 Perform your procedure completion actions.

Figure 9-6 Keep your back straight and gently lower the resident into the chair.

PERFORMANCE PROCEDURE

17 Ambulating the Resident with a Gait Belt

1 Perform your beginning procedure actions.

2 Assist the resident to sit on the side of the bed.

3 Assist the resident to put on shoes or other footwear with nonslip soles.

4 Explain to the resident that the gait belt is a safety device that will prevent pulling and tugging on the resident. It allows you to guide and support the resident during the ambulation procedure.

5 Always apply the belt over the resident's clothing.

6 Place the belt around the resident's waist and buckle it in the front.

7 Thread the belt through the teeth side first. Place the end of the belt through both openings so that it is double locked.

8 The belt should fit snugly, but you should check it by slipping your fingers comfortably underneath to be sure it is not too tight. Monitor female residents to be sure that the breasts are not under the belt.

9 Using an underhand grasp, insert your hands under the belt on each side and assist the resident to stand.

10 Walk behind and slightly to one side of the resident during ambulation. Maintain a firm, underhand grasp at the center back of the gait belt (Figure 9-7).

(continues)

17 *continued*

Figure 9-7 Walk behind and slightly to the side of the resident, maintaining an underhand grasp on the gait belt.

11 Encourage the resident to use handrails in the hallway.

12 Walk the distance recommended by the care plan or the nurse's instructions.

13 Monitor the resident for signs of fatigue. If this occurs, assist the resident to sit in a chair.

14 After ambulating the resident, return to the resident's room.

15 Assist the resident to sit in the chair or return to bed.

16 Remove the gait belt.

17 Perform your procedure completion actions.

PERFORMANCE PROCEDURE

18 Ambulating the Resident With a Cane or Walker

1 Perform your beginning procedure actions.

2 Assist the resident to sit on the side of the bed.

3 Assist the resident to put on shoes or other footwear with nonslip soles.

4 Check the tips of the cane and walker for safety.

5 Place the gait belt around the resident's waist and check the fit.

6 Place the cane in the resident's hand or the walker in front of the resident.

7 Help the resident stand. Grasp the gait belt underhand at the resident's sides.

8 When the resident is standing and is balanced, ask her if she feels dizzy or weak.

9 Walk behind and slightly to one side of the resident during ambulation. Maintain a firm, underhand grasp at the center back of the gait belt.

10 Walk the distance recommended by the care plan or the nurse's instructions.

11 Monitor the resident for signs of fatigue. If this occurs, assist the resident to sit in a chair.

12 After ambulating the resident, return to the resident's room.

13 Assist the resident to sit in the chair or return to bed.

14 Remove the gait belt.

15 Perform your procedure completion actions.

PERFORMANCE PROCEDURE

19   Transferring the Resident from Wheelchair to Toilet

1 Perform your beginning procedure actions.

2 Make sure the bathroom is empty.

3 Bring the resident in a wheelchair to the bathroom.

4 Close the bathroom door.

5 Position the wheelchair at right angles to the toilet.

6 Place the transfer belt around the resident's waist.

7 Lock the wheelchair brakes.

8 Tell the resident to push up from the wheelchair while you lift her with the transfer belt. Count to three to match movements.

9 Ask the resident to hold the bathroom grab bar.

10 Help the resident stand, giving her time to get balanced.

11 Pivot the resident so she is standing in front of the toilet, facing you.

12 Lower the resident's underwear.

13 Help the resident sit on the toilet.

14 Be sure the call light is close to the resident. Instruct the resident to call when she is finished.

15 Wash your hands and leave the bathroom if doing so is safe for the resident. Close the door behind you.

16 Return when the resident calls.

17 Put on gloves if helping the resident wipe excess urine or bowel movement is necessary.

18 Remove the gloves and discard according to facility policy.

19 Wash your hands.

20 Assist the resident to stand by using the gait belt. Tell the resident to hold onto the bathroom grab bar and pull herself up. Match movements on the count of three.

21 Pull the resident's underwear up.

22 Smooth the resident's clothing.

23 Pivot and seat the resident in the locked wheelchair. Flush the toilet. If abnormalities are noted in the urine or stool, do not flush. Save the specimen for the nurse to see.

24 Help the resident wash her hands.

25 Remove the resident from the bathroom.

26 Remove the transfer belt.

27 Perform your procedure completion actions.

The Mechanical Lift

The mechanical lift is used when a resident is heavy, helpless, unbalanced, or has a condition, such as amputated legs or **paralysis,** that makes transfer with a belt difficult or impossible. Many facilities use beds with frames that are 5 to 7 inches above the floor. If the resident falls from bed, the chance of injury is less than falling from a regular hospital bed. Unfortunately, transferring residents into and out of such low beds increases the risk of back injuries for nursing assistants. Using a mechanical lift for this type of transfer reduces the risk of injury. Know and follow your facility policy for use of the mechanical lift. Most facilities require two or more nursing assistants to operate the lift safely.

The mechanical lift is a hydraulic unit. Always check the floor near the lift before using it. If an oily substance is on the floor, do not use the lift until it is checked and repaired. Always check the sling, release mechanisms, straps, and chains for safety problems before using the lift. If anything is in need of repair, do not use it. Follow your facility policy for removing the lift from service. Obtain safe equipment before taking the lift to the resident's room.

20   Transferring the Resident Using a Mechanical Lift

Supplies needed:

- mechanical lift
- straps or chains for mechanical lift
- seat for mechanical lift
- disposable underpad for lift seat, if needed
- disposable exam gloves if contact with body fluids, secretions, or excretions is likely

1 Perform your beginning procedure actions.

2 Place the wheelchair at right angles to the foot of the bed, facing the head. Lock the wheelchair and elevate or remove the footrests.

3 Elevate the bed to a good working height for you. Lock the wheels of the bed.

4 Lower the side rail on the side nearest you.

5 Roll the resident on her side (Figure 9-8A).

6 Position the lift seat under the resident's body so that it supports the resident's shoulders, buttocks, and thighs. Smooth out the sling (Figure 9-8B).

7 Roll the resident back onto the sling and properly position it on the other side.

8 Position the frame of the lift over the bed. Spread the legs of the lift to the widest open position to maintain a broad base of support (Figure 9-8C).

9 Attach the suspension straps or chains to the sling. The "S" hook should face *away* from the resident's body, to prevent injury.

10 Position the resident's arms comfortably inside the sling.

11 Attach the straps or chains to the lift frame.

12 While talking to and reassuring the resident, slowly raise the boom of the lift until the resident is above the bed (Figure 9-8D).

13 Slowly guide the lift away from the bed.

14 Position the lift over the chair.

Figure 9-8A Roll the resident on her side, and position the sling from the shoulders to just below the hips.

Figure 9-8B Smooth the sling. Wrinkles are uncomfortable and increase the risk of skin breakdown.

(continues)

20 *continued*

15 The second nursing assistant holds the sling and helps lower the resident slowly into the chair, keeping the hips back while the first nursing assistant slowly lowers the lift.

16 Monitor the location of the resident's feet and arms to prevent injury.

17 Unhook the straps or chains and remove the lift.

18 Support the resident's feet with footrests.

19 Perform your procedure completion actions.

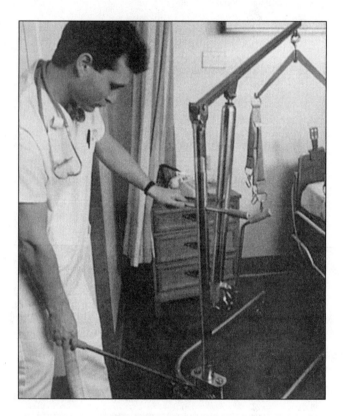

Figure 9-8C Position the lift over the bed and open the legs of the lift to provide a wide base of support.

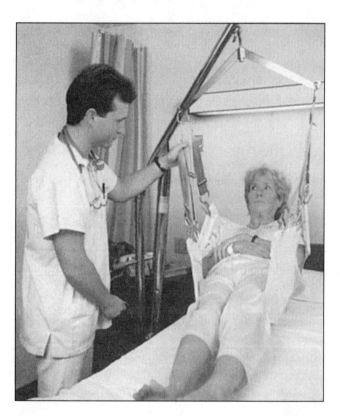

Figure 9-8D Slowly raise the sling until the resident is suspended above the bed.

RANGE-OF-MOTION EXERCISES

Range of motion is how far a joint can be moved. Active range of motion is when the resident can move her joints by herself. Passive range of motion is when the resident is unable to move her joints, so the nursing assistant moves them for her. A person's range of motion is affected by many things, such as age, body size, genetics, and the presence or absence of disease. You will help residents do range-of-motion exercises each day. Follow the directions on the care plan. Ask for help if you are not certain how to do this procedure.

You must become familiar with several terms regarding range-of-motion exercises. **Abduction** is moving the resident's extremity away from the body. **Adduction** is moving an extremity toward the body. **Flexion** is bending a joint. **Extension** is straightening a joint.

Purpose of Range-of-Motion Exercises

Range-of-motion exercises are done for residents who are unable to move their own joints. There are several reasons for these exercises. Muscles that are not used atrophy, become weak, and develop contractures. Contractures are deformities that cannot always be reversed.

Reasons for passive range-of-motion exercises include:

- preventing deformities.
- preventing pain.
- maintaining normal joint function.
- increasing joint motion.
- improving circulation.
- promoting a sense of well-being.

✓ GUIDELINES for Doing Range-of-Motion Exercises

- ☐ Follow the care plan instructions.
- ☐ Explain the procedure to the resident.
- ☐ Use good body mechanics.
- ☐ Expose only the part of the body being exercised.
- ☐ Know your facility policy for exercising the head and neck. This is not done without a doctor's order in some facilities.
- ☐ Support the limbs above and below the joint being exercised.
- ☐ Do not push the joint past the point of pain or resistance.
- ☐ Watch the resident's face for an indication of pain or discomfort.
- ☐ Stop at the end of each motion before repeating it again.
- ☐ Do each exercise three to five times, or as indicated in the care plan.
- ☐ Encourage the resident to help with the exercises as indicated on the care plan.
- ☐ Report and record how the resident tolerated the procedure, the degree of joint movement, which extremity was exercised, and type of exercise.

PERFORMANCE PROCEDURE

21   Giving Passive Range-of-Motion Exercises

1   Perform your beginning procedure actions.

2   Position the resident in the supine position.

3   Exercise the extremities as indicated on the care plan, supporting the extremity at the closest joints.

Head and Neck

Perform range of motion in this area only if it is your facility policy or if you have a physician's order:

1   Lean the head forward, bringing the chin to the chest.

2   Lean the head backward, with the chin up.

3   Turn the head from side to side.

4   Turn the head back and forth in a circular motion.

Shoulders, Arms, and Elbows

1   Move the arm over the head, with arm touching the top of head.

2   Return the arm to the side.

3   Move the arm across the chest.

4   Return the arm to the side.

5   Move the arm straight up.

6   Return the arm to the side.

7   Bring the arm away from body at the side to the shoulder level.

8   Return the arm to the side.

9   With the arm straight out at the side, bend at the elbow and rotate the shoulder.

10   Return the arm to the side.

(continues)

21 *continued*

11 Bend at the elbow and bring hand to chin (Figure 9-9A).

12 Return the arm to the side.

Wrists, Fingers, and Forearms

1 Bend the hand backward at the wrist (Figure 9-9B).

2 Bend the hand forward at the wrist.

3 Clench the fingers and thumb slightly, as if making a fist.

4 Extend the fingers and thumb (Figure 9-9C).

5 Move fingers and thumb together and then apart.

6 Flex and extend joints in the thumb and fingers.

7 Move each finger in a circular motion.

8 Extend the arm along the side of the body with the palm facing upward.

9 Rotate the forearm with the palm facing upward, then downward.

Legs, Hips, and Knees

1 Stretch the leg out from the body. Return the leg to the other leg, crossing over the other leg only at the ankle.

2 Bend and straighten the knee (Figure 9-9D).

3 Roll the knees inward and outward.

Ankles, Feet, and Toes

1 With the leg straight on the bed, push foot and toes toward front of the leg (Figure 9-9E).

2 Push the foot and toes out straight. Point toward the foot of the bed.

3 With the leg straight, turn the foot and ankle from side to side.

4 Curl toes downward and upward.

Figure 9-9A When exercising the elbow, support the arm above and below the joint.

Figure 9-9B Range-of-motion exercises for the wrist.

(continues)

21 *continued*

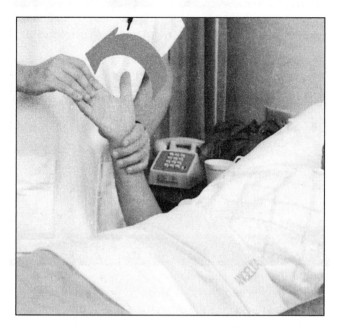

Figure 9-9C Range-of-motion exercises for the fingers.

Figure 9-9D Range-of-motion exercises for the hip and knee. Support the knee joint during this activity.

5 Spread the toes and move each toe away from the second toe, then toward the second toe.

6 Repeat each exercise as indicated on the care plan.

7 Note the resident's response to exercise.

8 Perform your procedure completion actions.

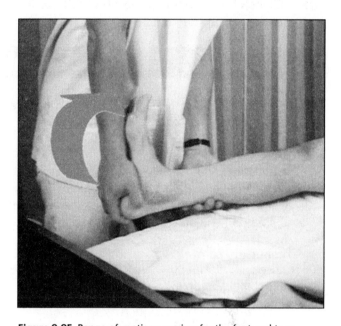

Figure 9-9E Range-of-motion exercises for the foot and toes.

KEY POINTS IN THIS CHAPTER

▲ Rehabilitation and restorative nursing are designed to restore and maintain the resident's highest level of ability.

▲ Immobility leads to complications in all body systems.

▲ Proper body alignment is necessary for the resident while sitting or lying down.

▲ Using a transfer belt helps prevent injury to the nursing assistant and the resident.

▲ Always follow the care plan when moving and lifting residents.

▲ Range-of-motion exercises are done to prevent deformities and increase circulation and joint motion.

▲ Safety is important when moving or lifting residents.

REVIEW QUIZ

1. The process designed to help a person restore and maintain her highest level of ability is:
   a. range of motion.
   b. rehabilitation.
   c. activities of daily living.
   d. assistance.

2. Maintenance, prevention, and restoration of abilities are the principles of:
   a. adaptive devices.
   b. nursing care.
   c. rehabilitation.
   d. activity therapy.

3. What is a prosthesis?
   a. a mechanical lift
   b. a walker or cane
   c. an adaptive tool
   d. an artificial body part

4. All of the following are true statements *except*:
   a. Immobility affects the resident physically.
   b. There are mental effects from the resident's inability to move about.
   c. Only the circulatory system is affected by immobility.
   d. Residents may feel frustrated when they must rely on others to move about.

5. An effect of immobility on the circulatory system may be:
   a. swelling of the tissues due to poor blood flow.
   b. constipation and loss of appetite.
   c. development of a bladder infection.
   d. loss of calcium in the bones.

6. Proper body mechanics includes:
   a. having a wide base of support.
   b. using the strong back muscles to lift.
   c. keeping the feet close together when lifting.
   d. keeping the object to be lifted at arm's length from the body.

7. Using good body mechanics does all of the following *except*:
   a. prevent fatigue in the nursing assistant.
   b. reduce injury to the nursing assistant.
   c. reduce the risk of injury to the resident.
   d. increase the resident's strength.

8. Body alignment is:
   a. lifting and moving residents.
   b. positioning the body correctly.
   c. comfortable positioning for the nursing assistant.
   d. using the muscles the best way.

9. What is the correct positioning for the resident when sitting in a chair?
   a. The feet should be dangling.
   b. The hips should be at right angles in the chair.
   c. The knees should be extended.
   d. The spine should be slanted as much as possible.

10. A resident in the supine position is lying on the:
    a. side.
    b. abdomen.
    c. back.
    d. side with pillows supporting the spine.

11. When a resident is in the prone position, she is lying on the:
    a. abdomen.
    b. side.
    c. back.
    d. back and side.

12. When moving a resident up in bed, ask the resident to help by:
    a. pulling on the side rails.
    b. pushing the pillow up.
    c. straightening the legs and pushing with the feet.
    d. bending the knees, placing feet flat on the bed, and pushing.

13. Using a draw sheet when moving residents helps prevent:
    a. infections.
    b. friction and shearing.
    c. contractures.
    d. atrophy.

14. When moving a resident up in bed, the pillow should be:
    a. placed against the headboard.
    b. placed on the chair.
    c. kept at the foot of the bed.
    d. left under the resident's head.

15. A belt that is placed around the resident's waist when transferring is called a:
    a. lifting belt.
    b. transfer or gait belt.
    c. mechanical lifter.
    d. lifting and moving belt.

16. Which of the following is *not* a true statement regarding lifting and moving residents?
    a. There is no need to explain procedures to confused residents.
    b. Refer to the care plan for special instructions.
    c. Make sure the equipment used for lifting and moving is working properly.
    d. Get help, if necessary.

17. When the resident has a weak side, it is best to move her:
    a. weak side first.
    b. with either side moving first.
    c. toward the weaker side.
    d. toward the stronger side.

18. Before assisting a resident to ambulate with a cane or walker, you should:
    a. check the tips of the cane or walker.
    b. place a gait belt around the resident's waist.
    c. make sure that the resident has on shoes with nonslip soles.
    d. all of the above.

19. Passive range-of-motion exercises are done for the resident:
    a. who is up and about.
    b. who can move well without help.
    c. who cannot exercise herself.
    d. by licensed professionals only.

20. What are your major concerns when lifting or moving a resident?
    a. how good the resident looks when you are finished
    b. safety of the resident
    c. how quickly you can do the task
    d. all of the above

21. Mr. Macmillan is a 66-year-old resident who is 6 feet tall and weighs 210 pounds. He has had a stroke and requires total care. You have never transferred this resident before. The nurse assigns you to get this resident up in the chair for two hours after his bath. You should:
    a. do as you are told without asking questions.
    b. check the care plan for instructions on how to transfer the resident.
    c. tell the nurse that the resident is too big for you to move.
    d. report the nurse to the director of nursing for giving you such a difficult assignment.

22. You are assigned to care for Dr. Stuart, a 77-year-old retired professor. Dr. Stuart has had a respiratory infection and fever. She is taking antibiotics and has been in bed for three days. The nurse tells you in report that the resident's fever is normal and that it is time to get Dr. Stuart up in the chair for an hour. When it is time to get Dr. Stuart up, she tells you that "Sick people must stay in bed." Your best response would be to:
    a. inform Dr. Stuart that the nurse insists that she get up.
    b. leave Dr. Stuart in bed.
    c. advise Dr. Stuart that getting out of bed may help her to get well faster.
    d. call the resident's daughter and inform her that her mother will not cooperate.

23. You are assigned to bathe Michael Cleary, a 72-year-old resident with diabetes. Mr. Cleary walks about the facility at will. When you hand him the washcloth and ask him to wash his face, he says, "I am paying you to wash my face." Your best response would be to:
    a. wash the resident's face.
    b. ignore what Mr. Cleary said and leave the room.
    c. tell him that you are not paid to wash his face.
    d. consult the care plan or ask the nurse for advice.

24. You are caring for Mrs. Kaiser, an 88-year-old resident who is confined to bed. The nurse instructed you in report to make sure that the resident was turned every two hours. Mrs. Kaiser has a large pressure sore on her buttocks. You do not know whether you should position her on her back or not. You should:
    a. turn her on her back anyway because the nurse did not give you special instructions.
    b. ask another nursing assistant what to do.
    c. consult the care plan or ask the nurse for advice.
    d. leave Mrs. Kaiser on her side for four hours because you cannot turn her on her back.

25. Mrs. Ashe is a newly admitted resident whose daughter has been caring for her in the home. You are assigned to transfer Mrs. Ashe from the bed to the chair by using the transfer belt. When you explain the procedure to Mrs. Ashe, she says that her daughter always put her hands under her arms and lifted her. She says she does not think the belt is necessary. You should:
    a. place your hands under Mrs. Ashe's arms and lift her into the chair.
    b. continue to explain to Mrs. Ashe why the transfer belt is the safest method to use.
    c. tell Mrs. Ashe that her daughter transferred her improperly.
    d. leave Mrs. Ashe and care for the other residents you are assigned to.

CHAPTER 9
CROSSWORD PUZZLE

Directions: Complete the puzzle using these words found in Chapter 9.

ADL
alignment
ambulate
atrophy
contracture
contraindicated
edema
extend

flex
Fowler's
friction
hemiplegia
immobility
lateral
mechanics
paralysis

pressure
prone
prosthesis
range
rehabilitation
restorative
shearing
supine

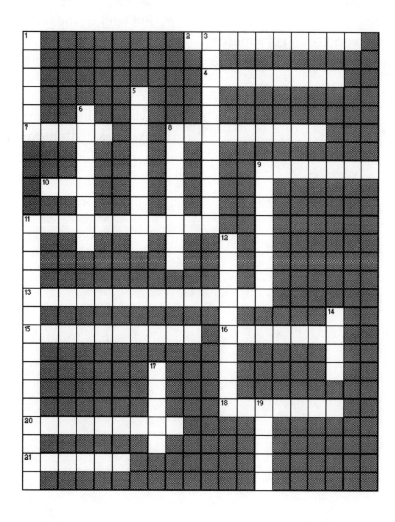

CHAPTER 9
PUZZLE CLUES

ACROSS

2. An artificial body part
4. Stretching the skin between the bone inside and the bed on the outside of the body is _____ .
7. Swelling
8. Loss of ability to move
9. Sitting in bed with the head elevated and knees bent is the _____ position.
10. Activities of daily living
11. Abnormal tightening or shortening of a muscle
13. Designed to restore and maintain the resident's highest level of ability
15. Inability to move
16. Side lying
18. Muscle wasting
20. Proper position in good posture
21. To straighten

DOWN

1. Lying on the back
3. Nursing care designed to assist the resident by restoring health and promoting independence is _____ nursing.
5. Proper use of the body is good body _____ .
6. To walk
8. Areas of skin redness or breakdown are _____ ulcers.
9. Rubbing on the resident's skin in a manner that irritates it
11. Improper or undesirable
12. Paralysis on one side of the body
14. To bend
17. Lying on the abdomen
19. Exercises that move muscles and joints are _____ of motion.

Personal Care Needs

OBJECTIVES

In this chapter, you will learn the importance of giving personal care to residents. After reading this chapter, you will be able to:

- Spell and define key terms.
- Describe the goals of skin care.
- Identify pressure ulcers and describe how they are caused and prevented.
- List guidelines for personal care of the resident.
- Perform oral hygiene for the resident.
- Bathe the resident.
- Perform perineal care.
- Help groom the resident.
- Describe care of a resident with a prosthesis.
- Demonstrate care of the hair and nails.
- Apply support hosiery.
- Make an occupied bed.

KEY TERMS

abrasion: a rubbing away or scraping of the skin

anti-embolism stockings: elastic stockings that improve circulation by compressing the veins in the legs

anus: the outlet for the rectum

axilla: the armpit

decubitus ulcer (plural: decubiti): a pressure sore, pressure ulcer, or bedsore

dentures: artificial teeth; may be partial or complete, upper or lower dentures

genital area: the area that includes the external sex organs and anus

incontinent: unable to control the discharge of urine or stool

perineal (peri) care: cleansing the genital area

SKIN CARE

The skin is the largest organ of the body, and it performs several necessary functions. The skin is an outer covering that protects a person from infection and injury. The skin also removes water, salt, and waste through sweat. At certain places the skin joins with mucous membranes to line body openings. The hair and nails are considered part of the skin system.

As a nursing assistant you will give skin care to residents (Figure 10-1). Knowing the changes caused by aging is important for you.

Age-Related Changes in the Skin

As in every body system, aging brings some changes in the skin, hair, and nails. The changes vary due to heredity and individual lifestyle, but generally the age-related changes in the skin are as follows:

- Skin becomes drier, scaly, thin, and wrinkled.
- Skin loses elasticity.

Figure 10-1 Nursing assistants provide most of the personal care to residents.

- The fatty tissue under the layer of skin decreases.
- Less oil and sweat are produced.
- Skin tags and moles are more common.
- The skin is less sensitive to heat, cold, and pain.
- The skin becomes fragile, easily damaged, and easily torn.
- Fingernails and toenails become thicker and brittle, cracking more easily.

Goals of Skin Care

The resident's care plan will state specific skin care goals, but some general goals are important to observe when giving skin care.

An elderly person's skin produces less oil, so the skin is often dry and flaky. Therefore, having a full bath everyday is not necessary for most elderly persons. In fact, bathing everyday often makes the skin drier. Most residents will have a partial bath at least once a day, but a full bath or shower is usually given only twice a week. The resident's care plan states the bathing schedule. In residents with dry skin, the care plan may direct you to apply a moisturizing lotion.

When a person perspires, or sweats, the drops on the surface of the skin can pick up dirt and dust that mix with tiny flakes of skin. Some diseases also cause flaking and cracking of the skin. Some residents are incontinent of bowel and bladder. These excretions are very irritating to the skin. The warm, dark, and damp skin area gives bacteria the chance to grow and spread. Therefore, cleaning the resi-

dent's skin is one of your major responsibilities. Know the major goals of bathing or cleaning the resident.

- Cleanliness
  - removes bacteria on the skin
  - removes sweat and other body secretions
  - removes body odors
  - promotes a sense of well-being
- Stimulate circulation
  - Warm water on the surface of the skin increases blood flow.
  - Light skin stroking during washing helps blood flow.
  - Massage soothes and stimulates the skin.
- Mild exercise for the resident
  - Moving the body, trunk, arms, and legs is mild exercise.
  - Mild exercise gives the resident the opportunity to do range-of-motion exercises.
- Observation. Bath time is an opportunity to inspect the resident's skin. Report:
  - irritation
  - texture change
  - color change
  - lumps under the skin or areas of new growth
  - injury
  - pressure ulcers
  - drainage
  - rashes
  - any resident complaint
- Other benefits of bathing
  - Bath time provides the nursing assistant an opportunity to have personal, therapeutic communication with the resident.
  - The feeling of being clean and attractive is refreshing and adds to the dignity, self-worth, and sense of well-being of the resident.

PRESSURE ULCERS

Bedsores are called pressure sores, pressure ulcers, **decubitus ulcers,** or decubiti. The most accurate name for this problem is "pressure ulcer." Pressure ulcers develop quickly in the immobile, elderly resident because of prolonged pressure and lack of blood flow to an area. The name "bedsore" is de-

Figure 10-2 A pressure ulcer can progress from a reddened area to a deep, serious ulcer very quickly. (Courtesy of Emory University Hospital, Atlanta, GA.)

ceiving. Pressure ulcers can develop anytime that the resident has pressure on the skin. Pressure ulcers may develop even when the resident is sitting up in a chair. Your observation and reporting skills must be very sharp in this area. A reddened area can progress to a deep ulcer very quickly (Figure 10-2). Deep ulcers are painful and difficult to heal. Infections and other complications may develop. Prevention is the best treatment for pressure ulcers. Pressure ulcers frequently develop over areas of bony prominences (Figure 10-3):

* back of head
* side of head
* ears
* shoulder blades
* elbows
* breasts in women
* spine
* hips and buttocks
* sacrum and coccyx
* genitalia in men
* thighs in contact with catheter tubing
* knees
* ankles
* heels
* toes

Stages of Pressure Ulcers

Pressure ulcers progress in four stages, as follows:

* *Stage I.* Redness that does not go away within 30 minutes of the time that pressure is relieved. In a dark-skinned person, this may appear as a blue or black discoloration.

Figure 10-3 Areas where pressure ulcers can develop.

* *Stage II.* Partial skin loss, a blister, or a shallow crater.
* *Stage III.* A full layer of skin is lost, extending down into the subcutaneous fat layer.
* *Stage IV.* A full layer of skin is lost, and the damage extends down to muscle, tendon, and bone.

Observation and Reporting

Report immediately:

* redness of the skin that does not go away within 30 minutes after the pressure is relieved
* blisters

GUIDELINES for Preventing Pressure Ulcers

Use the following approaches to prevent pressure ulcers from beginning:

☐ Keep the resident up and walking for as long as possible.

☐ Change all residents' positions every two hours, more often if the care plan indicates, or if the resident is uncomfortable. Remember that this applies to residents sitting in chairs and those in bed.

☐ Keep the skin clean and dry. Prolonged moisture causes the skin to break down. Wash the resident immediately after each episode of incontinence. Use a cleansing agent that reduces skin irritation. Be sure to rinse and dry well.

☐ Use facility-approved moisture lotions if the resident's skin is dry.

☐ Help the resident drink enough liquids and eat correctly.

☐ Keep linens free of wrinkles and crumbs.

☐ Avoid friction and shearing when moving the resident.

☐ Use lifting devices to move residents whenever possible.

☐ If residents are sitting in chairs, teach them to shift their weight every 15 minutes.

☐ Use pressure-relieving pads in beds and wheelchairs.

☐ Position and pad the resident so that the skin at bony areas, such as the knees and ankles, does not rub together.

☐ If the resident is in bed with the head elevated, do not allow the resident to sit in this position for more than two hours.

☐ Follow the nurse's or care plan instructions for special treatment of pressure ulcers.

☐ Apply the principles of standard precautions when providing care.

- skin tears or **abrasions**
- pain or tenderness
- bruises
- rashes
- any skin color changes

Use pressure-relieving devices such as:

- sheepskin (Figure 10-4).
- protective elbow and heel pads (Figure 10-5).
- pillows.
- foam wedges.
- alternating-pressure mattress.
- special gel-, water-, and foam-filled mattresses, cushions, and overlays (Figure 10-6).
- low air loss and other therapeutic beds (Figure 10-7).
- other devices used by your facility.

Follow the care plan when using these devices. Although the resident may be using a pressure relieving device, changing position is still necessary.

Nursing Measures

Certain nursing measures are used to prevent pressure ulcers from developing. These include changing the resident's position every two hours, or more often if necessary, and assisting the resident to maintain good nutrition and hydration.

Figure 10-4 A sheepskin may be used to prevent friction and shearing. (Courtesy of J.T. Posey Co., Arcadia, CA.)

PERSONAL CARE

Personal care of the resident includes care of the mouth, teeth, hair, nails, and feet. It is also bathing, dressing, and grooming the resident. You will be responsible for helping the resident with these activities of daily living. A well-groomed appearance affects the resident's self-esteem.

The resident has done his own care all his life. It may take longer to let the resident wash his own face and brush his own teeth, but you will add to the resident's self-worth by helping the resident, rather

Figure 10-5 Heel and elbow protectors provide padding and prevent pressure on these high-risk areas.

Figure 10-6 Gel mattresses are commonly used to relieve pressure.

Figure 10-7 Low air loss therapy beds are beneficial for residents with severe skin breakdown. Residents using these beds must be turned regularly because breakdown can still occur. (Courtesy of National Patient Care Systems.)

than doing it for him. Helping the resident be as independent as possible is one goal of restorative nursing care. Refer to the following guidelines for personal care:

ORAL HYGIENE

Oral hygiene is the cleaning of the mouth, teeth, gums, and tongue. The purpose of oral hygiene is to remove food particles and reduce the amount of bacteria in the mouth. One of your responsibilities is to provide good mouth care and cleanliness for the resident. A clean mouth helps prevent mouth odor and tooth decay. A feeling of well-being is created when a person has good oral hygiene.

Another purpose of providing oral hygiene is observation. While brushing the resident's teeth, you have an opportunity to observe the mouth. Remember when giving oral hygiene:

- Encourage self-care if consistent with the care plan.
- Let the resident brush his own teeth. Get supplies ready, and take the resident into the bathroom in a wheelchair.
- Wear gloves when doing oral hygiene.
- Observe and report any signs of irritation, sores, loose teeth, and pain to the nurse.

Special Situations

Some residents need frequent mouth care because of special medical problems. These include residents who are receiving tube feedings and those who are in a coma. Many of these residents breathe through the mouth. The mucous membranes of the mouth and nose dry out quickly. The mouth needs to be cleaned frequently to keep it moist, prevent caking of secretions, and to make breath feel and smell fresh. Follow your facility policy and the care plan for cleaning and moisturizing the resident's mouth. Some comatose residents require mouth care as often as every one or two hours. These points are important to remember when giving special mouth care:

- Always explain the procedure to the resident even if the resident appears unresponsive.
- Turn the resident's head to the side when cleaning the mouth of an unconscious resident to avoid getting liquids into the lungs.
- Moisten the resident's lips with lip balm or other lubricant according to facility policy.

DENTURE CARE

Many residents in a long-term care facility have **dentures** (false teeth). Dentures may be the entire set of teeth or only a few teeth. Dentures are necessary for eating, retaining the shape of the face and jaw, and for giving the resident a sense of well-being.

GUIDELINES for Providing Personal Care

☐ Bathing should be a good cleaning of the body in a pleasant, relaxed area. Refer to the care plan for special bathing instructions.

☐ Assist the resident with toileting before beginning a procedure.

☐ Give the resident choices. Schedule time for personal care according to the resident's needs and desires.

☐ Independence promotes positive self-esteem. Allow the resident to do as much self-care as possible. Follow the care plan.

☐ Use adaptive devices that promote independence, such as:

— long-handled shoe horn

— long-handled grippers

— adaptive brushes and combs

— other devices used by your facility to promote independence

☐ Protect the resident's privacy.

— Close the door, window curtain, and privacy curtain.

— Expose only the part of the body on which you are working.

☐ Dress the resident in appropriate clothing. Clothing should be appropriate for the season and the resident's age, and be color-coordinated. Clothing should be of the proper size and fit and in good repair.

☐ Avoid cold or exposure.

— Make sure the room is warm enough.

— Use a bath blanket to keep the resident covered if the body will be exposed. This is a modesty and dignity issue, in addition to providing warmth.

☐ Avoid the overuse of powders or talc. Too much powder is not good for the skin. Know and follow your facility policy. Some facilities do not allow the use of body powder unless the resident requests it.

☐ Dry the resident well.

— Pay special attention to skin folds, creases, and the skin between the toes.

— Drying the resident helps prevent infection and skin breakdown. Do not rub the resident vigorously. Pat and gently rub the skin dry.

☐ Be alert to safety concerns.

— Use the transfer belt to move the resident.

— Test the temperature of the bath water.

— Use safety belts on tub lifts and shower chairs.

— Make certain that bath mats are secure.

— Help residents in and out of the tub and shower.

— Stay with the resident in the tub and shower.

— Observe the resident for shortness of breath or complaints of feeling dizzy.

— Report anything unusual to the nurse.

— Record the procedure according to facility policy.

☐ Be alert to infection control issues.

— Apply the principles of standard precautions when providing personal care.

— Always wash from the cleanest area to the dirtiest.

— Change water, washcloth, and gloves after washing a contaminated or dirty area.

— Disinfect the tub, shower chair, or whirlpool after each use.

— Handle soiled towels and linen properly.

PERFORMANCE PROCEDURE

22   Brushing the Resident's Teeth

Supplies needed:
- toothbrush
- toothpaste
- water
- mouthwash
- straw
- emesis basin
- towel
- disposable exam gloves

1 Perform your beginning procedure actions.

2 Place a towel across the resident's chest.

3 Help the resident in self-care, if possible.

4 Moisten the toothbrush. Apply toothpaste.

5 Brush the resident's teeth using a circular motion on all surfaces. Brush gums, tongue, sides, and roof of the mouth.

6 Let the resident rinse the mouth with water or mouthwash.

7 Hold the emesis basin while the resident spits.

8 Wipe the mouth with a towel.

9 Check the mouth for sores, redness, or irritation.

10 Perform your procedure completion actions.

PERFORMANCE PROCEDURE

23   Special Oral Hygiene

Supplies needed:
- special mouth applicators or swabs used by your facility
- water
- plastic bag
- lubricant for lips
- emesis basin
- two towels
- disposable exam gloves

1 Perform your beginning procedure actions.

2 Cover the pillow with a towel and turn the resident's head to the side. Position the head forward so that any fluid and secretions will not run down the resident's throat.

3 Place the emesis basin against the resident's chin.

4 Gently open the resident's mouth.

5 Dip the premoistened applicators into water, mouthwash, or solution used by the facility.

6 Wipe the gums, teeth, and inside of the mouth with applicators.

7 Discard the used applicators in the plastic bag.

8 Apply lubricant to the resident's lips.

9 Perform your procedure completion actions.

Losing teeth is depressing to some people. Many residents will try to keep others from seeing them without their dentures in place. Always respect the resident's privacy when giving denture care. Be very careful when handling dentures. Dentures are very expensive and can break easily if dropped. Follow these important considerations in caring for dentures:

- Wear gloves and apply the principles of standard precautions.
- Remove dentures carefully. Let the resident remove them, if possible. Place the dentures in an emesis basin lined with a paper towel.
- Fill the sink with water and line the bottom of the sink with a paper towel or washcloth so that the dentures do not break if they slip.
- Brush dentures very well with a denture brush and the cleaning agent used by your facility. Hold them securely.
- Rinse the dentures.
- Check the dentures for cracks, chips, or loose teeth.
- Let the resident clean and rinse the mouth before replacing dentures.
- Store dentures in a marked denture cup according to facility policy. Some facilities store dentures dry. Others put water or denture cleaning tablets in the cup.
- Always respect the resident's privacy during this procedure.

BATHING THE RESIDENT

The resident in a long-term care facility usually needs help bathing. Most residents receive a full bath or shower once or twice a week. A partial bath is given at least once a day. The care plan and assignment sheet will tell you what type of bath to give the resident and when to give the bath. Bathing assignments may be flexible depending on resident requests and needs.

Types of Baths

Residents who are able will get a tub, shower, or whirlpool bath. Many long-term care facilities have a bathroom that has a whirlpool tub, which cleans as well as tub or shower bathing and is very relaxing for the resident. A special shower chair is used for residents who are getting showers. A shampoo is often given as part of the bathing procedure. Refer to the care plan if the resident is to have the hair washed while having a bath.

Follow your facility policy for transporting residents to the tub or shower room. Make sure that they are not exposed while transporting them in the hallway.

Residents who are either too weak or ill to receive a tub bath or shower are given a bed bath. A nursing assistant cleans the resident's entire body, one part at a time while the resident remains in bed.

A partial bath is usually given to residents at least once a day. A partial bath includes washing the face, hands, underarms, back, and genital area. The procedures for giving a bed bath and partial bath follow later in this chapter. Most facilities also assist residents to wash their face and hands before and after meals.

Perineal Care

Perineal care is also called **peri care** and refers to the thorough washing of the **genital area.** In the female the genital area includes the urinary opening, the vaginal area, and the rectum. In the male, the penis, scrotum, and rectum are included. For the resident who is **incontinent,** peri care must be given frequently. Urine or stool on the skin causes the already frail skin of the elderly person to break down more quickly. Practice peri care keeping these considerations in mind:

- Apply the principles of standard precautions during this procedure.
- Realize that many older people are modest and may be embarrassed by having others clean their genital area.
- Give care that protects the resident's modesty by giving privacy and exposing only the body part you are cleaning. Cover the resident with a bath blanket and be sure that the privacy curtain, window curtain, and door are closed during this procedure.
- Wash properly, using warm soapy water. Always wash the cleanest area first. This means that you always wash from the front to the back of a female. In the male resident, begin at the end of the penis and move down toward the body, under the scrotum, then back to the rectum. Do not rub back and forth. Rinse and dry thoroughly. Some nursing facilities may use special products for peri care. Follow your facility policy.
- For the catheterized resident, wash the catheter gently to remove urine, stool, or mucus.
- Wash away from the resident's body. Begin at the urinary meatus and wash downward on the catheter. Do not rub back and forth.
- You will be expected to give perineal care to both male and female residents in most cases.

PERFORMANCE PROCEDURE

24   Giving a Bed Bath

Supplies needed:
- washbasin
- soap
- washcloth
- bath blanket
- two or more towels
- clean gown or clothing
- lotion
- comb or brush
- deodorant
- disposable exam gloves

1 Perform your beginning procedure actions.

2 Remove the bedspread and blanket. Fold them and place on the chair.

3 Place the bath blanket over the top sheet. Remove the sheet without exposing the resident. Place the soiled sheet in the hamper or dispose of it according to facility policy.

4 Remove the resident's gown.

5 Raise the side rail.

6 Fill the basin with warm water. Check the temperature with a thermometer. It should be 105°F. Changing the water during the procedure may be necessary. Add more hot water if it becomes too cool.

7 Return to the bedside and lower the side rail.

8 Place a towel under the resident's chin.

9 Offer the resident the washcloth to wash his own face, if possible.

10 Make a mitten by folding the washcloth around your hand.

11 Wash the resident's eyelids from the inner side of the eye to the outer side of the eye, using plain water without soap. The eyes have a mucous membrane, so you should wear gloves during this part of the procedure.

12 Rinse the washcloth.

13 Dry the washed area.

14 Wash the remainder of the resident's face, neck, and ears. Ask the resident if he prefers to use soap. Some elderly residents do not use soap on the face.

15 Place a towel under the resident's arm farthest from you.

16 Hold the resident's arm up. Wash the whole arm from the shoulder to the wrist and fingertips.

17 Rinse and dry the arm.

18 Wash, rinse, and dry the **axilla** or armpit.

19 Repeat for the other arm.

20 If possible, place the resident's hands in water. Wash, rinse, and dry hands, fingers, and nails.

21 Place the towel across the chest. Pull the bath blanket down to the abdomen.

22 Move the towel to expose half of the chest.

23 Wash, rinse, and dry the chest. In the female resident, dry the area under the breasts well. Repeat for the other side of the chest.

24 Cover the chest with the towel.

25 Pull the bath blanket down to expose the abdomen.

26 Wash, rinse, and dry the abdomen.

27 Return the bath blanket to the resident's shoulders.

28 Remove the towel from under the blanket.

29 Uncover the leg farthest from you. Place the towel under the leg.

30 Wash, rinse, and dry the leg from the groin area to the toes.

31 Repeat for the other leg.

32 If possible, place feet in a basin one at a time.

33 Wash, rinse, and dry the feet. Make sure that you dry well between the toes.

(continues)

24 *continued*

34 Cover the legs with the bath blanket.

35 Raise the side rail.

36 Empty the basin and refill with clean water.

37 Lower the side rail.

38 Ask the resident to turn with his back toward you. Assist if necessary.

39 Wash, rinse, and dry the back.

40 Put lotion on back, massaging the entire back.

41 Use gloves to wash the genital area. Wash from the front of the genital area to the rectal area.

42 Dispose of soiled linen according to facility policy.

43 Remove gloves and dispose of them according to facility policy.

44 Put the side rail up.

45 Wash your hands.

46 Return to the bedside and put the side rail down.

47 Help the resident into a clean gown or other clothing of choice.

48 Comb the resident's hair. Help with other grooming requests.

49 Replace bed linens, if indicated, or straighten the bed.

50 Perform your procedure completion actions.

PERFORMANCE PROCEDURE

25   Giving a Partial Bath

Supplies needed:
- washbasin
- soap
- washcloth
- two towels
- clean gown or clothing
- bath blanket
- lotion
- comb or brush
- deodorant
- disposable exam gloves

1 Perform your beginning procedure actions.

2 Place a towel under the chin.

3 Offer the resident the washcloth to wash her own face, if possible.

4 Make a mitten by folding the washcloth around your hand.

5 Wash the resident's eyelids from the inner side of the eye to the outer side of the eye, using plain water without soap. Wash the eye on the opposite side first, then the eye closest to you. The eyes have mucous membranes, so you should wear gloves for this part of the procedure.

6 Rinse the washcloth.

7 Dry the washed area.

8 Wash the remainder of the resident's face, neck, and ears. Ask the resident if she prefers to use soap. Some elderly residents do not use soap on the face.

9 Dry the washed area.

10 Place the towel under the hand farthest from you.

(continues)

25 *continued*

11 If possible, place resident's hand in the basin. Wash, rinse, and dry hand.

12 Repeat for other hand.

13 Wash, rinse, and dry axilla (armpit).

14 Repeat for the other axilla.

15 Ask the resident to turn with her back toward you. Assist if necessary.

16 Wash, rinse, and dry the back.

17 Put lotion on back, massaging the entire back lightly.

18 Use gloves when washing the genital area. Wash from the front of the genital area to the rectal area.

19 Put side rail up.

20 Remove gloves and dispose of them according to facility policy.

21 Wash your hands.

22 Return to the bedside and put side rail down.

23 Help the resident into a clean gown or other clothing of choice.

24 Comb the resident's hair. Help with other grooming requests.

25 Replace bed linens, if indicated, or straighten the bed.

26 Perform your procedure completion actions.

PERFORMANCE PROCEDURE

26 Female Perineal Care

Supplies needed:
- washbasin
- soap
- washcloth
- two towels
- clean gown or clothing
- bath blanket
- bed protector
- disposable exam gloves

1 Perform your beginning procedure actions.

2 Remove the bedspread and blanket. Fold them and place on the chair.

3 Place the bath blanket over the top sheet. Fanfold the sheet to the foot of the bed without exposing the resident. If the sheet is soiled, dispose of it according to facility policy.

4 Ask the resident to raise her hips while you place a bed protector under her buttocks.

Remove the soiled bed protector, if present. (Apply the principles of standard precautions during this activity.)

5 Raise the side rail.

6 Fill the basin with warm water.

7 Return to the bedside and lower the side rail.

8 Position the bath blanket so that only the area between the legs is exposed.

9 Ask the resident to separate and bend her knees.

10 Put on disposable gloves.

11 Wet the washcloth and make a mitten out of it.

12 Apply soap to the washcloth. Use caution. Too much soap can be irritating.

13 With one hand, separate the labia.

(continues)

26 *continued*

14 With the other hand:

a Wash the far side of the labia from top to bottom, using a single downward stroke.

b Rinse the washcloth (Figure 10-8).

c Wash the near side of the labia from top to bottom, using a single downward stroke.

d Rinse the washcloth.

e Wash the center of the labia from top to bottom, using a single downward stroke.

f Rinse the area well with the washcloth.

g Gently dry the area with a towel.

15 Turn the resident away from you. Flex the upper leg slightly, if possible.

16 Wet washcloth and make a mitt. Apply soap.

17 Expose the **anus.**

18 Wash the area, stroking from the perineum to the coccyx (Figure 10-9).

19 Rinse the area well with the washcloth.

20 Gently dry the area with a towel.

21 Return the resident to her back.

22 Remove and dispose of the bed protector according to facility policy.

23 Raise the side rail.

24 Dispose of soiled linen according to facility policy.

25 Remove gloves and dispose of them according to facility policy.

26 Wash your hands.

27 Lower the side rail. Replace the top covers and remove the bath blanket.

28 Help the resident into a clean gown or other clothing of choice.

29 Perform your procedure completion actions.

Figure 10-8 Wash the labia from front to back using downward strokes.

Figure 10-9 Wash from the perineum to the coccyx.

PERFORMANCE PROCEDURE

27   Male Perineal Care

Supplies needed:
- washbasin
- soap
- washcloth
- two towels
- clean gown or clothing
- bath blanket
- bed protector
- disposable exam gloves

1   Perform your beginning procedure actions.

2   Remove the bedspread and blanket. Fold them and place on the chair.

3   Place the bath blanket over the top sheet. Fanfold the sheet to the foot of the bed without exposing the resident. If the sheet is soiled, dispose of it according to facility policy.

4   Ask the resident to raise his hips while you place a bed protector under his buttocks. Remove the soiled bed protector, if present. Apply the principles of standard precautions during this activity.

5   Raise the side rail.

6   Fill the basin with warm water.

7   Return to the bedside and lower the side rail.

8   Position the bath blanket so that only the area between the legs is exposed.

9   Ask the resident to separate and bend his knees.

10 Put on disposable gloves.

11 Wet the washcloth and make a mitten out of it.

12 Apply soap to the washcloth. Use caution. Too much soap can be irritating.

13 With one hand, grasp the penis gently and wash. Begin washing at the urinary meatus and wash the penis in a circular motion toward the base of the penis (Figure 10-10).

14 If the resident is not circumcised, pull the foreskin back to wash it. Rinse the penis, dry, and replace the retracted foreskin.

15 Wash the scrotum, then gently lift it and wash the perineum.

16 Rinse the washcloth, make a mitten, and rinse the entire area, beginning with the penis.

17 Gently dry the area with a towel.

18 Ask the resident to turn so his back is facing you. Assist if necessary.

19 Expose the anus.

20 Wash the area, stroking from the perineum to the coccyx.

21 Rinse the area well with the washcloth.

22 Gently dry the area with a towel.

23 Return the resident to his back.

24 Remove and dispose of the bed protector according to facility policy.

25 Raise the side rail.

26 Dispose of soiled linen according to facility policy.

27 Remove gloves and dispose of them according to facility policy.

28 Wash your hands.

29 Return to the bedside and lower the side rail.

30 Replace the top covers and remove the bath blanket.

31 Help the resident into a clean gown or other clothing of choice.

32 Perform your procedure completion actions.

Figure 10-10 Wash from the tip of the penis down to the scrotum, then underneath the scrotum.

PERFORMANCE PROCEDURE

28   Giving a Back Rub

Supplies needed:
- basin of water (105°F)
- soap
- washcloth
- towel
- disposable exam gloves
- lotion of resident's choice

1 Perform your beginning procedure actions.

2 Place the bottle of lotion in the basin of water to warm it.

3 Expose the resident's back and upper buttocks.

4 Wash, rinse, and dry.

5 Pour a small amount of lotion into one hand.

6 Warm the lotion by holding it between your hands, if necessary.

7 Apply lotion to the back.

8 Rub the back with gentle but firm strokes with both hands in a circular motion from buttocks to shoulders:

   a Begin at the base of the spine and rub up the center of the back with long, soothing strokes (Figure 10-11).

   b Use a circular motion with your hands as you bring them down from the shoulders back to the buttocks.

   c Repeat this procedure for three to five minutes.

9 Remove excess lotion from the back.

10 Straighten and tighten the bottom sheet and draw sheet.

11 Change the resident's gown, if necessary.

12 Perform your procedure completion actions.

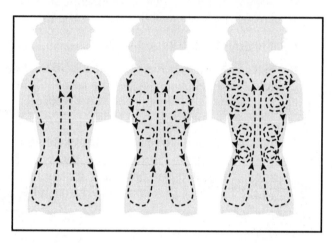

Figure 10-11 Rub the resident's back using gentle, circular motions.

APPLYING LOTION TO THE RESIDENT

Another part of good skin care is massaging the skin with lotion. Always refer to the care plan. If indicated, massage the resident's skin with light, smooth strokes. Massage can stimulate circulation and is often recommended. It is soothing and refreshing to the resident. If the resident uses lotion on the legs, pat it in gently. Do not massage the legs. Massaging the legs may cause complications due to blood clots. Avoid placing lotion between the toes.

GROOMING THE RESIDENT

Grooming the resident includes combing hair, shaving, caring for nails, and putting glasses or hearing aids in place. Self-esteem is increased when one is well groomed (Figure 10-12). Follow these rules for grooming residents:

- Give the resident choices, if possible.
- Encourage self-care, if possible.
- Provide privacy.
- Dress and groom the resident appropriately.
- Do not share grooming items with other residents.
- Clean all grooming items after using them: razor, comb, brush.
- Help the resident clean eyeglasses. Handle the glasses with care.
- Care for the resident's hearing aid, if necessary.

PERFORMANCE PROCEDURE

29   Combing the Resident's Hair

Supplies needed:
- towel
- comb
- hair brush

1 Perform your beginning procedure actions.

2 Cover the pillow with a towel. If the resident is sitting in a chair, place the towel over the shoulders.

3 Section the resident's hair with one hand between the scalp and the ends of the hair.

4 Brush the hair thoroughly.

5 Have the resident turn so that you can comb and brush the back of the hair.

6 If the hair is tangled, use the comb to separate it. Take a small section of hair. Beginning at the end, comb downward. Support the hair above where you are combing with the fingers of your other hand so that you do not pull on the resident's scalp. Continue working upward until you reach the scalp.

7 Style the hair attractively and in a style appropriate for the resident's age. If the resident has long hair, consider braiding it or putting it up. Coarse, tightly curled hair may require special treatment.

8 Perform your procedure completion actions.

Figure 10-12 A well-groomed appearance promotes a positive self-esteem.

Shaving the Male Resident

Men should be shaved every day as part of the morning care procedure. Honor the resident's preference to grow a mustache or beard. Since the probability of contacting blood during this procedure is fairly high, you should wear gloves.

PROSTHESIS CARE

A *prosthesis* is an artificial body part. Prosthetic devices such as artificial legs, arms, or breasts can make life much more enjoyable for the person using the device. You will find some residents in the long-term care facility who wear a prosthesis. Understand these considerations when caring for a resident who uses a prosthesis:

- Refer to the care plan for special instructions.
- Remember that this is part of the resident's body and should be cared for as such. Be aware of confidentiality issues. The resident may not want others to know of the prosthesis.
- Keep the prosthesis clean.
- Be alert to pressure areas under the prosthesis. Check for redness, irritation, and blisters. Listen carefully to resident complaints of discomfort.
- Keep the skin under the prosthesis clean and dry.
- Dress the resident wearing the prosthesis properly. Stockinette may be worn under artificial limbs.
- Report to the nurse if you feel that the prosthesis needs repair.
- An artificial eye is usually cared for by the nurse. If you are instructed to care for a resident with an artificial eye, handle it carefully. The artificial eye socket and the eye must be cleaned as indicated

PERFORMANCE PROCEDURE

30   Shaving the Resident

Supplies needed:
- washcloth
- towel
- electric or safety razor
- shaving cream or preshave lotion
- basin of water (105°F)
- mirror
- aftershave lotion
- disposable exam gloves

1 Perform your beginning procedure actions.

2 Cover the resident's chest with the towel.

3 Soften the resident's beard by placing a warm washcloth over it for two to three minutes. Moisten the face with water and apply shaving cream.

4 Put on disposable gloves.

5 Beginning in front of the ear, hold the skin taut.

6 Bring the razor down from the cheek to the chin in one-half- to one-inch increments.

Continue until the entire cheek has been shaved. Rinse the razor between strokes.

7 Repeat with other cheek.

8 Ask the resident to tighten his upper lip. Shave from the nose to the upper lip in short, downward strokes.

9 Ask the resident to tighten his chin. Shave the chin in downward strokes in one-half- to one-inch increments.

10 Ask the resident to tip his head back.

11 Apply shaving cream to the neck area.

12 Hold the skin taut. Shave the neck area in smooth, upward strokes in one-half- to one-inch increments.

13 Wash the resident's face and neck. Dry the area well.

14 Apply aftershave lotion if resident prefers.

15 Perform your procedure completion actions.

---

on the care plan. Apply the principles of standard precautions during this procedure.
- Maintain a professional attitude when caring for a resident with a prosthesis.

FOOT CARE

Special care is sometimes part of caring for the resident's feet. Because poor blood circulation to the feet is common, the skin on the resident's feet heals slowly if injured. Injury prevention is often the best treatment in caring for the feet. Know and follow your facility policy for foot and toenail care. Many facilities do not allow the nursing assistant to trim toenails. In these facilities, the nursing assistant is responsible for keeping the feet clean and dry. Report to your supervisor if the nails need to be cut or if other abnormalities are noted. Note these considerations in giving foot care:

- Follow the care plan.
- Soak the feet often.

- Dry the feet well, especially between the toes.
- Apply lotion to clean feet, but do not put lotion between the toes.
- Follow your facility policy for clipping toenails.

APPLYING SUPPORT HOSIERY

Support hosiery is for the resident who has circulation problems. The hose provide some pressure on the legs, which helps increase the blood flow. These stockings are made of stretchable elastic and fit very closely. Support stockings may be knee length or cover the entire leg. These types of hosiery are called **anti-embolism stockings,** and are often referred to by the brand name, such as TED® Hose. Practice the following rules when using support hosiery:

- Follow the care plan regarding when the stockings are to be put on and for how long the resident is to wear the hosiery.
- Put stockings on the resident before he gets out of bed in the morning. Elevate the legs before applying the hosiery, if this is your facility policy.

PERFORMANCE PROCEDURE

31   Hand and Fingernail Care

Supplies needed:
- soap
- towel
- bed protector
- basin of water (105°F)
- lotion
- nail clippers
- orange stick
- nail file or emery board
- disposable exam gloves if contact with non-intact skin is likely

1   Perform your beginning procedure actions.

2   Adjust the height of the overbed table and place it in front of the resident. Cover the overbed table with the bed protector.

3   Place the basin of water on the table.

4   Instruct the resident to place hands in the water (Figure 10-13A).

5   Soak the hands for approximately 10 minutes. Cover the resident's hands and the basin with a towel to keep the water warm. Add more warm water if necessary.

6   Wash the resident's hands. Push the cuticles back gently with the washcloth or an orange stick.

7   Lift the resident's hands out of the water and dry them with the towel.

8   Clip the nails if permitted by facility policy (Figure 10-13B):

    a   Cut the nails straight across.

    b   Do not trim the nails below the fingertips.

    c   Keep the nail clippings on the bed protector to be discarded later.

9   Shape the nails with the nail file or emery board (Figure 10-13C). Apply fingernail polish if requested by a female resident.

10   Pour a small amount of lotion into your hands and rub it into the resident's hands.

11   Perform your procedure completion actions.

Figure 10-13A Soak the resident's hands in warm water.

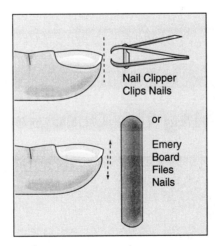

Figure 10-13B Clip the nails straight across, then smooth the corners and edges.

Figure 10-13C Gently clean under the nails.

- The stockings must be applied smoothly with no wrinkles.
- If your facility policy allows, a light dusting of powder on the feet and legs will make it easier to apply the hosiery.
- Make sure that the hosiery is the correct size.
- The hosiery must fit well to be effective.
- A plastic sandwich bag placed over the foot allows the hosiery to slide on easily. Remove the bag through the opening in the toe area.

MAKING THE OCCUPIED BED

There may be times when you must change the sheets or make the entire bed while the resident is in it. This is done for residents restricted to bed rest; that is, those who are too weak or ill to get out of bed. Other times you will change only some linens while the resident remains in bed. Follow your facility infection control policies and procedures for placement of clean and dirty linen. Apply the principles of standard precautions during this procedure.

PERFORMANCE PROCEDURE

32   Applying Support Hosiery

Supplies needed:
- anti-embolism hosiery of proper size

1 Perform your beginning procedure actions.

2 Expose one leg at a time.

3 Grasp the stocking with both hands at the top opening and roll or gather toward the toe end.

4 Apply the stocking to the leg by rolling or pulling upward over the leg.

5 Make sure the stocking is on evenly. Be sure there are no wrinkles.

6 Expose the other leg.

7 Grasp the stocking with both hands at the top opening and roll or gather toward the toe end.

8 Apply the stocking to the leg by rolling or pulling upward over the leg.

9 Make sure the stocking is on evenly. Be sure there are no wrinkles.

10 Perform your procedure completion actions.

PERFORMANCE PROCEDURE

33   Making the Occupied Bed

Supplies needed:
- two large sheets
- linen draw sheet, if used
- plastic or rubber draw sheet, if used
- bed protector, if used
- pillowcase
- bath blanket
- laundry bag or hamper
- clean bedspread and blanket, if needed
- disposable exam gloves

1 Perform your beginning procedure actions.

2 Remove the bedspread and blanket. Fold them and place on the chair.

3 Place the bath blanket over the top sheet. Remove the sheet without exposing the resident. Place the soiled sheet in the hamper, or dispose of it according to facility policy.

4 Help the resident to turn on the side away from you.

5 Loosen bottom linens.

6 Roll the soiled draw sheet and rubber sheet, and tuck along resident's back.

7 Place the clean sheet on the bed with the center fold at the center of the bed.

(continues)

33 *continued*

8 Unfold one-half of the sheet.

9 Place the bottom hem of the sheet even with the edge of the mattress, or fit the corner of the fitted sheet.

10 Tuck the top of the sheet under half of the head end of the mattress.

11 Miter the corner.

12 Tuck the sheet under the side of the entire mattress, working from the head to the foot of the bed.

13 Roll the remaining half sheet and tuck it under the soiled sheet.

14 Place the rubber draw sheet in the middle of the bed. Tuck in at the side.

15 Place a clean linen draw sheet over the rubber draw sheet. Tuck in at the side. If a bed protector is used, place it on top of the draw sheet and roll it inside the draw sheet.

16 Roll the remaining halves of draw sheets and tuck them along the resident's back under the soiled sheets.

17 Help the resident roll over the linen pile on his side facing you.

18 Raise the side rail.

19 Go to the other side of the bed.

20 Lower the side rail.

21 Loosen and remove soiled linens from under the mattress.

22 Raise the side rail if leaving the bedside.

23 Dispose of soiled linens according to facility policy. *Do not put soiled linen on the floor. Hold soiled linen away from your uniform.*

24 Remove gloves and dispose according to facility policy.

25 Wash your hands.

26 Return to the bedside and lower the side rail.

27 Pull the clean bottom sheet over the mattress.

28 Tuck the bottom sheet tightly under the head of the mattress.

29 Miter the corner of the sheet at the head of the bed or fit the corner of the fitted sheet.

30 Pull the bottom sheet tight and tuck under the side of the mattress, working from head to foot.

31 Pull the rubber sheet tight and tuck over the bottom sheet at the side of the mattress.

32 Pull the draw sheet tight and tuck over the rubber sheet at the side of the mattress. If a bed protector is used, smooth and straighten it.

33 Help the resident to roll on his back. Cover the resident with the bath blanket.

34 Place the clean sheet over the bath blanket, centering the center fold of the sheet.

35 Pull the bath blanket from under the clean sheet.

36 Place the blanket and bedspread over the sheet.

37 Fold the top sheet over the edge of the blanket. Spread to make a cuff with the sheet.

38 Tuck the top linens under the foot of the mattress, allowing room for the resident's toes. Follow the care plan instructions for special devices, such as bed cradles and footboards.

39 Miter the corner of top linens at the foot of the bed.

40 Raise the side rail.

41 Go to the other side of the bed.

42 Lower the side rail.

43 Miter the corner of the top linens at the foot of the bed.

44 Remove the pillow and soiled pillowcase.

45 Place a clean pillowcase on the pillow.

46 Perform your procedure completion actions.

KEY POINTS IN THIS CHAPTER

▲ The skin of the elderly is more fragile, tears and breaks readily, and is much more easily damaged compared with younger adults.

▲ The skin in the elderly produces less oil, which causes dry, flaky skin.

▲ Pressure ulcers are breaks in the skin caused by unrelieved pressure.

▲ Changing the resident's position is often the best prevention for pressure ulcers.

▲ Encourage residents to do as much of their personal care as possible.

▲ Allow the resident choices over routines and procedures.

▲ An important responsibility of the nursing assistant is observing and reporting any redness or other signs of skin irritation.

▲ The resident's self-esteem can be increased by appropriate clothing and attractive grooming.

▲ Anti-embolism stockings, which must be applied when the resident is lying down, must fit very well and smoothly to be effective.

REVIEW QUIZ

1. Which organ of the body provides it with a protective covering?
   a. skin
   b. hair
   c. nails
   d. heart

2. Age-related changes in the skin include:
   a. dry skin.
   b. thick nails.
   c. less oil.
   d. all of the above.

3. Which of the following are goals of skin care?
   a. removal of bacteria on the skin
   b. removal of perspiration and other body discharges
   c. stimulating blood circulation
   d. all of the above

4. Another term for pressure ulcers is:
   a. mucous membranes.
   b. decubiti.
   c. cyanosis.
   d. edema.

5. Which of the following help prevent pressure ulcers?
   a. changing the resident's position every shift
   b. giving adequate amounts of food and fluids
   c. using alcohol to toughen the resident's skin
   d. all of the above

6. A sign of a pressure ulcer developing is:
   a. an area of redness on the skin.
   b. foul-smelling breath.
   c. change in bowel habits.
   d. pain in the chest.

7. What is included in oral hygiene?
   a. a complete bed bath and linen change
   b. cleaning of the mouth, teeth, and gums
   c. helping the resident ambulate
   d. all of the above

8. Which of the following is true about dentures?
   a. Dentures should be cleaned while in the resident's mouth.
   b. Dentures should be removed when eating.
   c. Dentures are expensive and can break if dropped.
   d. Only the nurse should handle the resident's dentures.

9. You are assigned to care for Mrs. White. She cannot walk, spends most of her day in the wheelchair, and is able to use her hands and arms well. What is the best way for you to help her brush her teeth?
   a. Brush her teeth for her while she is in bed.
   b. Brush her teeth for her when she is up in the wheelchair.
   c. Get the nurse to help her brush her teeth.
   d. Help her brush her own teeth by taking her in the bathroom and getting the supplies she needs.

10. Which of the following should be done when giving a partial bath to Mrs. White?
    a. Take her to the shower room to give the partial bath.
    b. Let her do as much of the bath as possible.
    c. Wash Mrs. White's hands and feet as part of the procedure.
    d. All of the above.

11. What is perineal care?
    a. cleaning the genital area
    b. washing the resident's hair
    c. cleaning the tub and bathroom
    d. cleaning the fingernails and toenails
12. Anti-embolism stockings should be put on the resident:
    a. after the resident has been walking about.
    b. so the stockings fit loosely.
    c. when the resident is lying down.
    d. only at night when the feet are elevated.
13. When is an occupied bed made?
    a. whenever the resident is in the room
    b. when the resident is on bed rest
    c. when all the linens are changed
    d. when the resident has a complete bath
14. A prosthesis is:
    a. a part of your body.
    b. the medical term for a disease.
    c. an artificial body part.
    d. none of the above.
15. When giving perineal care to a female resident, you should:
    a. wash from back to front.
    b. wash from front to back.
    c. wash back and forth vigorously.
    d. not use soap.
16. When giving perineal care to a male, you should:
    a. wash the scrotum and anus only.
    b. wash from the anus toward the penis.
    c. wash from the penis to the anus.
    d. wash the scrotum and penis only.
17. You are assigned to care for Mr. Caldwell, a 71-year-old alert resident with Parkinson's disease. Mr. Caldwell's hands shake because of his illness. Mr. Caldwell is able to wash his face and upper body. You finish the rest of his bath. It is time to shave the resident. He uses a safety razor and shaving cream. When Mr. Caldwell begins to shave his cheek, his hand is shaking badly. He seems embarrassed. You should:
    a. leave the room so that the resident is not embarrassed.
    b. ask Mr. Caldwell if he would like you to shave him.
    c. take the razor from Mr. Caldwell so he does not cut himself.
    d. tell the resident that he does not have to shave today.
18. Mrs. Beverlin is a 57-year-old comatose resident. She is fed by tube because she cannot eat. You are assigned to do special oral hygiene for this resident. You should:
    a. turn the resident's head to the side when doing mouth care.
    b. explain what you are going to do even though you are not sure if the resident can hear you.
    c. observe the resident's mouth for signs of irritation.
    d. all of the above.
19. Mrs. Sinski is an 84-year-old resident being treated for pressure ulcers on her hips. The nurse tells you in report that Mrs. Sinski is at high risk for further skin breakdown, so you must give her good skin care. You should:
    a. turn Mrs. Sinski at least every two hours.
    b. bathe Mrs. Sinski with a large amount of soap to be sure she is clean.
    c. massage her arms and legs well.
    d. all of the above.
20. Mrs. Hyde is a 71-year-old alert resident who is on complete bed rest. You are assigned to give her a bed bath and oral hygiene. Mrs. Hyde wears dentures. She insists on removing them from her mouth herself. When she hands them to you, her hand bumps the overbed table and the dentures fall to the floor, breaking in half. Mrs. Hyde begins yelling that you are careless and that you broke her dentures. You should:
    a. hide the dentures and tell everyone that the resident is confused.
    b. explain what happened to your supervisor.
    c. glue the dentures together.
    d. tell the resident it was her fault.

CHAPTER 10
CROSSWORD PUZZLE

Directions: Complete the puzzle using these words found in Chapter 10.

abrasion	dentures	perineal
anus	embolism	pressure
axilla	genital	prosthesis
decubitus	incontinent	ulcer

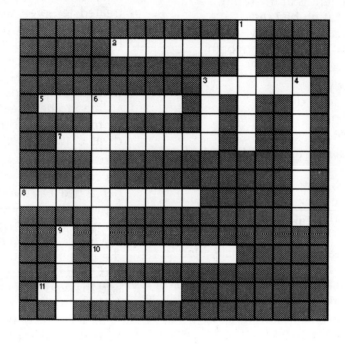

CHAPTER 10
PUZZLE CLUES

ACROSS

2. Bedsores are the direct result of _____.
3. The armpit
5. Cleansing the genital area is called _____ care.
7. A pressure sore or pressure ulcer may also be called a _____ ulcer.
8. An artificial body part is a _____.
10. Elastic stockings that improve circulation are called anti-_____ stockings.
11. Artificial teeth

DOWN

1. The area that includes the external sex organs and anus
3. The outlet for the rectum
4. A rubbing away or scraping of the skin
6. Unable to control the discharge of urine or stool
9. Pressure sore or pressure _____

11

Nutrition and Fluid Needs

OBJECTIVES

In this chapter, you will learn the importance of your role in helping the resident with good nutrition and hydration. After reading this chapter, you will be able to:

- Spell and define key terms.
- Describe proper nutrition.
- Identify factors affecting the resident's nutrition.
- Describe special diets and alternative nutrition.
- Describe the importance of fluid balance.
- Demonstrate how to help with meals and feed a resident.
- Identify alternative means of meeting residents' nutritional needs.
- Record intake and output.

KEY TERMS

aspiration: breathing liquid or food into the air passages

constipation: difficult or infrequent bowel movements.

cubic centimeter (cc): a metric unit of measurement; 30 cc equals one ounce

dehydration: a condition in which the body has less than the normal amount of fluid

digestion: the process by which food is broken down in the body and changed into usable forms

emesis: vomiting or what is vomited

enteral feeding: feeding liquid nutrients through a tube; this procedure is done by the nurse

essential nutrients: substances in food that are necessary for a well-balanced diet and good nutrition

food pyramid: a guide to proper nutrition that helps you select the foods you need to eat a well-balanced diet

force fluids: an order to encourage the resident to drink as much fluid as possible

gastrostomy (G) tube: a feeding tube that is surgically placed in the stomach to feed the resident a liquid formula diet

graduate: a pitcher used to measure liquids

infusion site: the location at which the intravenous needle or cannula is inserted

intake and output (I & O): the recording of the amount of fluid taken and fluid eliminated by a person

intravenous feeding: a liquid feeding given directly into a vein

lethargic: abnormal sleepiness or drowsiness

milliliter (mL): a metric unit of measurement; 30 mL equals one ounce

nasogastric (NG) tube: a method of feeding liquid nutrition to a resident in which a tube is passed through the nose into the stomach

nutrients: chemical substances necessary for life found in food

ounce: a unit of measurement equal to 30 cc or 30 mL

restrict fluids: an order to restrict the resident's fluid intake to a specific amount each shift because of a medical condition

therapeutic diet: a special or modified diet designed to meet the resident's medical needs.

PROPER NUTRITION

Proper nutrition is important for everyone. An adequate intake of proper foods and fluids is necessary to live and grow. The **nutrients** in foods provide the elements we need for growth, energy, and repair of tissues. Nutrients essential for good nutrition include:

- proteins.
- carbohydrates.
- fats.
- water.
- vitamins.
- minerals.

Proper nutrition is when you take in an adequate amount of these nutrients. The **food pyramid** serves as a guide to proper nutrition (Figure 11-1).

The Food Pyramid

A balanced diet contains the **essential nutrients.** Eating the right number of servings from each food group is a balanced diet. The following sections contain a listing of the food groups, number of servings per day, and why these nutrients are necessary. The amount of each serving is listed. People with lower calorie needs should select the lower number of servings from each group. People with higher calorie needs should select the higher number of servings. If you eat more than the amount listed, it counts as more than one serving. For example, a piece of bread is one serving. If you eat a sandwich, this counts as two servings of bread. For mixed foods, estimate the food groups of the main ingredients. For example, beef stew would count in both the meat and vegetable group. Sausage pizza would count in the bread group (crust), meat group (sausage), milk group (cheese), and vegetable group (tomato sauce).

- Bread, cereal, rice, and pasta group

  — Six to eleven servings per day are needed.

  — Foods from this group are needed for energy, cell development, and to fight infection.

  — One serving is the same as one slice of bread, three crackers, one-half cup cooked pasta or rice, one ounce of ready to eat cereal, or one pancake.

- Vegetable group

  — Three to five servings a day are needed.

  — Foods from this group are needed for energy, healthy tissues, bones, and teeth.

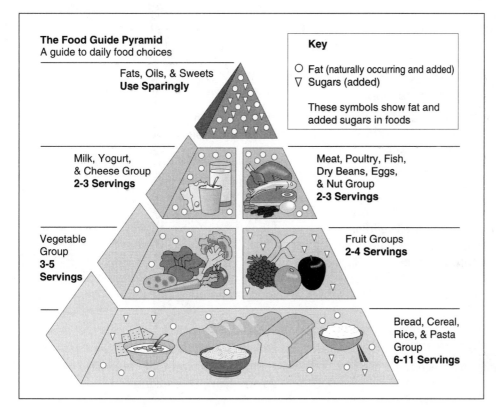

The Food Guide Pyramid
A guide to daily food choices

Fats, Oils, & Sweets
Use Sparingly

Key

○ Fat (naturally occurring and added)
▽ Sugars (added)

These symbols show fat and added sugars in foods

Milk, Yogurt, & Cheese Group
2-3 Servings

Meat, Poultry, Fish, Dry Beans, Eggs, & Nut Group
2-3 Servings

Vegetable Group
3-5 Servings

Fruit Groups
2-4 Servings

Bread, Cereal, Rice, & Pasta Group
6-11 Servings

Figure 11-1 The USDA food guide pyramid serves as a guide for menu planning. (Courtesy of the U.S. Department of Agriculture.)

— One serving is equal to one-half cup chopped raw or cooked vegetables; one cup raw, leafy vegetables; or three-quarters cup vegetable juice.

- Fruit group

  — Two to four servings a day are needed.

  — Foods from this group are needed for energy, healthy tissues, bones, and teeth.

  — One serving is equal to one piece of fruit or melon wedge; three-quarters cup fruit juice; one-half cup cooked or canned fruit; or one-quarter cup dried fruit.

- Milk, yogurt, and cheese group

  — Two to three servings a day are needed.

  — Foods from this group are needed for healthy bones and teeth.

  — One serving is equal to one cup milk or yogurt; one and one-half ounces of natural cheese; or two ounces processed cheese.

- Meat, poultry, fish, dry beans, eggs, and nuts group

  — Two to three servings a day are needed.

  — Foods from this group are needed for growth, and to build and repair body tissues.

  — One serving is equal to two and one-half to three ounces cooked lean beef, pork, poultry, or fish; one-half cup cooked beans; one egg; two tablespoons peanut butter; or one-third cup nuts.

- Fats and sweets

  — Use foods containing fats or sugar sparingly.

  — Fats and sweets come mostly from animal fats, oils, and sugars, but can be part of or added to foods from other food groups as well.

Water

Water is necessary to life. A person can live only a few days without water. Water is necessary for all cellular functions in the body. An adequate intake of fluids is required to replace fluids lost through urine, stool, sweat, and evaporation through skin. The normal adult intake of fluids should be two to three quarts a day.

Offering liquids to the resident frequently is extremely important for the following reasons:

- Many residents are not able to drink liquids without your help.

- The sense of thirst is less in the elderly.
- An adequate fluid intake is necessary to prevent urinary problems and constipation.

Vitamins and Minerals

A person must have enough vitamins and minerals to stay healthy. Therefore, a regular diet should provide the necessary vitamins and minerals for a healthy adult. A balanced diet contains all of the vitamins and minerals needed to stay healthy. Some elderly and ill people also take vitamin pills to give them extra nutrients. Signs of good nutrition include:

- shiny hair.
- bright, clear eyes.
- alert mind.
- healthy sleep patterns.
- good appetite.
- normal elimination.
- healthy skin, nails, and teeth.

FACTORS THAT AFFECT RESIDENT NUTRITION

Nutritional needs of the older person are the same as the younger adult. However, meeting these needs can be more difficult for the elderly person. Often the resident in the long-term care facility depends on your help to receive proper nutrition. Know these considerations for nutritional care:

- General factors

  — fatigue level

  — level of alertness

  — absence or presence of disease

  — medical conditions affecting the appetite.

  — some medications affect the appetite

- Sensory loss

  — Sensory loss can mean decreased taste, smell, and vision. Meals may need to be enhanced with proper seasonings unless this is against the diet ordered by the resident's physician.

  — Sight, smell, taste, and even the sound of food preparation affect appetite.

- Physical comfort

  — Assure the resident's comfort.

  — Position the resident properly to prevent **aspiration,** or choking, on food.

— Position residents so they can reach their food.

- Dentures
  — Improperly fitting dentures impair the resident's ability to enjoy mealtime.
  — Be sure the resident has dentures properly in place at mealtime.

- Ability to chew and swallow
  — Residents who cannot chew or swallow require special diets or procedures such as pureed foods or tube feeding.
  — Residents who cannot swallow easily have a hard time eating.

- Cultural influences. Culture may affect the resident's nutrition. The following are some common cultural influences that affect the food choices of the resident:
  — religion
  — national culture
  — family customs
  — economic background
  — personal tastes

- Emotional factors. These common emotional states can affect the resident's eating habits:
  — loneliness
  — depression
  — anger, frustration
  — eating disorders

- Environmental factors. The environment in which food is served can affect nutrition:
  — Mealtime is a source of social contact.
  — All staff members can make mealtime pleasant.
  — Pleasant table companions and conversation at mealtime are important.
  — Too much noise in the dining room can be a problem. Avoid shouting and clanging dishes.
  — Eliminate unpleasant odors, sights, and smells; these can cause the resident to lose her appetite quickly.
  — The food served should be attractive and appetizing in appearance.
  — Food served should be the correct temperature. Hot foods should be served hot and cold foods served cold.

SPECIAL DIETS

Most residents will be on a general or regular diet. The dietitian in the long-term care facility plans meals for the residents. The dietitian makes menu changes for residents on special diets. Knowledge of various special and **therapeutic diets** will help you understand their effect on the disease process and know if the resident is allowed to have certain food items.

Common Therapeutic Diets

Clear Liquids. The clear liquid diet is used for persons who have stomach or intestinal distress or as first foods after surgery.

- Clear liquids include tea, broth, gelatin, some fruit juices, and some soft drinks (Figure 11–2).
- This diet is not generally used for residents with swallowing problems.
- This diet is usually only served for short periods because it does not contain adequate nutrients.

Full Liquid. The full liquid diet is given to residents who have digestive disorders.

- Full liquid is clear liquid plus milk, custards and puddings, cream soups, ice cream and sherbet.
- This diet is usually only served for short periods because it does not contain adequate nutrients.

Puree or Mechanical Soft. This diet is used for residents who cannot chew well or those who have missing teeth.

Figure 11-2 Items found on a clear liquid tray.

- The diet is used for residents who have difficulty chewing or swallowing solid foods.
- The diet is the same as a regular diet, but the food has been ground in a blender or chopped finely. The foods should be prepared so that a plastic spoon stands straight up in them. They should not be watery.

Diabetic, No Concentrated Sweets, or Calorie-Controlled Diet. These diets are ordered for residents who have diabetes or who must lose weight.

- No sugar is included on the tray.
- No foods with high sugar content:

  — honey
  — syrup
  — regular soft drinks
  — jelly, jams
  — candy

- Residents may have sugar-free substitutes, if indicated on the diet plan.
- Snacks are very important for residents on this diet. If snacks are ordered, they are part of the calorie count upon which the resident's medication is based.

Low Sodium (Low Salt). Low sodium diet is ordered for persons with high blood pressure, heart, or kidney disease.

- No salt is included on the tray.
- Foods that are high in salt are limited (Figure 11-3):

  — bacon
  — ham
  — luncheon meats
  — canned meats and fish
  — some cheeses and soups
  — some soft drinks
  — many common snack food items
  — pickles and olives

Pureed Diets. Pureed diets have been mechanically altered so they are the consistency of baby food. These diets contain the same foods as the diets listed, but they have been blended so they are easy to swallow. They are given to people who have problems chewing and swallowing regular foods. If a pureed food is the correct consistency, a plastic spoon will stand up in it. If the food will not support the spoon, it may be too watery to feed the resident.

Figure 11-3
Foods that are high in sodium.

FLUID BALANCE

Proper fluid balance occurs when the loss of body fluids is about the same as fluid taken in. The nursing assistant has an important role in helping the resident maintain proper fluid balance.

Reasons for Proper Fluid Balance

Water makes up more than one-half of body weight. Maintaining the proper fluid balance is important because it:

- helps proper blood flow.
- helps food **digestion.**
- improves removal of body waste.
- protects cells by keeping:

  — skin moist.
  — mouth and throat moist.
  — eyeballs moist.

- regulates body temperature.

Dehydration

Dehydration occurs when there is not enough fluid in the body. This condition may cause serious harm to vital body organs. Death occurs when loss of body fluid is severe.

Signs of Dehydration. Be aware of these signs of dehydration:

- Mouth becomes dry. The resident may have trouble swallowing.
- Tongue becomes thick and coated.
- Skin becomes dry, itches, or cracks. It may tear easily and show evidence of "tenting" when it is

pinched lightly. If the tent does not go away immediately, this should be reported to the nurse.

- Urine output decreases.
- Urine is darker and cloudy, and may have a strong odor.
- The resident may be tired or **lethargic.**
- Confusion and mental impairment may develop.
- The resident may show signs of **constipation.**

Edema

Edema may occur as the result of poor circulation, heart, or kidney disease. *Edema* is swelling or the retention of fluid in the tissues. The nursing assistant must be alert for signs of edema in the resident. Indications of edema are:

- swelling or puffiness, usually in feet, ankles, hands, eyes, face, and abdomen.
- difficulty breathing, such as:
  — congestion or cough.
  — wheezing when breathing.
- the resident gains weight quickly.
- urine output decreases.

Providing Adequate Hydration

Assist residents to take enough fluids in the following ways:

- Refer to the care plan. Know which fluids are restricted or encouraged. Some may be given between meals.
- Offer fluids every time you are in the room. Give the resident fluids that she likes, if allowed on her diet.
- Fluids are especially important in hot weather or when the resident has a fever.
- Help the resident drink properly. Hold the glass and straw if necessary.
- Encourage the resident to help herself. Use hand-over-hand technique or adaptive cups.
- Be sure that the resident always has fresh drinking water available in the room.
- Record all fluid intake and output accurately when ordered.

Special Situations

Sometimes the physician writes special fluid orders because of the resident's disease or condition. Special fluid orders are noted on the care plan. **Force fluids** is ordered for residents who do not take in an adequate amount of fluid each day. The title "force fluids" is deceiving. You do not really force the resident to drink. Rather, you must encourage the resident to drink as much as possible. Sometimes it helps to offer the resident many beverages. If you offer fluids frequently in small cups, the resident may drink more than if you give her a large glass and instruct her to drink it all. Getting to know the resident's patterns, likes, and dislikes is important. Give her fluids that she likes in quantities that she will drink. It may be necessary for you to stay in the room while the resident drinks the liquids. Residents who have orders to force fluids are often on intake and output. This means their fluid intake is measured to be certain that they drink enough.

An order to **restrict fluids** is sometimes written for residents with heart or kidney disease. Orders to restrict fluids are highly individualized. Instructions for the amount of fluids that the resident is allowed are written on the care plan. Often this amount is restricted to what is on the meal trays, with some additional liquids for the nurses to give medications. Residents who have orders to restrict fluids are usually on intake and output so that their fluid intake can be measured. They often have orders for frequent weights. If they gain weight rapidly, this may be because they have consumed too much liquid. If you observe a resident with a fluid restriction order drinking extra liquids, notify your charge nurse.

HELPING WITH MEALS

You will be responsible for helping the residents eat. This may include spoon-feeding some residents. You have already learned many factors that affect residents' overall nutrition. Making mealtime pleasant and enjoyable should be your goal. Encourage proper nutrition by helping residents as follows:

- Pleasant environment
  — Most residents eat their meals in the dining room.
  — If the resident stays in her room, be sure the room is clean and neat. Remove objectionable items such as commodes, bedpans, and urinals.

- Social concerns
  — Ask residents where and with whom they wish to eat, if consistent with the care plan.
  — If facility policy permits, encourage the resident's family to occasionally eat a meal with the resident.

— Realize that the resident may feel resentment or be embarrassed if she is unable to feed herself.

— Remember that eating is a social occasion. Residents usually eat better in a group than they do when they are alone.

— If the resident must have her clothing protected because of spills, do not call the clothing protector a "bib." Some elderly residents feel that this is degrading and childlike. Call this garment an "adult clothing protector" or "apron."

• Resident comfort

— Be sure the resident is clean and has recently toileted.

— Dress the resident in comfortable clothing.

— Be sure the resident is wearing dentures, eyeglasses, and hearing aid at mealtime.

• Proper positioning

— Be sure the resident is not too low to reach the table, or too far away because of the arms of a wheelchair.

— It is the policy in many facilities to seat residents in regular dining room chairs instead of wheelchairs at mealtime.

• Adaptive equipment (Figure 11-4)

— plate guards

— adaptive silverware

— special cups or glasses

• Serving trays

— Be sure that the resident receives the right tray.

— Visually check the items on the tray to be sure that they are allowed on the resident's diet. Ask if you are unsure.

Figure 11-4 Adaptive devices that enable residents to eat and drink independently.

— Be sure food is served at the proper temperature. Hot foods should be served hot and cold foods cold.

— Notice and report the resident's likes, dislikes, and techniques that do and do not help the resident meet nutritional needs.

— Offer substitutes if the resident does not eat. A substitute should always be available for the meat and vegetable. Follow your facility policy.

— Accurately record how much the resident eats, if this is the policy of your facility. Report any changes in appetite to your charge nurse.

— Record fluid intake if the resident is on intake and output.

— Be aware that residents with some medical conditions, such as a stroke, may not have a full field of vision. If the resident does not eat the food on a certain area of the tray, turn the tray around so the food is on the opposite side.

Feeding Techniques

Proper Positioning. Various feeding techniques encourage optimal nutrition in residents. Position is important to prevent aspiration and choking.

• The resident's head should be elevated as much as possible.

• Feeding the resident with the head in a flat position creates a risk of choking. If the resident's head cannot be elevated, position the resident on her side.

Prepare the Food. Cut food, open cartons, and assist in other ways according to the resident's needs. In addition:

• Season food if the resident wishes.

• Tell the resident which items are hot.

• Use a clock description for the resident with a visual impairment. For example, the meat is on the plate at the six o'clock location.

• Remind and encourage residents to eat. Assist if they are unable to feed themselves.

Encourage Self-Care.

• Let the resident feed herself foods that can be handled easily.

• If the resident eats slowly, reheating some food may be necessary. When the resident is eating independently, do not feed her even though she is slow. Assist only when she is unable to feed herself.

- Use adaptive equipment to enable the resident to be independent.

Feeding Residents.
- Check the temperature of foods before feeding.
- Explain what foods are on the tray. Ask the resident what she would like to eat first.
- Do not mix foods together when feeding.
- Feed residents who are unable to feed themselves. Check the care plan goals.

Many residents who must be spoon-fed are encouraged to eat their own finger foods, such as bread.

- Check the temperature of a hot food by placing a drop on your wrist. If it feels too hot, wait a few minutes before feeding (Figure 11-5).
- Use hand-over-hand technique to help residents feed themselves.
- Offer liquids at intervals.
- Use a straw or spouted cup for liquids.
- Make pleasant conversation, but do not ask the resident questions that take a long time to answer.
- Never rush the resident.

- Sitting next to the resident conveys a relaxed feeling and is less intimidating than standing over the resident to feed her.
- Sit at or below eye level to prevent the resident from bending her head backward, which may cause choking.

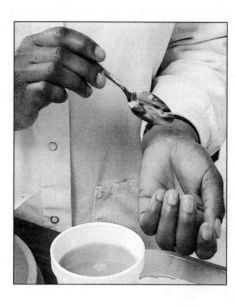

Figure 11-5
Test hot foods by placing a drop on your wrist.

PERFORMANCE PROCEDURE

34   Feeding the Resident

Supplies needed:
- adult clothing protector
- napkin or towel
- adaptive equipment as needed

1 Perform your beginning procedure actions.
2 Check the name on the tray and the diet served.
3 Check the meal tray for silverware and spilled foods.
4 Place the tray on the table. Remove food covers.
5 Sit near the resident.
6 Explain what is on the tray.
7 Ask the resident what foods she would like to eat first.

8 Encourage the resident to feed herself, if able, by using finger foods or adaptive equipment.
9 Use hand-over-hand technique to help the resident feed herself, if consistent with the care plan.
10 Fill the fork or spoon only half full or less, according to the resident's ability to swallow.
11 Use a straw for liquids.
12 Encourage the resident to eat. Talk pleasantly. Do not rush.
13 Wipe the resident's mouth.
14 Offer liquids between bites of solid food.
15 Remove the tray when the resident is finished.
16 Wash the resident's hands, if necessary.
17 Perform your procedure completion actions.

TUBE FEEDING

Some residents are unable to eat solid food and are fed in different ways. The nursing assistant does not usually give these types of feedings, but an understanding of the techniques will help you care for the resident.

A feeding tube may be used for residents who have difficulty swallowing. Tube feeding may also be called **enteral feeding.** Some tubes are inserted through the nose and threaded through the throat and into the stomach. This type of tube is called a **nasogastric (NG) tube.** Most residents who receive tube feedings in the long-term care facility have permanent tubes surgically placed into the stomach. The most common type of permanent feeding tube is called a **gastrostomy (G) tube.** The resident is fed a liquid formula through the tube. The head of the bed should always be elevated when the tube feeding is running (Figure 11-6). The head should remain elevated for a specified period after the feeding stops. The care plan gives specific instructions. Residents who are tube-fed require frequent mouth care. Check your facility policy and the care plan for the type of solution to use and how often mouth care should be done.

When residents have feeding tubes in place, be very careful not to pull or tug on the tubing. Serious complications can occur if the tube becomes dislodged.

Safety Precautions

When caring for a resident who has a feeding tube, be sure to:

Figure 11-6 Always keep the head of the bed elevated during and after tube feeding.

- keep the skin around the tube clean.
- keep the head of the bed elevated.

Oral Hygiene

Residents with feeding tubes need frequent mouth care.

Nasogastric Tube

Follow these guidelines for residents with a nasogastric tube:

- Clean the nose around the tube.
- The tube is usually taped at the nose.
- The end of the tubing is pinned to the resident's clothing to prevent pulling.

Gastrostomy Tube

Follow these guidelines for residents using a gastrostomy tube:

- Clean the skin around the tube if it is open to the air.
- The nurse may place clean gauze around the wound opening. Do not remove gauze dressings.

Reporting

Report to the nurse immediately if the:

- alarm used to monitor the feeding solution sounds.
- tube becomes dislodged.
- resident begins to cough, choke, or vomit.
- feeding solution is not flowing properly.
- level of the formula in the bag is low or empty.
- feeding is leaking around the gastrostomy tube.
- skin appears irritated where the tube contacts the skin.
- resident has loose stools.

INTRAVENOUS FEEDINGS

Intravenous feedings, or IVs, are sometimes used to add to the resident's nutrition (Figure 11-7). Sometimes residents who receive intravenous feedings also receive a meal tray. Some residents receive only the intravenous solution. Check with the care plan and your charge nurse for instructions regarding a meal tray. The intravenous line can be placed in the veins of the arms or legs. Sometimes the intravenous line is in the neck or chest. When caring for the resident, be very careful not to dislodge the tubing. If you notice that the solution in the intravenous bag or bottle is running low, inform the nurse.

Figure 11-7 An intravenous infusion.

Safety Precautions

When caring for a resident who has an intravenous line, observe these precautions:

- Make sure the intravenous solution is flowing.
- Handle the **infusion site** carefully.
- Do not adjust the clamps on the tubing.
- Be careful when changing the resident's gown.

Reporting

Report to the nurse immediately if:

- the alarm used to monitor the intravenous solution sounds.
- there is swelling, redness, pain, or bleeding at the site of needle insertion.
- fluid is not dripping.
- the level of the fluid in the bag is low or empty.
- the needle or tubing becomes dislodged.
- there is blood in the tubing.

INTAKE AND OUTPUT

Intake and output is a procedure in which all liquids taken in by the resident and all liquids put out by the resident are recorded. This procedure is done to monitor the resident's fluid balance. Recording

---

PERFORMANCE PROCEDURE

35   Recording Intake and Output

Supplies needed:
- paper towel
- graduate pitcher
- disinfectant used by facility
- pen and paper or I & O worksheet
- disposable exam gloves

1 Perform your beginning procedure actions.

2 Check to identify equivalents used in your facility.

3 Identify foods considered to be liquid as taken by the resident.

4 Estimate liquid food taken.

5 Record how much liquid is taken by the resident in cubic centimeters.

6 Record amounts under the *intake* column.

7 Apply the principles of standard precautions when measuring output.

8 Measure output by pouring the contents of the bedpan, urinal, or emesis basin into the graduate. Remove one glove. Flush contents down the toilet after they are measured by holding graduate with gloved hand and pushing flush lever on toilet with ungloved hand.

9 Rinse and disinfect the graduate and bedpan, urinal, or emesis basin according to facility policy.

10 Perform your procedure completion actions.

intake and output is the nursing assistant's responsibility. Intake and output is abbreviated in most facilities as **I & O.** Note the following considerations for caring for a resident on I & O:

- Explain the procedure to the resident. Request the resident's cooperation if he is able.

- Record the information accurately.

- I & O worksheets are often kept at the bedside (Figure 11-8).

- Know your facility policy on I & O. Usually amounts taken by the resident are totaled at the end of shift and recorded on the medical record.

Recording Intake

- Remember that I & O includes *all liquid* that the resident takes in, including fluid consumed in the dining room and during activities.

- Foods that are liquid at room temperature are recorded on the I & O sheets. For example, ice cream and Jell-O® are recorded.

- Fluids from any source are recorded. The nurse records intravenous and tube feedings.

- Record amounts under the intake column in **cubic centimeters (cc)** or in **milliliters (mL)** according to facility policy.

- Some measurements to know are:

  — 1 **ounce** equals 30 cc (or mL).

  — 1 cup (8 oz.) equals 240 cc (or mL).

  — 1 teaspoon equals 5 cc (or mL).

- When measuring intake, remember that the measurements given are usually for containers filled to the top. Since most glasses and cups are not filled completely full, you should adjust how much fluid you record.

- The nursing assistant must learn the equivalents used in the facility. Most facilities provide conversion tables for recording intake.

- Record only the amount actually taken by the resident. For example, do not record a full glass of water if the resident drinks only half of the glass.

Recording Output

- Output includes all fluids lost from the body:

  — urine

  — blood or drainage

  — **emesis** (vomiting)

  — diarrhea

  — sweat

INTAKE – OUTPUT WORKSHEET

*INTAKE EQUIVALENTS

Medicine Cup – 30 cc	Soup Bowl – 8 oz./240 cc
Water Pitcher – 800 cc/1,000 cc	Ice Cream – 3 oz./90 cc
Water Glass – 8 oz. – 240 cc	Carton Milk – 8 oz./240 cc
Styrofoam Cup (hot) – 6 oz./180 cc	
Juice Glass – 4 oz./120 cc	*Chart in CC's

TIME	INTAKE	OUTPUT	
	NOC	URINE	Emesis
0200	150cc	300 cc	
0600	200cc	300 cc	BM
			Drainage
	AM	URINE	Emesis
0730	525cc		
0900		350 cc	
1000	100 cc		BM
1100		200 cc	
			Drainage
	PM	URINE	Emesis
			BM
			Drainage

*These are guidelines only, verify containers used in your facility.

Figure 11-8 An intake and output worksheet.

- Apply the principles of standard precautions when measuring output.

- Output is measured by pouring urine or other discharge into a **graduate** or measuring pitcher. Record the amount shown on the side of the pitcher.

- If the resident is incontinent, follow facility policy for recording urinary output. In some facilities, wet underpads are weighed on a scale. The weight is compared with the weight of a dry pad and the output is estimated.

- Report any blood or wound drainage to the nurse immediately.
- Report excessive perspiration.

KEY POINTS IN THIS CHAPTER

▲ A balanced diet containing the essential nutrients is necessary for good health.

▲ Many residents in the long-term care facility need some help getting proper nutrition.

▲ Many residents are on special diets. Make sure the resident receives the right tray at mealtime.

▲ Fluid balance occurs when fluid intake and fluid output are about equal.

▲ Dehydration occurs when there is not enough fluid in the body.

▲ Making mealtime as pleasant as possible is important.

▲ Residents should feed themselves whenever possible.

▲ Be alert to safety when caring for residents who have feeding tubes.

▲ The head of the bed should always be elevated when the resident is receiving a tube feeding.

▲ When the resident is on I & O, all liquids taken in are recorded. Also, all liquid output must be measured and recorded.

REVIEW QUIZ

1. What is the purpose of the food pyramid?
   a. to provide a guide to eating a well-balanced diet
   b. to list foods that people on special diets should not eat
   c. to provide a plan for eating two meals a day for those who skip breakfast
   d. to provide a plan for those who plan school menus only

2. What is the normal daily fluid intake for an adult?
   a. 1 quart
   b. 1 to 2 quarts
   c. 2 to 3 quarts
   d. more than 3 quarts

3. Which of the following statements is true?
   a. Everyone should take a vitamin pill every day.
   b. Proper nutrition can be obtained by eating proper amounts from the food pyramid.
   c. The elderly should take extra vitamins once a week.
   d. Most foods do not contain vitamins or minerals.

4. Which factors affect the resident's nutrition?
   a. sensory loss
   b. general health
   c. physical comfort
   d. all of the above

5. Which of the following are ways the nursing assistant can help residents at mealtime?
   a. Make sure residents are dressed in comfortable clothing.
   b. Help residents assume a comfortable position for eating.
   c. Remove unpleasant sights and odors from the area.
   d. All of the above.

6. Cultural influences that may affect eating habits are:
   a. religion and family customs.
   b. well-fitting dentures.
   c. the ability to chew or swallow.
   d. all of the above.

7. Making mealtime a pleasant experience is the responsibility of the:
   a. nursing assistant only.
   b. dietary staff only.
   c. housekeeping staff.
   d. entire facility staff.

8. The person responsible for planning meals for residents is the:
   a. nursing assistant.
   b. dietitian.
   c. head nurse.
   d. administrator.

9. Which of the following would *not* be included on a clear liquid diet?
   a. tea
   b. milk
   c. broth
   d. gelatin (Jell-O®)

10. When serving a tray to a resident on a diabetic diet, you should make sure:
    a. there is no salt on the tray.
    b. the resident does not have coffee.
    c. there is no sugar on the tray.
    d. the tray has no fruit or vegetables on it.

11. Some residents must have a low salt diet. A food that is high in salt content is:
    a. ham.
    b. milk.
    c. bread.
    d. fruit.

12. Dehydration occurs when:
    a. there is too much fat in the body.
    b. there is not enough fluid in the body.
    c. one has overeaten.
    d. the body is at rest.

13. When feeding a resident:
    a. turn on your favorite television program.
    b. feed the resident all solids before giving liquids.
    c. give all foods at room temperature.
    d. avoid rushing the resident.

14. A feeding tube may be inserted for residents who:
    a. are on a low-calorie diet.
    b. are on salt-restricted diets.
    c. have problems swallowing.
    d. have dentures that do not fit well.

15. When a resident is on intake and output, you must record:
    a. all the food eaten by the resident.
    b. the liquids the resident drinks.
    c. all liquids served to the resident.
    d. both liquids and solids taken by the resident.

16. You are assigned to work in the dining room. Mrs. Martinez is feeding herself very slowly. Several of the other residents have finished eating, and Mrs. Martinez is still eating. You should:
    a. feed Mrs. Martinez so that she gets done quickly.
    b. ask Mrs. Martinez if she would like any of the food heated again.
    c. leave Mrs. Martinez alone and check on her again later.
    d. remove Mrs. Martinez's tray.

17. Mr. Burns is an 83-year-old resident who has had a stroke and is not able to swallow. He is fed through a nasogastric tube. Mr. Burns's tube feeding is administered by a pump that runs all the time during your shift. When you go to Mr. Burns's room at 10:00, you notice that he is coughing and choking. You should:
    a. ask another nursing assistant what to do.
    b. leave the room and check on Mr. Burns later to see if he is still coughing.
    c. stay with Mr. Burns and call for the nurse immediately.
    d. pull the nasogastric tube out.

18. Mrs. Carroll has an order on her care plan to force fluids. Mrs. Carroll is on a regular diet. You know that she does not like to drink water. In order to be sure that she takes enough liquid on your shift, you should:
    a. ask Mrs. Carroll what kinds of fluids she likes and offer them.
    b. provide fluids that you like.
    c. offer Mrs. Carroll water each time you are in the room.
    d. all of the above.

19. Mrs. Carroll drinks 3 ounces of the beverage that you offer her. You should record her fluid intake as:
    a. 3 cc.
    b. 30 cc.
    c. 60 cc.
    d. 90 cc.

20. At the end of the day shift, Mrs. Carroll has consumed 1,500 cc of liquid. You know that this is:
    a. not enough liquid.
    b. an adequate amount of liquid.
    c. too much liquid.
    d. enough fluid to meet her needs for 24 hours.

CHAPTER 11
CROSSWORD PUZZLE

Directions: Complete the following puzzle using the following words found in Chapter 11.

aspiration	gastrostomy	ounce
centimeter	graduate	output
dehydration	infusion	pyramid
digestion	intake	restrict
edema	intravenous	therapeutic
emesis	milliliter	
force	nutrients	

CHAPTER 11
PUZZLE CLUES

ACROSS

6. "cc" is the abbreviation for cubic _____.
9. _____ and output
10. "mL" is the abbreviation for _____.
12. A special or modified diet used to treat a disease
14. A pitcher used for measuring drainage
15. Abnormal swelling
16. Chemical substances found in food that are necessary for life
17. Process by which food is broken down and changed into nutrients
19. Intake and _____

DOWN

1. The location where the intravenous tubing is inserted is the _____ site.
2. A unit of measurement equal to 30 cc
3. An order to _____ fluids means to encourage the resident to drink.
4. A resident whose doctor has ordered a limited amount of fluids has an order to _____ fluids.
5. Breathing liquid into the air passages
7. A feeding tube that is surgically placed in the stomach
8. The food _____ provides a guide to eating a balanced diet
11. Less than adequate amount of fluid
13. A liquid feeding given into a vein
18. Vomiting or what is vomited

Elimination Needs

OBJECTIVES

In this chapter, you will learn how to help the resident with elimination needs. After reading this chapter, you will be able to:

- Spell and define key terms.
- Describe normal elimination.
- Describe factors that interfere with normal elimination.
- Describe bowel and bladder management guidelines.
- Position a resident on a bedpan.
- Assist a resident with the urinal.
- List observations of elimination that should be reported to the nurse.
- Perform catheter care.
- Empty a catheter bag.
- Describe ostomy care.
- List guidelines for enema administration.

KEY TERMS

bedpan: a container used by bedridden residents to discharge body waste

bladder: a hollow muscle that stores urine until it is eliminated from the body

bowel: the same as intestine; part of the digestive system extending from the stomach to the rectum

catheter: a tube inserted into a body cavity; it is often inserted into the bladder to drain urine

colon: the large bowel or the lower part of the intestine

colostomy: a surgical procedure in which the colon is attached to the outside of the body and waste is eliminated into a plastic bag attached to the skin

commode: a portable toilet

defecate: to have a bowel movement

diarrhea: multiple loose bowel movements

enema: administration of fluid into the rectum; usually done to cleanse the bowel

feces: waste products from the bowel; the same as stool or bowel movement

homeostasis: a constant state of balance within the body

impaction: mass of hard feces that cannot be passed from the rectum normally

incontinence: inability to control the passage of urine or stool

involuntary: done without choice; often refers to inability to control stool passage

kidneys: organs that filter the blood, removing waste products

ostomy: a surgically created opening through the abdominal wall into the intestines; body waste passes through this opening

stoma: the opening in the abdomen created by an ostomy

stool: feces or bowel movement

ureters: tubes that connect the kidneys to the urinary bladder

urethra: the body tube through which urine passes from the body

urinal: a container used by males for urination

urinate: to pass urine

void: to pass urine

NORMAL ELIMINATION

Elimination is the body's way of removing waste products and toxic substances through the digestive and genitourinary system. A review of these systems follows.

Genitourinary System

The genitourinary system eliminates waste products from the blood, forms urine, and allows for the discharge of urine. The genitourinary system is very important in maintaining **homeostasis,** or stable body function.

Organs in the Genitourinary System.

- **Kidneys**
  — filter the blood
  — return necessary water and chemicals to the blood after filtering out waste
  — form urine from waste products taken from the blood

- **Bladder**
  — stores urine in a hollow muscle until it is passed out of the body

- **Ureters**
  — tubes that connect the kidneys to the bladder

- **Urethra**
  — tube through which urine passes out of the body

Characteristics of Normal Urine.

- clear or yellow-golden color
- nearly odorless, but smells like ammonia if it stands over time
- free from sediment or mucus
- urge to **urinate** is usually felt when the bladder contains 150–200 cc

Digestive System

In the digestive system, food is chemically broken down so it can be absorbed by the blood as nutrients.

Main Organs of the Digestive System.

- Mouth
  — Food is chewed and mixed with saliva. This causes the food to break down.

- Esophagus
  — the tube connecting the mouth to the stomach

- Stomach
  — a muscular organ where food is churned and mixed with digestive juices

- Intestines
  — large and small tube-like canals that extend from the stomach to the rectum
  — nutrients are absorbed into the blood as food passes through the intestine
  — undigested food passed on as **stool (feces)** into the rectum

- Rectum
  — the last five to six inches of the **colon**
  — feces stored in the rectum until the urge to move the **bowel** is felt
  — feces are eliminated from the anus, or outlet to the rectum

Characteristics of Normal Feces.

- light to dark brown color
- soft and formed
- frequency from daily bowel movement to every three days
- no difficulty in passing normal stool

INTERFERENCE WITH NORMAL ELIMINATION

When caring for the elderly, you must be aware of things that can cause elimination problems.

Aging

- Normal aging slows all body functions, including the digestive and urinary systems.
- Feeling thirsty decreases with age. Many elderly do not take enough liquids to allow for proper elimination.
- Blood flow to the kidneys is decreased. Urine, therefore, is not produced as often.
- Feeling of a full bladder and bowel is reduced. Elderly residents often feel urgency only when actually eliminating.

- Incontinence is not a part of normal aging.

Disease and Disability

- Many residents have chronic illnesses that affect elimination.
- Residents may have nerve damage. The nerve damage causes limited, reduced, or no feelings of urgency.

Inactivity

- The elimination systems rely on the stimulation from muscle movements to function effectively.

Medication

- Many residents take medications that affect the elimination systems. Medications may cause **diarrhea,** constipation, or urinary problems.
- Many elderly persons have a history of taking laxatives. Laxatives affect normal intestinal function.

Improper Diet

- An inadequate fluid intake can cause elimination problems.
- Food should have sufficient bulk or roughage.

Lack of Privacy

- Many persons need privacy to have normal elimination.

Stress

- This emotion may cause diarrhea, constipation, or urinary frequency.

Abnormal Body Position

- Using a **bedpan** is often difficult.
- When the resident remains in bed, urine pools, making voiding difficult. This often leads to urinary tract infections.

Time

- A sufficient amount of time is needed.

BOWEL AND BLADDER MANAGEMENT

Many residents who are incontinent or **involuntary** can relearn to control urine and stool passage. Bowel and bladder training plans take time and attention of the entire nursing staff. A plan to retrain may require scheduling changes and a lot of effort by the nursing assistant (Figure 12-1). Once the process is relearned, however, it will become part of the daily routine and will save you time and energy.

The resident, of course, benefits from any bowel and bladder plan. Control of one's body functions adds to self-esteem, dignity, happiness, and health.

Considerations for Care

- Establish regularity and prevent **incontinence.**
- Set plans according to each resident's pattern. You will collect information about the resident's pattern of elimination. The nurse will use this information to write the toileting plan.
- Explain the procedure to the resident. This helps ensure resident cooperation.
- Refer to the care plan about:
  - fluid intake.
  - recording fluid output.
  - positioning the resident.
  - the schedule of voiding intervals.
- Reporting and recording your observations is very important.
- Treat incontinence in a matter-of-fact manner. Never scold, yell at, or ridicule the resident.

Special Guidelines for Toileting

- Some residents cannot tell you they need to use the toilet. They may become restless or irritable instead.
- Loss of appetite and small, watery rectal discharge may indicate a fecal **impaction.** Report to the nurse immediately.
- Pressure or a full feeling in the lower abdomen may suggest a full bladder or a hard fecal mass. Report to the nurse immediately.
- The urge to eliminate may occur quickly and suddenly. Respond promptly.
- Many residents must void more often at night.

Help with Elimination Needs

Some ways you will help the resident with elimination needs include helping the resident to the bathroom or commode. A **commode** is a portable toilet. You will also be giving the resident the bedpan or **urinal.** These are specially shaped containers designed to help the bedridden resident urinate (**void**) or **defecate.** Other duties you will perform are observing and reporting unusual output, providing catheter care, helping with care for an ostomy, and giving enemas.

INITIAL INCONTINENCE EVALUATION 2 DAY VOIDING PATTERN ASSESSMENT

N615

O O Ø ... incontinent SMALL amount
O Ø O ... incontinent MODERATE amount
Ø O O ... incontinent LARGE amount

● Dry When Checked
(/) Stool Present
(/) Resident Asked to Use Toilet

Day _Wed._   Date _9_ / _1_ / _2000_

AIDE	TIME	INCONTINENT	DRY	STOOL	PATIENT REQUESTED	TOILETED
Ellen Stacey	24 Midnite	Ø O O	●	( )	( )	cc
Ellen Stacey	1 AM	O O O	●	( )	( )	cc
Ellen Stacey	2 AM	O O O	●	( )	( )	cc
Ellen Stacey	3 AM	O O Ø	●	( )	( )	cc
Ellen Stacey	4 AM	O O O	●	( )	( )	cc
Ellen Stacey	5 AM	O O O	●	( )	( )	cc
Ellen Stacey	6 AM	O O O	●	( )	( )	cc
Ellen Stacey	7 AM	O O O		( )	(/)	cc 300
Audrey King	8 AM	O O O	●	( )	( )	cc
Audrey King	9 AM	O O O	●	( )	( )	cc
Audrey King	10 AM	O O Ø	●	( )	( )	cc
Audrey King	11 AM	O O O		( )	(/)	cc 200
Audrey King	12 PM	O O O	●	( )	( )	cc
Audrey King	13 PM	O O O	●	( )	( )	cc
Audrey King	14 PM	O O O	●	( )	( )	cc
Audrey King	15 PM	O Ø O	●	( )	( )	cc
Carlos Ramos	16 PM	O O O	●	( )	( )	cc
Carlos Ramos	17 PM	O O Ø	●	( )	( )	cc
Carlos Ramos	18 PM	O O O	●	( )	( )	cc
Carlos Ramos	19 PM	O O O	●	( )	( )	cc
Carlos Ramos	20 PM	O O O	●	( )	( )	cc
Carlos Ramos	21 PM	O O O	●	( )	(/)	cc 150
Carlos Ramos	22 PM	O O O	●	( )	( )	cc
Carlos Ramos	23 PM	O O O	●	( )	( )	cc
TOTALS						

RESIDENT NAME _Martin, Frank_   ROOM NO. _409_

Figure 12-1 Accurate recordkeeping is an important nursing assistant responsibility in a bowel and bladder management program. The nurse uses this information to develop a toileting schedule for the resident.

PERFORMANCE PROCEDURE

36   Giving a Bedpan

Supplies needed:
- bedpan
- bedpan cover or disposable bed protector for cover
- bed protector
- toilet tissue
- washbasin
- soap
- washcloth
- towel

1 Perform your beginning procedure actions.

2 Ask the resident to flex his knees and rest weight on his heels, if able.

3 Help the resident to raise his buttocks:

   a Put one hand under the small of the resident's back, and gently lift while the resident pushes with his feet.

   b With the other hand, insert the bed protector under the resident.

4 If the resident is unable to lift his buttocks:

   a Help the resident to turn on his side, with his back toward you.

   b Place the bed protector on the bed.

   c Place the bedpan flat against the resident's buttocks (Figure 12-2).

   d Roll the resident on his back, while holding the bedpan in place.

Figure 12-3 Elevate the head of the bed so that the resident is comfortable.

5 Cover the resident with the top sheet.

6 Raise the head of the bed slightly for comfort (Figure 12-3).

7 Remove the disposable gloves.

8 Raise the side rail.

9 Dispose of gloves according to facility policy.

10 Wash your hands.

11 Give the resident the call signal and toilet tissue. Instruct him to use the signal when he is done. Leave the room.

Figure 12-2 Position the bedpan flat against the resident's buttocks, then roll him back toward you while holding the pan in position.

(continues)

36 *continued*

12 Return immediately when the resident calls.

13 Put on disposable gloves.

14 Lower the side rail.

15 Remove the bedpan by asking the resident to raise his hips.

16 If the resident is unable to raise hips, hold the bedpan securely while the resident rolls to his side with back facing you (Figure 12-4). Remove the bedpan. Cover the pan with a bedpan cover or other cover according to facility policy.

17 Place the bedpan on a bed protector on the chair in the room, or according to facility policy. It is usually not placed on the overbed table or bedside stand.

18 Fill the washbasin with water (105°F). Help the resident to clean his perineal area, if necessary. Dispose of toilet tissue in the bedpan. Cover the bedpan.

19 Wash the resident's perineal area with soap and water. Rinse and dry.

20 Remove one glove and raise the side rail with the ungloved hand.

21 Take the covered bedpan to the bathroom (Figure 12-5). Empty and disinfect it according to facility policy. Use the ungloved hand to turn on faucets and flush the toilet. Store the bedpan in its proper location.

22 Remove the other glove and dispose according to facility policy.

23 Wash your hands.

24 Help the resident to wash his hands. Clean and return the basin to its proper location.

25 Perform your procedure completion actions.

Figure 12-4 Hold the bedpan securely while the resident turns on his side.

Figure 12-5 Cover the bedpan after you remove it.

OBSERVING AND MEASURING OUTPUT

Nursing Alert

Apply the principles of standard precautions when measuring residents' output.

Urine

- Measure and record in cubic centimeters or milliliters as indicated by facility policy.
- If the resident is incontinent, or unable to control the passage of urine, follow facility procedure by

PERFORMANCE PROCEDURE

37   Giving a Urinal

Supplies needed:
- urinal with cover
- washbasin
- soap
- washcloth
- towel
- disposable exam gloves

1 Perform your beginning procedure actions.

2 Lift the top covers and hand the resident the urinal under the covers. If the resident is unable to take the urinal, place the urinal in the bed and insert the resident's penis into the opening.

3 Remove the disposable gloves and dispose according to facility policy.

4 Raise the side rail.

5 Wash your hands.

6 Give the resident the call signal and instruct him to use it when he is done. Leave the room.

7 Return immediately when the resident calls.

8 Put on one disposable glove.

9 Ask the resident to hand you the urinal. Remove it if he is unable.

10 Take the urinal to the bathroom, and empty and disinfect it according to facility policy. Use the ungloved hand to turn on faucets and flush the toilet. Store the urinal in its proper location.

11 Remove the glove and dispose according to facility policy.

12 Wash your hands.

13 Fill the washbasin with water (105°F).

14 Lower the side rail.

15 Help the resident to wash his hands.

16 Raise the side rail.

17 Lower the height of the bed.

18 Clean and return the basin to its proper location.

19 Perform your procedure completion actions.

Figure 12-6 Pour the specimen into the graduate to measure the output.

measuring the size of the urine puddle or weight of the pad.
- Record amounts in drainage bags by measuring in a graduate (Figure 12-6). Do not use the markings on the drainage bags, as the marks are estimates only.

Feces (Bowel Movements)

- Recording bowel movements is very important to ensure that elimination is adequate.
- Most facilities use checklist charting for recording bowel movements.

Observe and Report Abnormalities

These abnormalities should be reported to the nurse immediately:

- blood
- mucus

- liquid stool
- very hard stool
- stool that is very dark in color
- undigested food or pills in the stool
- unusual color (clay color, black, etc.)

Record on I & O Sheet

Accurate reporting requires you to be observant. Be sure to record:

- amount of urine
- profuse perspiration or sweat
- time of output, if required
- amounts of emesis and liquid stools.

CATHETERS

A **catheter** is a tube inserted into a body cavity, usually for draining liquids. The most commonly used catheter is the indwelling urinary catheter, which is inserted by the nurse. You may hear this catheter called a "Foley." The catheter is usually left in the bladder, where it is held in place by a small, inflatable balloon (Figure 12-7). The catheter is attached to tubing that connects to the drainage bag that collects the urine.

Because the catheter opens into a body cavity, the resident is at high risk of infection. Many facilities have policies stating that the tubing and catheter are not to be disconnected. Some facilities use leg bags to collect the urine when the resident is out of bed during the day. The leg bag is worn under the clothing and is not as obvious as the regular

catheter bag. Know and follow your facility policies and procedures for disconnecting the tubing and handling the catheter. This is a very important responsibility.

Catheter Care

This procedure may vary from one facility to another. Always refer to the care plan for specific instructions. Refer to the guidelines on page 199 for catheter care.

OSTOMIES

An **ostomy** is a surgical opening made through the abdomen for excretion of body waste (Figure 12-9). This procedure is done when disease or injury prevents normal elimination. An ostomy may be done to allow for urinary or fecal waste discharge. The opening of the ostomy is called the **stoma**. Ostomies may be temporary or permanent. The most common type of ostomy is the **colostomy**, an opening into the colon to allow for feces to be eliminated. Many people live well with ostomies. They work and are very active. Many people care for their own ostomy. The resident in a long-term care facility may need some assistance caring for the ostomy. Procedures vary from one facility to another. However, some general guidelines apply.

Caring for the Resident with an Ostomy

Although policies vary, practice ostomy care carefully, and follow the guidelines on page 201.

Figure 12-7 Placement of an indwelling catheter in the female and male resident

✔ GUIDELINES for Catheter Care

❑ Apply the principles of standard precautions when providing catheter care.

❑ Gently wash the genital area around the catheter with warm water.

❑ Wash the perineal area. Wash from front to back on females, and from the tip of the penis to the scrotum on males.

❑ Rinse and dry well.

❑ Some facilities include washing the catheter close to the body as part of this procedure. Follow your facility policy. If you are washing the catheter, always wash in the direction away from the body. Avoid rubbing back and forth.

❑ Make sure that the catheter tubing is without kinks.

❑ Make sure that all connections are tight.

❑ Make sure that the resident is not lying or sitting on the catheter tubing.

❑ Position the catheter to avoid pulling. Pulling the catheter is irritating to the resident. It is very painful for the resident if the catheter is accidentally dislodged. Use a Velcro strap or tape to secure the catheter to the leg to prevent pulling.

❑ Attach the drainage tubing to the sheet to allow the urine to drain well.

❑ The drainage bag should be below the level of the bladder at all times. If the bag is raised above the bladder, the urine will drain back into the body, causing the potential for an infection to develop.

❑ The catheter bag should never touch the floor.

❑ Attach the catheter bag to the bed frame, not the side rail.

❑ Take care when moving or transferring residents so that you do not pull on the catheter.

PERFORMANCE PROCEDURE

38 Giving Catheter Care

Supplies needed:
- bath blanket
- bed protector
- tape or catheter strap
- rubber band
- pin
- washbasin
- soap
- washcloth
- towel
- disposable exam gloves

1 Perform your beginning procedure actions.

2 Cover the resident with a bath blanket.

3 Fanfold the upper linen down to the foot of the bed.

4 Ask the resident to raise hips and place the bed protector under the resident.

5 Position the bath blanket to expose the resident's catheter.

6 Wash the urethra area around the catheter entrance.

7 Wash the genital area from front to back. Rinse well.

8 Dry the area well.

9 Secure the catheter with a catheter strap or tape.

10 Place the drainage tubing over the resident's leg.

11 Place the rubber band around the tubing and pin it to the sheet at the edge of the mattress to make sure that the tubing stays on the bed.

12 Cover the resident. Replace the bedding and remove the bath blanket.

13 Perform your procedure completion actions.

PERFORMANCE PROCEDURE

39 Emptying a Catheter Bag

Supplies needed:
- graduate pitcher
- paper towel
- alcohol sponge
- disposable exam gloves

1 Perform your beginning procedure actions.

2 Place a paper towel on the floor and place the graduate on top of it.

3 Remove the drainage spout from the bag and center it over the graduate (Figure 12-8). Be careful not to touch the tip of the drainage spout. Do not let the tip or the sides of the drainage spout touch the graduate.

4 Open the clamp on the drainage spout and allow the urine to drain into the graduate.

5 After the urine has drained into the graduate, wipe the spout with the alcohol sponge, if this is your facility policy. Some facilities do not wipe the tip of the spout unless it has contacted your hands or the graduate.

6 Replace the drainage spout into the holder on the side of the catheter bag. Pick up the graduate. Dispose of the paper towel.

7 Note the amount, color, and character of urine.

8 Discard urine and disinfect the graduate according to facility policy. Store the graduate in its proper location.

9 Perform your procedure completion actions.

Figure 12-8 Center the tip of the tubing over the graduate. Avoid touching the tubing against the sides of the container.

ENEMAS

An **enema** is the injection of fluid into the rectum. This is usually done to empty the rectum of feces. You may be responsible for giving a resident an enema. In some facilities nursing assistants are not allowed to give enemas. Know and follow your facility policy.

There are two types of enemas: a cleansing enema and a retention enema. The cleansing enema is given to clean the rectum. The retention enema is given to soften the feces or to administer medication.

The type of enema nursing assistants usually administer is the cleansing enema. The solution for enemas may be plain water, a soap or salt solution, or a commercial preparation.

Figure 12-9 An ostomy bag in place on the resident's abdomen.

GUIDELINES for Ostomy Care

- ☐ Apply the principles of standard precautions when caring for an ostomy.
- ☐ Realize that the resident with an ostomy may feel a great loss of control and have a poor body image and low self-esteem. Be aware of your own body language during this procedure so that you do not further lower the resident's self-esteem.
- ☐ Be a good listener. Allow the resident to talk about his feelings.
- ☐ Report signs of depression to the nurse.
- ☐ Remove the soiled bag.
- ☐ Wash the area around the ostomy according to directions on the care plan.
- ☐ Observe and report any redness or irritation of the skin around the stoma.
- ☐ Apply protective cream around the stoma, if indicated on the care plan.
- ☐ Apply a clean bag.
- ☐ Change ostomy bags often to reduce odors. Some residents use deodorizer tablets or drops in the ostomy bag.
- ☐ Dispose of soiled bags according to facility policy.

 GUIDELINES for Giving Enemas

Policies of long-term care facilities vary regarding who is responsible for giving enemas. Check with the nurse before giving a resident an enema.

- ☐ Apply the principles of standard precautions when giving an enema.
- ☐ Check with the nurse about which solution to use.
- ☐ Enema solutions should be warm, about 105°F. Check the temperature with a bath thermometer.
- ☐ The amount of solution in a cleansing or tap water enema is usually 700 cc to 1,000 cc.
- ☐ Have the resident's bathrobe, slippers, bedpan, or commode nearby. The resident will feel urgency after the enema.
- ☐ When administering the enema solution, the resident should be lying on his left side in the Sims' position, with the right knee drawn toward the chest.
- ☐ Always lubricate the rectal tube of the enema.
- ☐ Before inserting the tubing into the rectum, clear air from the tubing by running water through the tubing. Clamp the tubing.
- ☐ Insert the tube about two to three inches.
- ☐ Raise the container of solution 12 to 18 inches above the rectum.
- ☐ Allow the solution to run in slowly.
- ☐ If the resident complains of cramping, clamp the tubing and instruct him to take deep breaths. Then open the tubing and continue the procedure.
- ☐ Give the amount of solution ordered by the physician and as tolerated by the resident.
- ☐ Ask the resident to hold the solution in the rectum for a few minutes, if possible.
- ☐ Help the resident to the bathroom, commode, or onto the bedpan.
- ☐ Make sure the resident's call light is in reach.
- ☐ Observe and report the results of the enema. Instruct the resident not to flush the toilet until results have been observed. If blood or other abnormalities are noted, do not flush the toilet until you have notified the nurse.

KEY POINTS IN CHAPTER

▲ Elimination of body waste is done through the body's digestive and genitourinary systems.

▲ Due to reduced sensitivity, the elderly person often feels urgency just when the elimination is felt.

▲ Some factors affecting normal elimination in the resident may be disease, inactivity, medications, and lack of privacy.

▲ Bowel and bladder management programs can help the resident regain control over these body functions.

▲ Catheter care includes cleaning the genital area and watching for proper urine drainage.

▲ Enemas are the administration of fluid into the rectum, usually to remove feces.

▲ An ostomy is an opening into the abdomen to allow body waste to come out.

REVIEW QUIZ

1. The body's way of removing waste products is called:
   a. digestion.
   b. circulation.
   c. elimination.
   d. impaction.

2. The organs of the urinary system that filter the blood and form urine are the:
   a. bowels.
   b. kidneys.
   c. bladders.
   d. intestines.

3. Normal urine is:
   a. clear.
   b. dark yellow.
   c. foul-smelling.
   d. streaked with mucus.

4. What are the intestines?
   a. tubes connecting the kidneys and bladder
   b. tubelike canals extending from the stomach to the rectum
   c. a storage place for urine before discharge
   d. the tubes through which blood circulates throughout the body

5. In normal aging, the blood flow to the kidneys is:
   a. lessened.
   b. increased.
   c. stimulated.
   d. unchanged.

6. Which of the following may be factors causing elimination problems in the elderly?
   a. normal aging
   b. improper diet
   c. lack of activity
   d. all of the above

7. Bowel and bladder training plans should include:
   a. the resident only.
   b. only the nursing staff on the night shift when the resident is incontinent.
   c. the entire nursing staff involved with the resident's care.
   d. facility administration.

8. All of the following statements are true *except:*
   a. Many residents will have the urge to urinate more frequently at night.
   b. The need to eliminate will occur quickly and urgently in many residents.
   c. All residents are unable to control the passage of urine while sleeping.
   d. Some residents may be restless and irritable, which may indicate a need to eliminate urine.

9. What does the term *void* mean?
   a. to pass stool
   b. to urinate
   c. to insert a tube to drain urine
   d. to end the passage of urine or stool

10. When placing a resident on a bedpan:
    a. make certain the resident has privacy.
    b. make certain the resident is positioned properly on the bedpan.
    c. place the call light within the resident's reach.
    d. all of the above.

11. After removing a bedpan from a resident, you notice some blood in the urine. What is your best response?
    a. Empty the bedpan, and clean and replace equipment.
    b. Empty the bedpan into the toilet, then record the incident on the resident's chart.
    c. Place the bedpan and contents in the bathroom. Report the appearance of blood in the urine to the nurse immediately.
    d. Pour the urine into a cup and take it to the doctor's office for examination.

12. Caring for the resident with a urinary catheter includes:
    a. securing the catheter to the resident's leg.
    b. inserting the catheter into the resident.
    c. removing the catheter at night.
    d. changing the catheter every other day.

13. An opening made through the abdomen to allow for discharge of body waste is a/an:
    a. enema.
    b. ostomy.
    c. catheter.
    d. defecation.

14. When placing a resident on a commode to defecate, you are:
    a. helping the resident to sit on a bedpan.
    b. helping the resident to use a portable toilet to urinate.
    c. placing the resident on a portable toilet to have a bowel movement.
    d. placing the resident on a bedpan to have a bowel movement.

15. When giving a cleansing enema, you should insert the tubing into the rectum:
    a. one inch.
    b. two to three inches.
    c. six to seven inches.
    d. eight to nine inches.

16. You are caring for Mrs. Hunter, a 67-year-old resident who has had a stroke and is mentally confused. Mrs. Hunter has been having loose stools all morning that are watery in appearance. Her abdomen is hard to touch. You know that:
    a. Mrs. Hunter has had too much water to drink.
    b. this is normal in residents who have had a stroke.
    c. this could indicate a fecal impaction and should be reported to the nurse.
    d. the loose stools will stop after the resident eats some solid food.

17. You are emptying catheter bags at the end of your shift. Mrs. McQueen's catheter bag only has 50 cc in it. You should:
    a. record the output on the flow sheet and go home.
    b. assume that another nursing assistant has emptied this catheter.
    c. do nothing, as the bag does not need to be emptied.
    d. report your observations to the nurse.

18. While you are emptying catheters, you accidentally touch the drain spout of Mr. Gates's catheter on the bed frame. You should:
    a. insert the drain spout back in the catheter bag immediately.
    b. wipe the drain spout with an alcohol sponge.
    c. remove the catheter.
    d. leave the drain spout exposed to the air after the bag is empty.

19. Miss Gunther is an 86-year-old resident who has Alzheimer's disease. She is confused. The resident requires total care and is usually incontinent of urine. Miss Gunther urinates 10 times on your shift. The urine has a strong odor. You know that:
    a. this may indicate a urinary tract infection and should be reported to the nurse.
    b. Miss Gunther has had too much liquid to drink.
    c. this is normal in Alzheimer's disease.
    d. the resident is urinating frequently to get extra attention.

20. Mr. Haley is a 75-year-old resident with a colostomy. You are assigned to bathe him and do his colostomy care. The area around the stoma appears very red. You should:
    a. wipe the area with an alcohol sponge.
    b. remove the used colostomy bag and place a new one on the area immediately.
    c. ask the nurse to look at the area before you reapply the bag.
    d. apply moisturizing lotion to the area around the stoma.

CHAPTER 12
CROSSWORD PUZZLE

Directions: Complete the puzzle using these words found in Chapter 12.

anus
bedpan
bowel
catheter
colon
commode
colostomy

defecate
enema
feces
homeostasis
impaction
incontinent
involuntary

stoma
stool
urethra
urinal
void

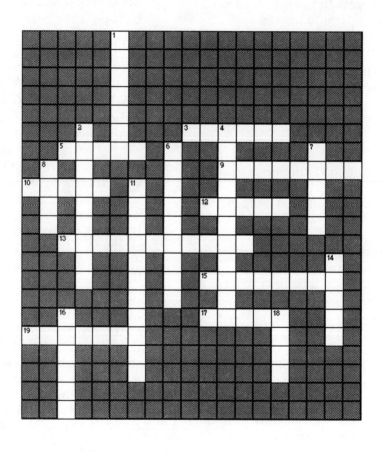

CHAPTER 12
PUZZLE CLUES

ACROSS

3. A container that men use for urination
5. The lower part of the intestine
9. A tube inserted into a body cavity to drain liquid
10. The large bowel or lower part of the abdomen
12. Administration of fluid into the rectum to cleanse the bowel
13. A constant state of balance in the body
15. To have a bowel movement
17. The opening in the abdomen created by an ostomy
19. The tube through which the urine passes as it leaves the body

DOWN

1. A portable toilet
2. A surgically created opening into the abdominal wall to eliminate feces from the body
4. Unable to control the passage of urine
6. A mass of hard feces that the resident is unable to pass normally
7. Bowel movement
8. To urinate
11. Done without choice; usually refers to inability to control the passage of stool
14. Another word for stool
16. A special container that the resident uses to discharge body waste when in bed
18. The opening of the rectum

13

Vital Signs, Height, and Weight

OBJECTIVES

In this chapter, you will learn how to measure and record the vital signs of body temperature, pulse, respiration, and blood pressure. You will learn how to measure the resident's height and weight. After reading this chapter, you will be able to:

- Spell and define key terms.
- Describe vital signs.
- List four pulse sites.
- Measure the resident's temperature, pulse, and respirations.
- Measure the resident's blood pressure.
- Identify abnormal vital signs.
- Record the resident's vital signs.
- Measure and record the resident's height and weight.

KEY TERMS

aural: concerning the ear

axillary: concerning the armpit area

blood pressure: the pressure of the blood against the walls of the arteries

body temperature: the amount of heat in the body measured by a thermometer

brachial pulse: the pulse felt on the inner side of the arm at the bend of the elbow

bradycardia: a pulse rate less than 60 beats per minute

Celsius: a metric unit of measuring temperature

cyanosis: a bluish color in the skin, lips, or fingertips due to lack of oxygen

diastolic pressure: the lower number of a blood pressure reading; the relaxing phase of the heartbeat cycle

dyspnea: difficult breathing; shortness of breath

exhalation: breathing air out

expiration: the same as exhalation; breathing air out

Fahrenheit: a scale for measuring temperature, commonly used in the United States

hypertension: abnormally high blood pressure

hypotension: abnormally low blood pressure

inhalation: breathing air in

inspiration: the same as inhalation; breathing air in

oral: concerning the mouth

palpated pressure: systolic blood pressure that is determined by palpating the brachial or radial pulse while the sphygmomanometer is deflated; diastolic blood pressure cannot be determined by using this method

pulse: the beat of the heart that is felt when an artery is compressed against a bone

radial pulse: the pulse felt at the radial artery on the inner side of the wrist

rate: the number of pulse beats or respirations per minute

rectal: concerning the anus or rectum

respiration: the exchange of oxygen and carbon dioxide in the body

rhythm: the regularity of the pulse

sphygmomanometer: the cuff used to take the blood pressure

stethoscope: the device used to listen to the resident's blood pressure, apical pulse, and other body sounds

systolic pressure: the top number of the blood pressure reading; the contraction phase of the heart cycle

tachycardia: a pulse rate more than 100 beats per minute

temperature: measurement of heat in the body

vital signs: the temperature, pulse, respirations, and blood pressure

volume: the strength of the blood flow through the blood vessels

VITAL SIGNS

The **vital signs** measure the functions of vital organs of the body. These four functions are temperature, pulse, respiration, and blood pressure. All are necessary for life. When the body is not functioning normally, the rates and character of vital signs change. The resident's condition can be monitored and evaluated by measuring the vital signs.

It is important for you to learn how to correctly take and accurately record vital signs. Whenever you are not sure of the readings, tell the nurse immediately. Accurate measurement of the vital signs takes learning and practice.

Abbreviations for Vital Signs, Height, and Weight

You must become familiar with the commonly used abbreviations for the vital signs, height, and weight. They are:

BP or B/P	blood pressure
V.S.	vital signs
TPR	temperature, pulse, and respiration
O or PO	oral temperature (taken in the mouth)
R	rectal temperature (taken in the anus)

A or AX	axillary temperature (taken in the axilla or armpit)
A or AU	aural, or taken in the ear; follow facility policy for recording
F	Fahrenheit measurement
C	Celsius measurement
Ht.	height
Wt.	weight

Facilities have different policies for recording the **aural** temperature, which is taken in the ear, and the **axillary** temperature, which is taken in the armpit. Because both begin with the letter "A," differentiating which temperature you have taken is important. Follow your facility policy for taking and recording these temperatures. Most aural thermometers can be set to provide the equivalent of an oral or rectal reading.

TEMPERATURE

The **temperature** measures body heat. Body heat is created by food changing into energy. Body heat is lost by perspiration, respiration, and excretion. The balance between heat produced by the body and the heat lost is the **body temperature.**

The normal aging process may interfere with the body's ability to regulate the temperature. Careful temperature monitoring is important for the resident in a long-term care facility. Other factors might affect the body temperature. Body temperature can be increased by:

- infection, illness, and disease.
- dehydration.
- physical exercise.
- intake of hot liquids, chewing gum, or smoking cigarettes.
- a very warm environment.

Body temperature can be decreased by:

- shock.
- a cold environment.
- cold fluids.
- medications.
- stress.

Thermometers

The temperature is taken using a thermometer. There are many types of thermometers, including:

- electronic (Figure 13–1).
- plastic or paper (Figure 13–2).
- glass (Figure 13–3).

Figure 13–1 An electronic thermometer. Plastic probe covers are placed over the probe tip, then the tip is placed under the resident's tongue.

Figure 13–2 Plastic and paper thermometers have small dots that change color to record the temperature. They are used once and discarded. Remove the thermometer slowly to prevent cutting under the resident's tongue.

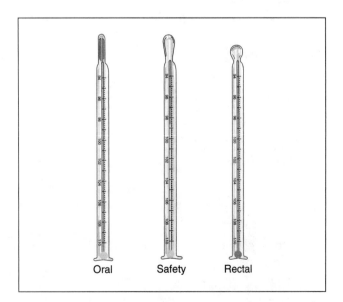

Oral   Safety   Rectal

Figure 13–3 Three types of glass thermometers. The thermometer with a blue dot on the end is for both oral and axillary use. The thermometer with the red dot on the end is for rectal use.

The glass and electronic thermometers are most commonly used in long-term care facilities. Follow your facility's policy when using paper or plastic thermometers.

Thermometers measure body temperature using either the **Fahrenheit** or the **Celsius** scale. Both scales are divided into units called *degrees.* Check which type of thermometer your facility uses.

On glass thermometers, each long line on the thermometer equals one degree, and each short line equals two-tenths of a degree. The thermometer is read by noting the point at which the mercury column ends. The temperature is read to the nearest two-tenths of a degree.

Many facilities use disposable sheaths to cover the thermometer when taking the temperature (Figure 13–4). These sheaths protect the resident because they contain the glass if the thermometer is accidentally broken (Figure 13–5). Some types of sheaths used for rectal temperatures are pre-lubricated. The sheath on a glass thermometer is used once and discarded. Become familiar with the type of sheath your facility uses.

Electronic Thermometers. The electronic thermometer is a battery-operated unit that shows the temperature reading on a lighted display. This type of unit eliminates human error that may occur with other types of thermometers.

Figure 13–4 A disposable plastic thermometer sheath.

Figure 13–5 The outer wrapper is removed and the plastic inserted into the resident's mouth. The plastic contains the glass if the thermometer breaks.

Two types of electronic thermometers are available. One type is used for oral, rectal, or axillary temperatures. This thermometer has a probe. A blue-colored probe is used for oral and axillary temperatures. A red-colored probe is used for the rectal temperature. This thermometer makes a "beep" sound when the temperature has been measured. The electronic thermometer usually has a cord to wear around your neck when you are walking down the hall or using the thermometer to take the temperature. Wear the thermometer like a necklace, and take care not to swing or drop it. The thermometer is very sensitive and will not work properly if it is banged or dropped.

Another type of electronic thermometer is used for taking the aural, or ear, temperature (Figure 13–6). This thermometer is inserted into the inner ear and records temperature very quickly. The aural thermometer also sounds a "beep" or the display screen blinks when the temperature has been measured.

Disposable plastic sheaths, called probe covers, are inserted over the electronic probe of both types of electronic thermometers. A clean probe cover must be used for each resident's temperature. The batteries of electronic thermometers must be charged regularly to stay accurate. Follow facility policy when using electronic thermometers.

Methods of Measuring Body Temperature

There are four methods of measuring a resident's body temperature. The **oral** method is done by inserting the thermometer under the resident's tongue. The **rectal** method is done by inserting the thermometer one inch into the resident's rectum. The axillary method is done by placing the thermometer in the resident's armpit. The aural temperature is taken by inserting the thermometer into the resident's ear. Always refer to the care plan to learn which method must be used for each resident. Apply the principles of standard precautions when taking temperatures. A brief overview of each of these methods follows.

Oral Temperature. The oral temperature is taken by mouth. It is used when the resident is alert and cooperative.

- Do not take an oral temperature on residents with known seizure disorders.
- The oral thermometer may have a bulb or slender tip with mercury. Sometimes the end of the thermometer is blue or green.
- Do not take the temperature by mouth if the resident has just taken hot or cold liquids, smoked a cigarette, dipped tobacco, or chewed gum. Wait 15 minutes before taking the oral temperature.
- Do not take the temperature orally if the resident is using oxygen.
- Follow your facility policy for using a disposable sheath to cover the glass thermometer.
- The oral thermometer should remain in place for three minutes, or according to facility policy.
- The normal oral temperature is 98.6°F.

Rectal Temperature. Note the following when using the rectal method.

- This thermometer has a shorter, rounded bulb tip with mercury.
- The tip opposite the mercury end of the rectal thermometer is usually red.
- Follow your facility policy for using a disposable sheath to cover the glass thermometer.
- Use for residents receiving oxygen ("mouth breathers"), confused or disoriented residents, and others who cannot keep the thermometer in the mouth.
- Do not take a rectal temperature on residents with hemorrhoids, diarrhea, fecal impaction, or a colostomy.
- The thermometer must always be lubricated before inserting into the rectum.
- Always hold the thermometer in place when taking rectal temperatures. Some rectal thermometer sheaths are pre-lubricated.
- This thermometer should remain in place for three minutes, or according to facility policy. Never leave the resident alone.
- The normal rectal temperature is 99.6°F.
- Record "R" if the temperature was taken rectally.

Figure 13–6 The electronic ear thermometer. A plastic probe cover is inserted into the resident's ear. The thermometer records the temperature in two to three seconds. For accuracy, position the thermometer correctly in the ear canal.

Axillary Temperature. Take the axillary temperature using an oral thermometer.

- Follow your facility policy for using a disposable sheath to cover the glass thermometer.
- This is the *least accurate* method of taking the temperature and should not be used if you can take the temperature by using another method.
- An axillary temperature may not be accurate on residents who are underweight.
- Remove perspiration by wiping the axillary area before placing the thermometer.
- Some facilities require the nursing assistant to hold this thermometer in place. Know and follow the policy of your facility.
- This thermometer should remain in place for 10 minutes, or according to facility policy.
- The normal axillary temperature is 97.6°F.
- Record "AX" when the axillary temperature is taken, or follow your facility policy.

Aural Temperature. This method of taking the temperature can be used for most residents.

- Use a special ear thermometer.
- Always use a disposable probe cover on the thermometer.
- Large amounts of ear wax may produce an inaccurate reading.

- Insert the thermometer securely in the ear canal to obtain an accurate reading.
- Most ear thermometers can be set to give the equivalent of an oral or rectal reading.
- Follow your facility policy for recording the oral or rectal equivalent.

PULSE

The **pulse** is the expansion and contraction of an artery. This rhythmic expansion and contraction in the artery indicates how fast or slow the heart is beating. It is felt in locations where an artery lies over a bone close to the surface of the skin (Figure 13–7). The pulse tells you how well the circulatory system is working. When you take the resident's pulse, be alert to the rate, rhythm, and volume of the pulse beat.

Pulse Rate

The pulse rate is the number of beats per minute. The pulse rate varies within individuals from time to time depending upon exercise or emotional state. The pulse should be counted while the resident is at rest. Guidelines for taking the pulse are as follows:

- The pulse rate varies. It depends on age, sex, body size, emotional state, and exercise.
- The pulse rate usually goes up as the body temperature increases.

✓ GUIDELINES for Taking Temperature

Some general rules are important to follow when taking the resident's temperature:

- ☐ Apply the principles of standard precautions when taking temperatures.
- ☐ Check the thermometer for chips and cracks.
- ☐ Follow facility procedure for wiping up broken thermometers. The mercury in the glass is poisonous, and your facility will have special policies for cleanup.
- ☐ Be alert to thermometers with both Celsius and Fahrenheit scales. The markings on this type of thermometer are very small. Be sure to read accurately.
- ☐ Shake the mercury down below 96° F before inserting the thermometer.
- ☐ Use care when shaking down the thermometer. Stand away from the resident or surfaces that the thermometer may hit.
- ☐ Follow your facility policy for using disposable thermometer sheaths.
- ☐ Lubricate the rectal thermometer before inserting.
- ☐ Hold the rectal thermometer in place with your gloved hand.
- ☐ Wipe the thermometer from the stem end to the mercury tip before inserting.
- ☐ Disinfect and store the thermometer according to facility policy.
- ☐ Never clean the mercury thermometer with hot water. The thermometer may break.
- ☐ Use a clean probe cover for each resident when using an electronic thermometer or ear thermometer.

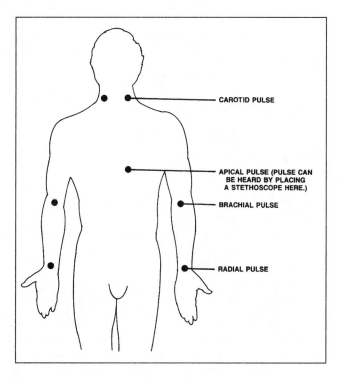

Figure 13–7 Locations where the pulse can be palpated.

- Pain usually increases the pulse rate.
- Medications may affect the pulse rate.
- The average adult pulse is 60 to 80 beats per minute.
- **Tachycardia** is a fast pulse rate greater than 100 beats per minute.
- **Bradycardia** is a slow pulse rate less than 60 beats per minute.

- Report pulse rates less than 60 or more than 100 to your charge nurse.
- The pulse is regular when the pulse beats are evenly spaced.
- The pulse is irregular when the beats are uneven or there are skipped beats.
- Report any irregular or unusual pulse beats.

Pulse Volume

The pulse volume is the forcefulness or degree of strength of the pulse. The volume of the pulse can be felt by noting how strong or weak the beat is when the artery is expanding and contracting. You will feel the pulse and note if it is:

- strong.
- weak.
- thready.

Pulse Location

Learn these facts so you can record the pulse accurately.

- The **radial pulse** is felt at the wrist. It is the most common location for taking the pulse.
- The carotid pulse is felt on either side of the neck.
- The apical pulse is heard at the base of the heart. A **stethoscope** must be used to take the apical pulse.
- The **brachial pulse** is felt on the inner arm at the elbow. This is the pulse used to take the blood pressure.

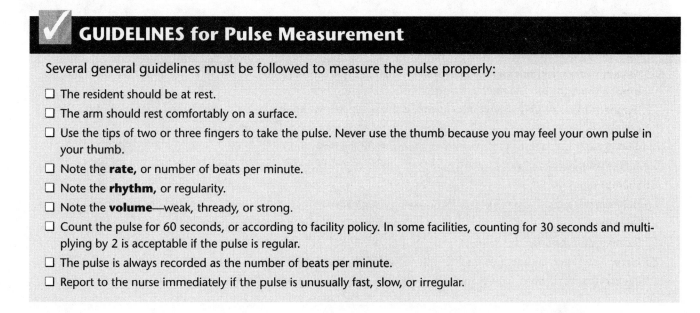

✓ GUIDELINES for Pulse Measurement

Several general guidelines must be followed to measure the pulse properly:

❑ The resident should be at rest.

❑ The arm should rest comfortably on a surface.

❑ Use the tips of two or three fingers to take the pulse. Never use the thumb because you may feel your own pulse in your thumb.

❑ Note the **rate,** or number of beats per minute.

❑ Note the **rhythm,** or regularity.

❑ Note the **volume**—weak, thready, or strong.

❑ Count the pulse for 60 seconds, or according to facility policy. In some facilities, counting for 30 seconds and multiplying by 2 is acceptable if the pulse is regular.

❑ The pulse is always recorded as the number of beats per minute.

❑ Report to the nurse immediately if the pulse is unusually fast, slow, or irregular.

RESPIRATION

Respiration is the process of breathing. It is this process that allows humans to take in oxygen and give off carbon dioxide. A single respiration or breath is one **inspiration** or **inhalation** (breathing air in) and one **expiration** or **exhalation** (breathing air out). As a nursing assistant you will be responsible for counting the resident's respirations.

Dyspnea is the medical term for shortness of breath. Shortness of breath always suggests a medical problem and should be reported to the nurse immediately. **Cyanosis** is a blue color of the skin, lips, or nail beds caused by a lack of oxygen.

The process of breathing is both voluntary and involuntary. You breathe without thinking about it. However, you can control your respirations by holding your breath. This is the reason you do not explain to the residents that you are counting the respirations. Counting respirations is usually done after counting the pulse. The resident will think you are taking the pulse while you are discreetly counting respirations.

Considerations for Care

Be aware of the following considerations regarding respiration:

- Normal respirations for adults are 12 to 20 per minute.
- Report respiratory rates below 12 or more than 20, or anything that differs from the normal range of the resident.

- Respirations increase with:
  - fever.
  - infection.
  - stress and emotional upsets.
  - exercise.

- Respirations decrease with:
  - some medications.
  - some diseases.
  - sleep.

BLOOD PRESSURE

Measuring **blood pressure** gives valuable information about how the heart and blood vessels are working. The heart pumps the blood throughout the body through the arteries. The arteries carry blood away from the heart. When you take a resident's blood pressure, you are measuring how much pressure is exerted on the artery walls as the blood passes through. There is always some blood in the arteries, so there is always some pressure on the walls of the blood vessels. As the heart contracts to send out blood, a force is felt on the artery. This working phase of the heartbeat is called the **systolic pressure.** When the heart relaxes between beats, the pressure is lower. This is called the **diastolic pressure.** You will be reading both pressures when you take a blood pressure measurement.

✔ GUIDELINES for Counting Respirations

Know the following information so you will count respirations accurately:

- ❑ Breathing can be controlled, so avoid telling the resident when respirations are being counted.
- ❑ One inspiration and one expiration of breath are counted as one respiration. Watch the rise and fall of the resident's chest.
- ❑ Count respirations immediately after counting the pulse. Remember the pulse count as you count the rise and fall of the chest.
- ❑ Keep your fingers on the pulse while you are counting the respirations.
- ❑ Note if respirations are:
  - regular.
  - shallow.
  - deep.
  - difficult or labored.
- ❑ Count the respirations for one minute or as indicated by your facility policy.
- ❑ Record the respirations. Report any abnormalities to your charge nurse.

The blood vessels of the older person are often thicker and less elastic, causing the heart to work harder to push blood through the arteries. Therefore, the blood pressure in the older resident is often higher than a younger adult's blood pressure.

Equipment Used to Measure Blood Pressure

The equipment used in measuring blood pressure varies from one facility to another. In all cases you will be using something called a **sphygmomanometer,** commonly called a blood pressure cuff (Figure 13–8). Unless you use an electronic digital recording sphygmomanometer, you will also use a stethoscope to listen to the reading. Handle the sphygmomanometer carefully when you walk down the hall. Take care not to hit it against a wall or drop it. The sphygmomanometer may not provide an accurate reading if it is banged or dropped. There are two types of sphygmomanometers used:

- Mercury sphygmomanometer
  - A column of mercury is observed as you read the blood pressure.

- This unit should be placed on a flat surface.
- Read the mercury column at eye level.

• Aneroid sphygmomanometer. A pointer on a dial is observed as you read the blood pressure.

Accuracy is very important in taking the blood pressure. It takes skill and practice to learn to take accurate blood pressure readings. Ask the nurse to recheck a reading if you are not sure.

Terms Associated with Blood Pressure

Understand the terms **hypertension** and **hypotension.**

Hypertension. High blood pressure, usually 140/90 or higher, is considered hypertension. An elderly person's blood pressure may be higher than 140/90.

Hypotension. Low blood pressure, usually 100/60 or less, is considered hypotension.

Know and follow your facility policy for reporting blood pressure that is too high or too low.

Figure 13–8 Equipment used to measure blood pressure.

✔ GUIDELINES for Taking Blood Pressure

Follow these points when taking blood pressure:

- ❏ Equipment should be in good working condition.
- ❏ Wipe the bell and ear pieces of the stethoscope with an alcohol sponge before and after use.
- ❏ Use a proper size cuff.
- ❏ Read the gauge at eye level.
- ❏ The resident should be sitting or lying in a relaxed, comfortable position, with the arm resting on a solid surface.
- ❏ Do not take blood pressure in an arm:
  - — with an intravenous feeding.
  - — with a dialysis shunt.
  - — weakened by a stroke.
  - — on the side where a breast has been removed.
- ❏ Do not reinflate the cuff immediately if you do not hear the blood pressure the first time. Let all of the air out, wait a minute, and take the blood pressure again.
- ❏ Record the blood pressure accurately in fraction form; for example, 120/80. Blood pressure is recorded as millimeters of mercury. For this reason, you may see the reading recorded as 120/80mm Hg.

REPORTING AND RECORDING VITAL SIGNS

It is a good idea to check the vital signs a second time if you think the values are abnormal. Report to the nurse any vital signs that are outside the normal range. Recording vital signs you have measured is an important part of your role as a nursing assistant. Accuracy and writing clearly are necessary. Your facility may require you to record the vital signs on a graphic sheet or on a daily flow sheet. Ask for help if you are unsure of the method your facility uses. Remember these abbreviations for vital signs:

T	temperature
P	pulse
R	respiration
BP	blood pressure
V.S.	vital signs (includes all of the above)

Proper Way to Record Vital Signs

Be sure to go about recording vital signs in the manner you have been trained:

1. List temperature first.
2. List the pulse count second.
3. List the respirations third.
4. Example: 98.6(O)- 80-16
5. Always write "R" after the temperature reading when the temperature is taken rectally.
6. Always write "A" or "AX" after the temperature reading when the temperature is taken by the axillary method.
7. Follow your facility policy for recording aural temperature readings.
8. Some facilities assume that the temperature is oral if no letter is written behind the reading. Other facilities use "O" to denote an oral temperature.
9. Write the blood pressure as a fraction, such as 120/80.
10. Record vital signs accurately.

MEASURING AND RECORDING HEIGHT AND WEIGHT

Measuring the resident's height and weight is the responsibility of the nursing assistant in the long-term care facility. Knowing the height and weight is very important to members of the interdisciplinary team. The dietitian uses the information to plan the diet. The physician uses the information to calculate doses of medications. If the resident has a heart or kidney condition, having an accurate weight is important so that gains or losses of fluid can be detected readily. The following points are important to remember when recording height and weight:

- Follow your facility policy to learn how often to weigh residents. Some residents are weighed daily or weekly. Most residents are weighed once a month.
- Obtaining the height and weight on the day of admission of a new resident is very important.

40 Taking the Oral Temperature with a Glass Thermometer

Supplies needed:
- oral thermometer
- tissue
- disposable thermometer sheath, according to facility policy
- watch with second hand
- pen
- paper
- tissues
- disposable exam gloves

1 Perform your beginning procedure actions.

2 Rinse the thermometer with cold water, and wipe with tissue from stem to the mercury bulb end, if the thermometer has been in disinfectant.

3 Read the thermometer. Shake down to 96°F.

4 Ask the resident if he has had hot or cold liquids or smoked a cigarette. If so, wait 15 minutes and return.

5 Cover the thermometer with a disposable sheath if this is your facility policy.

6 Apply gloves if contact with oral secretions is likely or if this is your facility policy.

7 Place the bulb of the thermometer under the resident's tongue.

8 Ask the resident to close his lips and breathe through his nose.

9 Note the time of insertion and remove the thermometer after three minutes, or time interval specified by your facility. Take pulse, respiration, and blood pressure.

10 Apply gloves if you are not already wearing them.

11 Remove the disposable sheath from the thermometer and dispose according to facility policy.
OR
Wipe the thermometer from stem to the bulb end with a tissue if a sheath was not used.

12 Read the thermometer to the nearest two-tenths of a degree.

13 Clean the thermometer, if indicated, or replace in container at bedside.

14 Perform your procedure completion actions.

Many individuals use this information when doing admission assessments.
- Refer to the care plan, or follow the nurse's instructions regarding the method and time.
- When recording weight, compare it with the previous month. If the difference is five pounds or more, recheck the weight.
- Follow facility policy for reporting changes in weight to the nurse. Usually, the nurse is notified if there is a difference of five pounds or more from the previous weight.

Methods of Weighing Residents
There are several ways to weigh residents.
- Balance scale (Figure 13-9). The resident must be able to stand without help to use this type of scale.

- Chair scale. The chair scale is manufactured with a chair permanently mounted on it. The resident sits in the chair while you obtain the weight.
- Wheelchair scale (Figure 13–10). You must weigh the wheelchair without the resident before weighing her in the wheelchair. The weight of the chair is subtracted from the total weight.
- Bed scale (Figure 13–11). Bed scales are commonly attached to a mechanical lifting device. Make sure that the resident is not touching the bed when you obtain the weight.

Methods of Measuring Height
- Balance scale. Most balance scales have a height bar that can be used for the resident who can stand. Follow your facility policy. In some facilities residents remove their shoes and stand on a paper towel.

PERFORMANCE PROCEDURE

41 Taking the Pulse and Respiration

Supplies needed:
- watch with second hand
- pen
- paper

1 Perform your beginning procedure actions.

2 Position the resident's arm on a flat surface. Ask the resident to relax.

3 Place the tips of two or three fingers on the palm and thumb side of the resident's wrist. Do not use your thumb.

4 Find the pulse with your fingers.

5 Press lightly with your fingers to feel the pulse.

6 Look at the position of the second hand on your watch.

7 Count and remember the pulse beats for 60 seconds. Note volume and rhythm.

8 Continue to hold the resident's wrist as if you are still taking the pulse count.

9 Observe the rising and falling of the resident's chest.

10 Count for 60 seconds or according to facility policy. Note regularity.

11 Perform your procedure completion actions.

PERFORMANCE PROCEDURE

42 Taking the Blood Pressure

Supplies needed:
- sphygmomanometer with proper size cuff
- stethoscope
- alcohol sponges
- pen
- paper

1 Perform your beginning procedure actions.

2 Clean the ear pieces and bell or diaphragm of the stethoscope with alcohol wipes.

3 Remove or loosen clothing from the resident's arm. If the resident is wearing long sleeves, push the sleeve up to expose the brachial area.

4 Place the arm in a comfortable position on a flat surface.

5 Locate the brachial artery.

6 Make sure that the cuff is decompressed.

7 Wrap the cuff snugly and smoothly around the upper arm. Place it about one to one-and-one-half inches above the bend of the elbow. The inflatable portion of the cuff must be over the brachial artery.

8 Make sure the tubing from the cuff is centered. An arrow or marking on the cuff will indicate exactly where to place it.

9 Find the radial artery at the wrist, and palpate it as you quickly inflate the cuff to 50mm Hg.

10 Continue to inflate the cuff in 10mm Hg increments until the radial pulse cannot be felt. When you can no longer feel the pulse, this number is known as the **palpated pressure.**

11 Deflate the cuff quickly. Ask the resident to raise his arm and flex his fingers.

12 Find the brachial artery inside the elbow area with your fingers.

13 Place the ear pieces of the stethoscope in your ears. Place the diaphragm or bell of the stethoscope over the brachial artery.

(continues)

42 *continued*

14   Reinflate the blood pressure cuff to 20mm Hg above the palpated pressure.

15   Slowly release the valve in the cuff and let the air escape slowly.

16   Listen carefully with the stethoscope until the first sound is heard. Remember this number. This is the systolic blood pressure.

17   Continue to release the air until the sound changes abruptly from very loud to soft and muffled. In some facilities, this number is recorded as the diastolic blood pressure. In other facilities, the diastolic blood pressure is recorded as the last sound that you hear before the sound completely disappears. Know and follow your facility policy.

18   Remember the diastolic reading while you rapidly deflate the blood pressure cuff.

19   Remove the stethoscope from your ears and wipe the ear pieces and bell or diaphragm with the alcohol sponges.

20   Perform your procedure completion actions.

Figure 13-9 A balance scale may be used for residents who can stand independently.

Figure 13-10 The wheelchair scale. Subtract the weight of the empty wheelchair from the total weight.

Figure 13-11 A hydraulic lift with scale attachment. The resident's body must be suspended completely above the bed for an accurate reading.

- Tape measure. A tape measure is used to measure the resident who cannot stand. The resident lies in bed. Place a pencil mark on the sheet even with the resident's head. Place another pencil mark at the level of the resident's heels. The distance between the two marks is measured with a tape measure to obtain the resident's height.

✓ GUIDELINES for Weight and Height Measurements

Follow these guidelines for taking accurate height and weight measurements:

☐ Weigh residents at the same time of day.

☐ Use the same scale each time the resident is weighed.

☐ Be certain scales are balanced before weighing the resident.

☐ Have the resident wear similar clothing each time he is weighed.

☐ There are electronic scales for standing weights, electronic chair scales, and electronic bed scales. Follow the manufacturer's directions for the type of scale you are using.

KEY POINTS IN THIS CHAPTER

▲ The vital signs tell you how well the body's vital organs are working.

▲ The body temperature can be measured using oral, rectal, or axillary methods.

▲ The most commonly used site for taking the pulse is the radial artery in the wrist.

▲ When taking the respirations of a resident, hold the wrist as if taking the pulse.

▲ While measuring the blood pressure, note the systolic and diastolic pressure.

▲ Always report any unusual vital signs to the nurse immediately.

▲ Accuracy is very important when taking and recording vital signs.

▲ The nursing assistant is responsible for obtaining and accurately recording the height and weight.

REVIEW QUIZ

1. Measuring the vital organs of the body is called taking:
   a. vital statistics.
   b. vital signs.
   c. blood pressure.
   d. pulse.

2. Which of the following may cause the body temperature to increase?
   a. infection
   b. dehydration
   c. exercise
   d. all of the above

3. When reading the glass thermometer, each long line represents:
   a. one degree.
   b. one-tenth of a degree.
   c. two-tenths of a degree.
   d. five-tenths of a degree.

4. An oral temperature should *not* be used for the resident who:
   a. has dentures.
   b. is a mouth breather.
   c. has eaten in the past hour.
   d. all of the above.

5. The thermometer must be lubricated before taking a/an:
   a. axillary temperature.
   b. oral temperature.
   c. rectal temperature.
   d. aural temperature.

6. The rhythmic expansion and contraction of an artery is called the:
   a. rate.
   b. pulse.
   c. volume.
   d. blood pressure.

7. What body system are you checking when you measure the pulse?
   a. respiratory
   b. digestive
   c. circulatory
   d. elimination

8. The pulse felt at the wrist is the:
   a. carotid.
   b. brachial.
   c. apical.
   d. radial.

9. Which of the following is *true* when counting the resident's respirations?
    a. Respirations are counted by watching the rise and fall of the chest.
    b. Counting of respirations is usually done when counting the pulse.
    c. Do not tell the resident that you are counting the respirations.
    d. All of the above.

10. Measurement of the amount of force exerted on the walls of the arteries as blood flows through is:
    a. pulse.
    b. blood pressure.
    c. pressure factor.
    d. arterial pulse.

11. The resident's blood pressure reading is 130/84. The diastolic reading is:
    a. 214.
    b. 130.
    c. 84.
    d. 56.

12. What is hypertension?
    a. high blood pressure
    b. low blood pressure
    c. nervousness
    d. rapid pulse

13. What is your best action when you have taken the blood pressure of a resident and are not sure of the reading?
    a. Tell another nursing assistant.
    b. Look up the last reading and record the same numbers.
    c. Tell the nurse about your uncertainty and ask her what to do.
    d. Forget the reading and try to take the resident's blood pressure the next day.

14. What should you do when the measurements of any vital sign are abnormally high or low?
    a. Record the measurements on the chart at the end of your shift.
    b. Alert the nurse immediately to the abnormal measurements.
    c. Tell the resident and ask what he would like you to do.
    d. Report to the nurse at the end of your shift.

15. The proper way to record the temperature, pulse, and respirations is to write the:
    a. temperature first, pulse second, respirations third.
    b. respirations first, pulse second, temperature third.
    c. temperature first, respirations second, pulse last.
    d. respirations first, temperature second, pulse last.

16. You have just taken Mrs. Heinrich's weight. Last month she weighed 120 pounds. This month her weight has dropped to 80 pounds. You should:
    a. notify the nurse immediately.
    b. record the 80-pound weight on the flow sheet.
    c. recheck the weight.
    d. order a high-calorie food for the resident from the kitchen.

17. You were assigned to take the TPR and B/P on Mrs. James, an 84-year-old resident who recently was admitted after a stroke. The readings were B/P 132/82, T 98.8, P 96, R 42. Which of these readings is *not* in the normal range?
    a. blood pressure
    b. temperature
    c. pulse
    d. respirations

18. Ramona Kelley is a 72-year-old resident with kidney disease. She is on a fluid restriction. She goes to the dialysis center three times a week. You must take her vital signs when she returns from dialysis. The care plan states you are to weigh her daily. Her weight on Monday is 133 pounds. On Tuesday, her weight is 140. You should:
    a. inform the nurse.
    b. record the weight on the flow sheet at the end of your shift.
    c. call the dialysis center and ask their advice.
    d. all of the above.

19. Mrs. Springer is a 92-year-old resident with a diagnosis of chronic obstructive pulmonary disease. When you enter her room to give her breakfast, you find her sitting up in bed. She has a blue color around her lips. You count her respirations and find that they are 40 and appear shallow. You should:
    a. feed Mrs. Springer breakfast.
    b. leave the breakfast tray in the room and continue your assignment.
    c. give the resident oxygen at 8 liters per minute.
    d. advise the nurse of Mrs. Springer's condition immediately.

20. You take Bill Walker's blood pressure and find that it is 220/160. Mr. Walker has hypertension and previously had a stroke. You know that the blood pressure reading is:
    a. too high.
    b. normal for a resident with hypertension.
    c. hypotensive.
    d. too low.

CHAPTER 13
CROSSWORD PUZZLE

Directions: Complete the puzzle using these words found in Chapter 13.

aural	hypotension	respiration
axillary	inhalation	rhythm
brachial	inspiration	sphygmomanometer
bradycardia	oral	systolic
cyanosis	oxygen	tachycardia
diastolic	palpated	temperature
dyspnea	pressure	vital
exhalation	pulse	volume
expiration	radial	weight
height	rate	
hypertension	rectal	

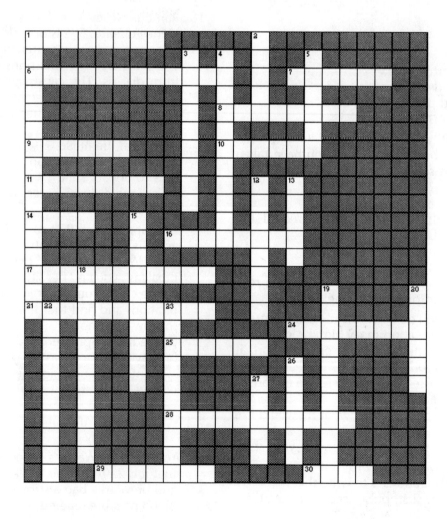

CHAPTER 13
PUZZLE CLUES

ACROSS

1. The top number of the blood pressure that is recorded when the heart is working
6. High blood pressure above 140/90
7. _____ can be taken on a standing scale or a chair scale.
8. The pressure indicated on the blood pressure gauge when the radial pulse can no longer be felt is the _____ systolic pressure.
9. A colorless, odorless, tasteless gas necessary for human life
10. The pulse at the wrist is the _____ pulse.
11. Having to do with the armpit
14. Having to do with the mouth
16. Bluish color
17. Pulse more than 100 beats per minute
21. The exchange of oxygen and carbon dioxide in the body
24. The pulse felt on the inner side of the elbow
25. Measurement of how tall the resident is
28. Measurement of heat in the body
29. Shortness of breath
30. The number of pulse beats or respirations in a minute

DOWN

1. The blood pressure cuff
2. Temperature, pulse, respirations, and blood pressure are known as _____ signs.
3. The lower number of the blood pressure taken when the heart is resting
4. Another word for inhalation
5. Temperature taken in the anus
12. Blood _____
13. The beat of the heart that is felt when an artery is compressed against a bone
15. Breathing air out
18. Low blood pressure below 100/60
19. A pulse rate less than 60 beats per minute
20. The force of the blood moving through the blood vessels
22. Another word for exhalation
23. Breathing in
26. The regularity of the pulse
27. Having to do with the ear

Anatomy Diagrams

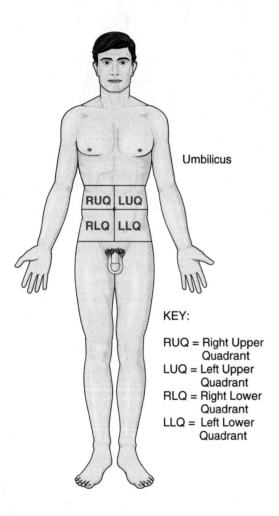

Umbilicus

RUQ | LUQ
RLQ | LLQ

KEY:

RUQ = Right Upper
Quadrant
LUQ = Left Upper
Quadrant
RLQ = Right Lower
Quadrant
LLQ = Left Lower
Quadrant

A-1A The four abdominal quadrants

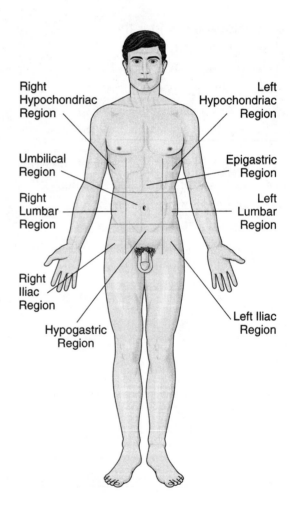

Right Hypochondriac Region

Left Hypochondriac Region

Umbilical Region

Epigastric Region

Right Lumbar Region

Left Lumbar Region

Right Iliac Region

Left Iliac Region

Hypogastric Region

A-1B The abdomen can be divided into nine regions.

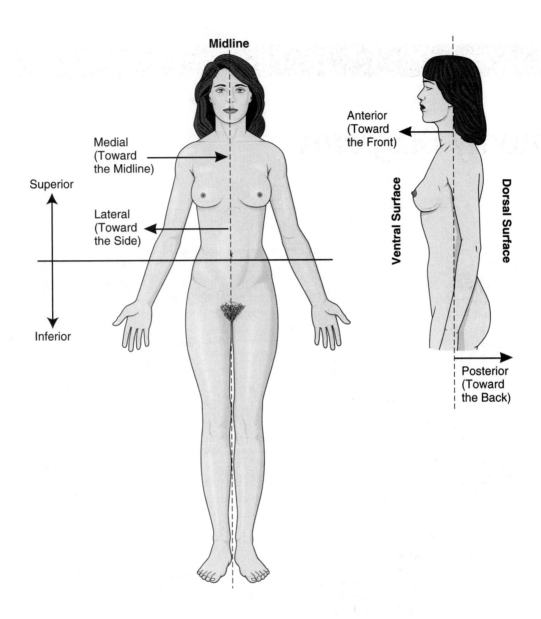

Midline

Medial
(Toward
the Midline)

Lateral
(Toward
the Side)

Superior

Inferior

Anterior
(Toward
the Front)

Ventral Surface

Dorsal Surface

Posterior
(Toward
the Back)

A-2 Imaginary lines are used to make it easier to refer to parts of the body.

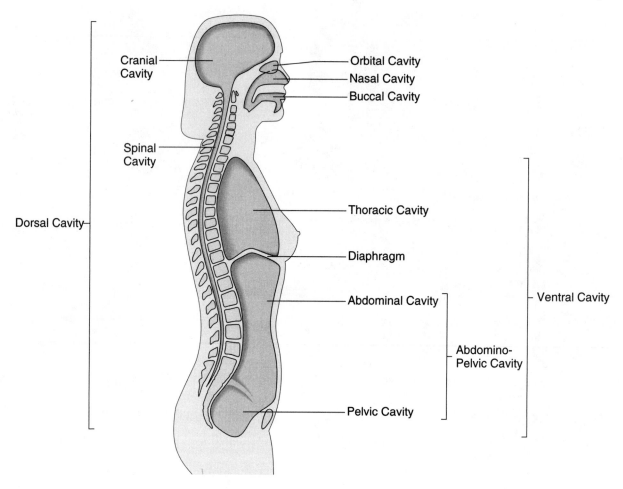

A-3 Lateral view of body cavities

Special senses
(controls pupil size)

Respiratory system
(controls respiratory rate)

Cardiovascular system
(controls heart rate and blood flow)

Digestive system
(controls functions of stomach and small
intestine)

Digestive system
(controls flow of pancreatic juices)

Endocrine system
(adrenal glands stimulate the sympathetic
nervous system)

Digestive system
(controls functions of large intestine)

A-4 The autonomic nervous system

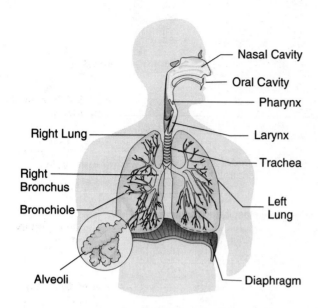

Nasal Cavity

Oral Cavity

Pharynx

Right Lung

Larynx

Trachea

Right Bronchus

Bronchiole

Left Lung

Alveoli

Diaphragm

A-5 The respiratory system

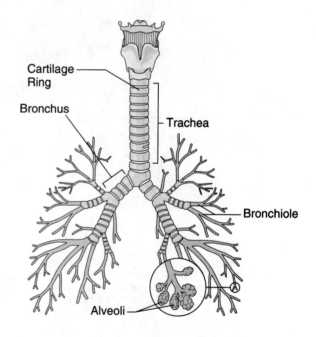

Cartilage Ring

Bronchus

Trachea

Bronchiole

Alveoli

A-6 Structures of the lower respiratory tract

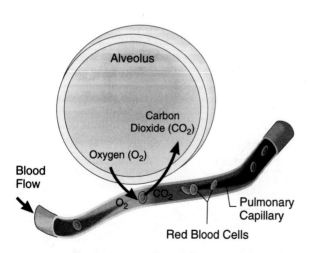

Alveolus

Carbon Dioxide (CO_2)

Oxygen (O_2)

Blood Flow

O_2

CO_2

Pulmonary Capillary

Red Blood Cells

A-7 Oxygen and carbon dioxide exchange in the capillaries of the alveoli.

Superior Vena Cava		Aorta
Right Pulmonary Artery		Left Pulmonary Artery
Right Pulmonary Veins		Left Pulmonary Veins
Right Atrium		Left Atrium
Right Coronary Artery		Left Coronary Artery
Right Coronary Vein		Left Coronary Vein
Right Ventricle		Left Ventricle

A-8 The heart and blood vessels

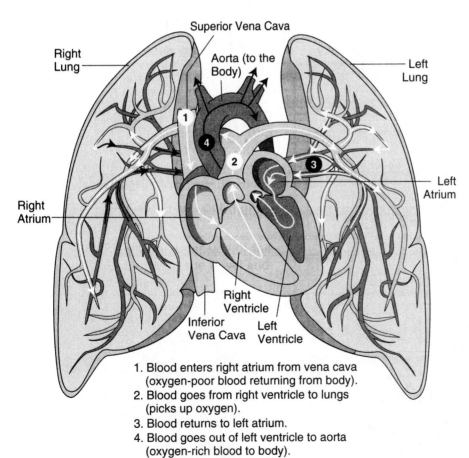

1. Blood enters right atrium from vena cava (oxygen-poor blood returning from body).
2. Blood goes from right ventricle to lungs (picks up oxygen).
3. Blood returns to left atrium.
4. Blood goes out of left ventricle to aorta (oxygen-rich blood to body).

A-9 Flow of blood from the heart to the lungs, to the body, and back to the heart where the cycle begins again.

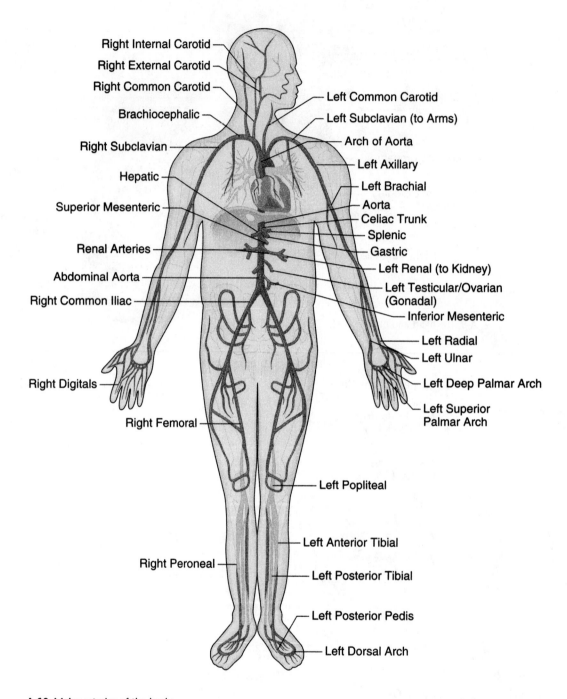

A-10 Major arteries of the body

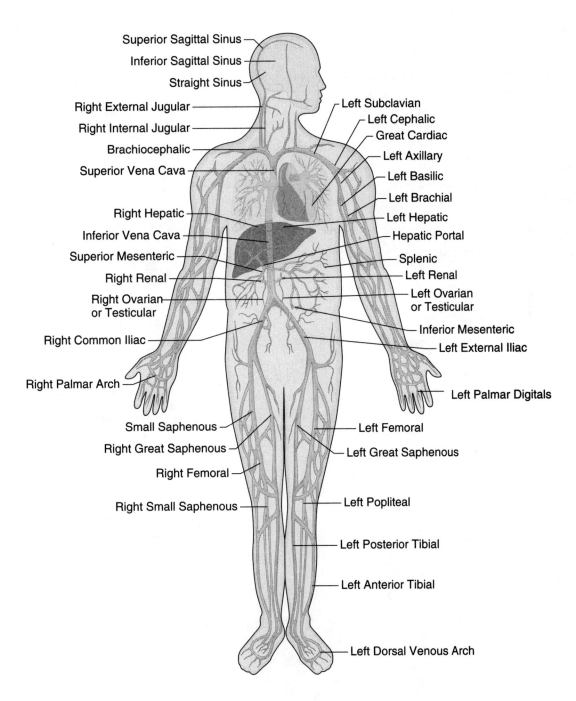

Superior Sagittal Sinus
Inferior Sagittal Sinus
Straight Sinus
Right External Jugular
Right Internal Jugular
Brachiocephalic
Superior Vena Cava
Right Hepatic
Inferior Vena Cava
Superior Mesenteric
Right Renal
Right Ovarian or Testicular
Right Common Iliac
Right Palmar Arch
Small Saphenous
Right Great Saphenous
Right Femoral
Right Small Saphenous

Left Subclavian
Left Cephalic
Great Cardiac
Left Axillary
Left Basilic
Left Brachial
Left Hepatic
Hepatic Portal
Splenic
Left Renal
Left Ovarian or Testicular
Inferior Mesenteric
Left External Iliac
Left Palmar Digitals
Left Femoral
Left Great Saphenous
Left Popliteal
Left Posterior Tibial
Left Anterior Tibial
Left Dorsal Venous Arch

A-11 Major veins of the body

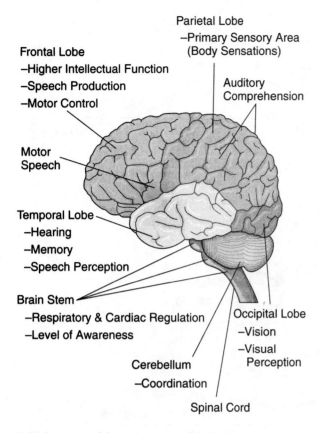

Parietal Lobe
–Primary Sensory Area
(Body Sensations)

Frontal Lobe
–Higher Intellectual Function
–Speech Production
–Motor Control

Auditory
Comprehension

Motor
Speech

Temporal Lobe
–Hearing
–Memory
–Speech Perception

Brain Stem
–Respiratory & Cardiac Regulation
–Level of Awareness

Occipital Lobe
–Vision
–Visual
Perception

Cerebellum
–Coordination

Spinal Cord

A-12 Functions of the various areas of the brain

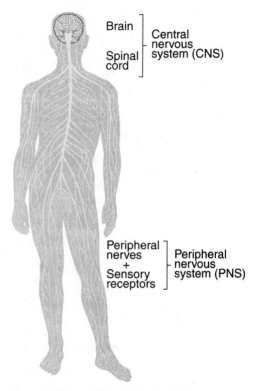

Brain
Spinal
cord
} Central
nervous
system (CNS)

Peripheral
nerves
+
Sensory
receptors
} Peripheral
nervous
system (PNS)

A-14 The peripheral nervous system connects the central nervous system to the various parts of the body. Messages are relayed to these structures through the brain and spinal cord.

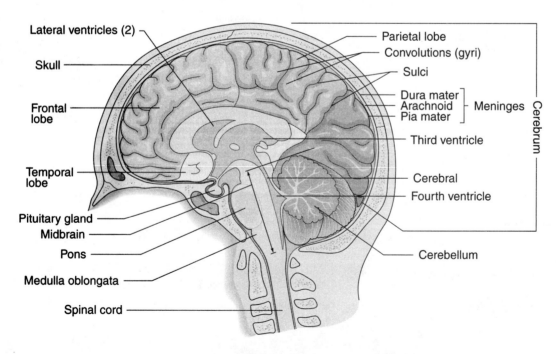

Lateral ventricles (2)

Skull

Frontal
lobe

Temporal
lobe

Pituitary gland

Midbrain

Pons

Medulla oblongata

Spinal cord

Parietal lobe

Convolutions (gyri)

Sulci

Dura mater
Arachnoid
Pia mater
} Meninges

Third ventricle

Cerebral

Fourth ventricle

Cerebellum

Cerebrum

A-13 The central nervous system consists of the brain and spinal cord.

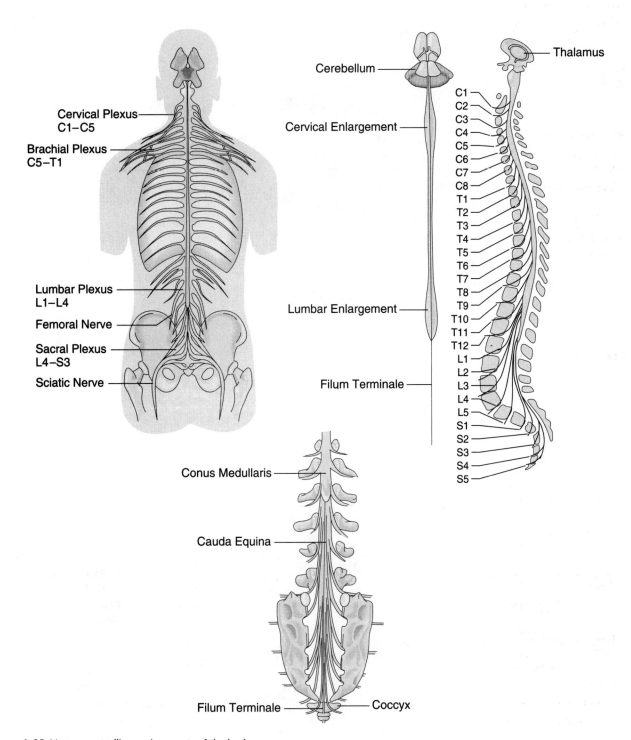

Cervical Plexus
C1–C5

Brachial Plexus
C5–T1

Lumbar Plexus
L1–L4

Femoral Nerve

Sacral Plexus
L4–S3

Sciatic Nerve

Cerebellum

Cervical Enlargement

Lumbar Enlargement

Filum Terminale

Thalamus

C1
C2
C3
C4
C5
C6
C7
C8
T1
T2
T3
T4
T5
T6
T7
T8
T9
T10
T11
T12
L1
L2
L3
L4
L5
S1
S2
S3
S4
S5

Conus Medullaris

Cauda Equina

Filum Terminale

Coccyx

A-15 Nerves controlling various parts of the body

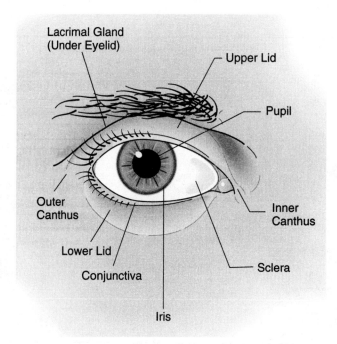

A-16 Structures of the external eye

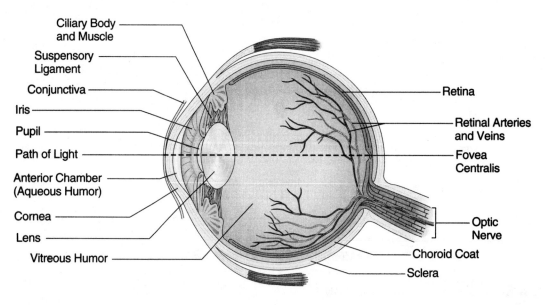

A-17 Internal structures of the eye

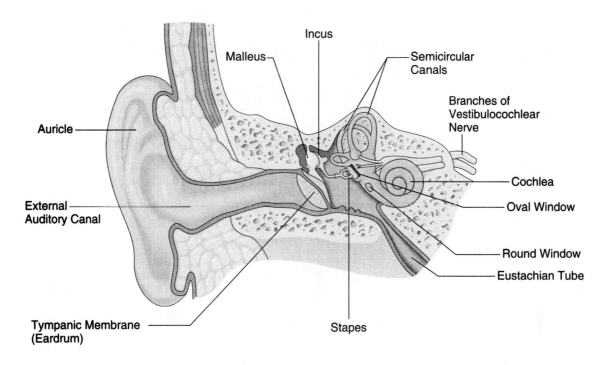

Incus

Malleus

Semicircular Canals

Branches of Vestibulocochlear Nerve

Auricle

Cochlea

Oval Window

External Auditory Canal

Round Window

Eustachian Tube

Tympanic Membrane (Eardrum)

Stapes

A-18 Internal structures of the ear

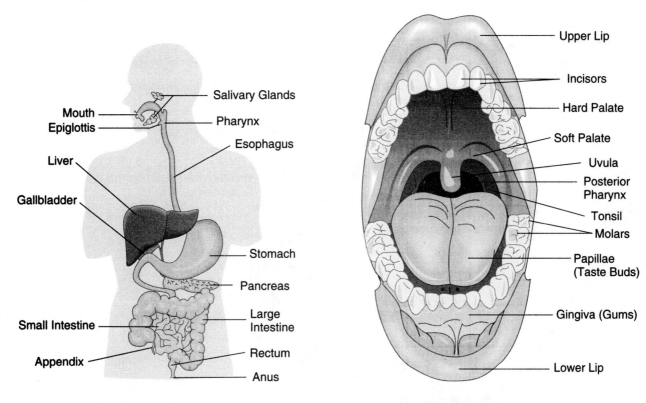

Salivary Glands

Mouth

Pharynx

Epiglottis

Esophagus

Liver

Gallbladder

Stomach

Pancreas

Small Intestine

Large Intestine

Appendix

Rectum

Anus

A-19A The digestive system

Upper Lip

Incisors

Hard Palate

Soft Palate

Uvula

Posterior Pharynx

Tonsil

Molars

Papillae (Taste Buds)

Gingiva (Gums)

Lower Lip

A-19B Structures of the mouth

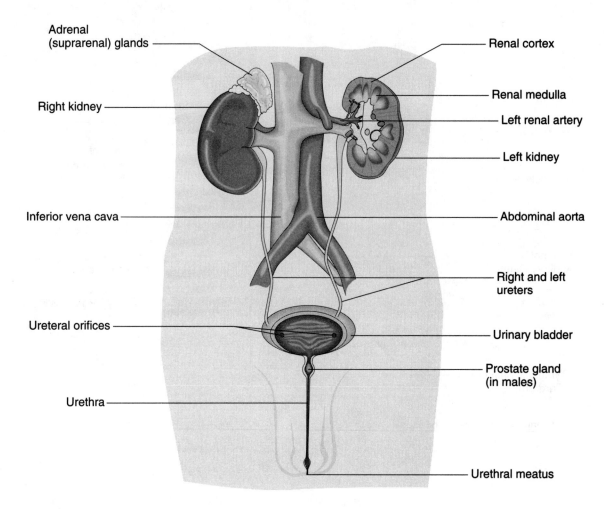

Adrenal (suprarenal) glands

Right kidney

Inferior vena cava

Ureteral orifices

Urethra

Renal cortex

Renal medulla

Left renal artery

Left kidney

Abdominal aorta

Right and left ureters

Urinary bladder

Prostate gland (in males)

Urethral meatus

A-20 The urinary system

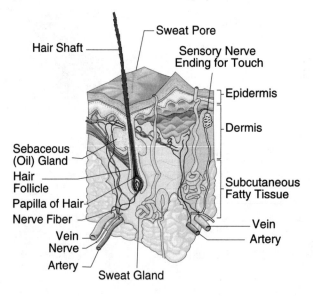

Hair Shaft

Sweat Pore

Sensory Nerve Ending for Touch

Epidermis

Dermis

Subcutaneous Fatty Tissue

Sebaceous (Oil) Gland

Hair Follicle

Papilla of Hair

Nerve Fiber

Vein

Nerve

Artery

Sweat Gland

Vein

Artery

A-21 Cross-section of the skin

A-22 The endocrine system

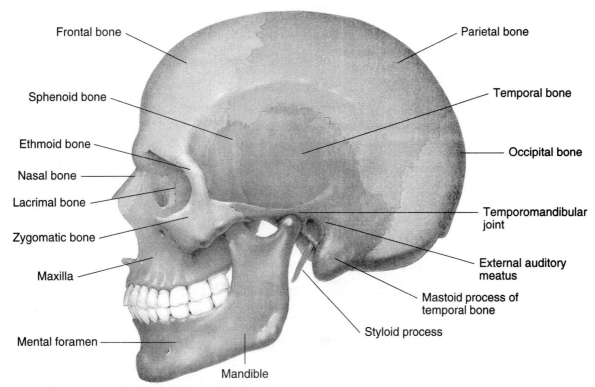

A-23 Bones of the skull

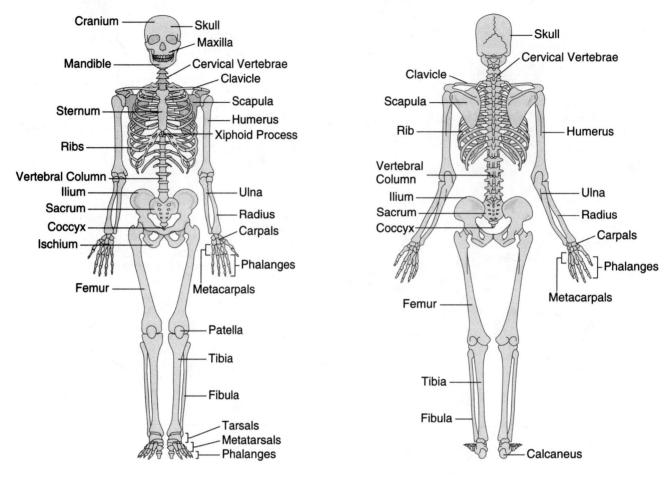

A-24 Major bones of the skeleton

A

A-25A Ball and socket joint

B

A-25B Hinge joints

C

A-25C Hinge joints

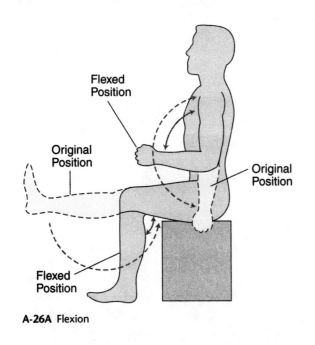

A-26A Flexion

- Flexed Position
- Original Position
- Original Position
- Flexed Position

A-26B Extension

- Original Position
- Extended Position
- Extended Position
- Original Position

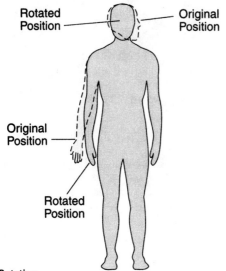

A-26C Rotation

- Rotated Position
- Original Position
- Original Position
- Rotated Position

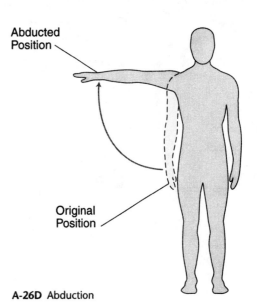

A-26D Abduction

- Abducted Position
- Original Position

A-26E Adduction

- Original Position
- Adducted Position

A-27A & B Major muscles of the body

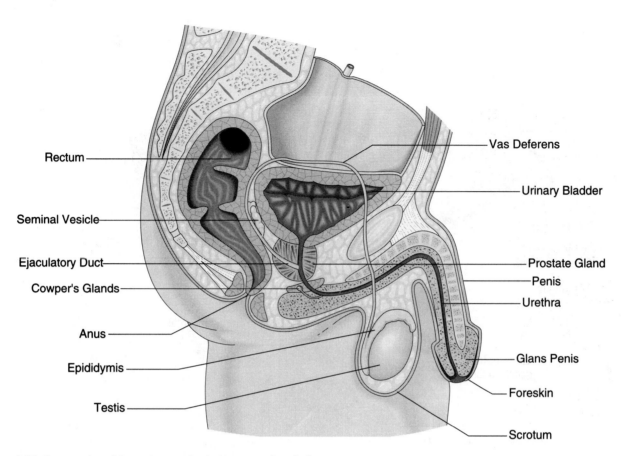

Rectum

Seminal Vesicle

Ejaculatory Duct

Cowper's Glands

Anus

Epididymis

Testis

Vas Deferens

Urinary Bladder

Prostate Gland

Penis

Urethra

Glans Penis

Foreskin

Scrotum

A-28 Cross-section of the male reproductive system and genitalia

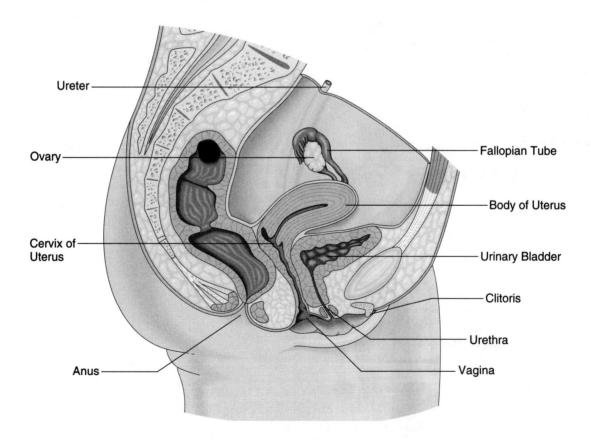

Ureter

Ovary

Cervix of
Uterus

Anus

Fallopian Tube

Body of Uterus

Urinary Bladder

Clitoris

Urethra

Vagina

A-29 Cross-section of the female reproductive system and genitalia

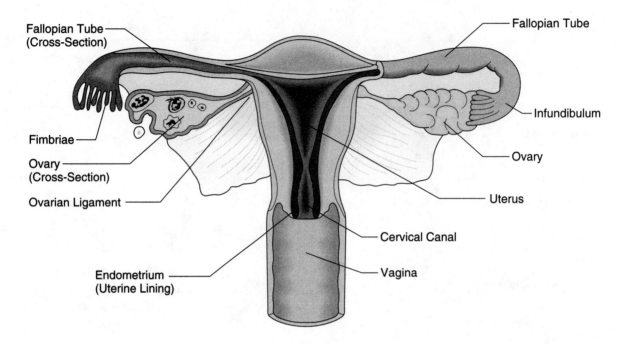

A-30 Internal female reproductive organs

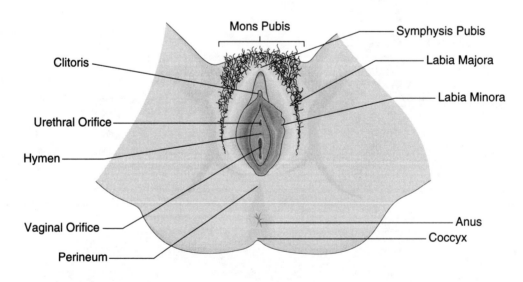

A-31 External female genitalia

Test-Taking Methods and Guidelines

As you know, the Nursing Home Reform Act was passed by Congress in 1987. It says that all people working as nursing assistants before July 1, 1989, must satisfactorily complete a competency evaluation program. Those employed after July 1, 1989, must first enroll in a nursing assistant training program and then successfully complete a competency exam. The competency exam is made up of written questions and performances. In some cases, an oral exam may be given instead of a written exam.

The 13 chapters in this training manual are designed to give the information and skills needed to complete the competency exam. We want you to become eligible for, or to continue, work as a nursing assistant. *We want you to be successful.*

The material covered in Appendix B will help you prepare for the written portion of the competency exam. No one was born knowing how to take a test. Your performance on an exam can be improved by learning some test-taking methods and guidelines. By learning what to expect and by developing test-taking skills, you will know more and be more confident when taking the exam.

THE TEST

Unexpected surprises can make you tense and confused. Avoid this by learning as much as possible about a test in advance.

Standardized Tests

The exam you will be taking is **standardized.** This means that it was planned and written in such a way that everyone who takes the exam will be tested fairly. A test becomes standardized after it has been used, revised, and used again until it shows consistent results. The purpose is to establish an average score on the exam. The average score, called a **norm,** allows the results of one person's performance to be compared with those of many others across the country who have taken the same test.

A standardized test must be given in the same way. The test examiner must follow the same plan, read the same directions, and give only certain kinds of help. The situation at all test sites should be as much alike as possible. Scoring is standardized also. Every answer is scored according to definite rules.

Overview of the Test

The content of the **Nursing Assistant Test** covers:
Physical care skills
- Activities of daily living
    - hygiene
    - dressing and grooming
    - nutrition and hydration
    - elimination
    - comfort, rest, and sleep

- Basic nursing skills
    - infection control
    - safety and emergency procedures
    - therapeutic and technical procedures such as bedmaking, specimen collection, and use of restraints
    - observation, data collection, and reporting

- Restorative skills
    - preventive health care, such as pressure ulcer and contracture prevention
    - promoting self-care and resident independence

Psychosocial care skills
- Emotional and mental health needs, including behavior management, needs of the dying resident, and sexuality needs

- Spiritual and cultural needs

Role of the nursing assistant

- Communication (includes verbal and nonverbal communication, listening, communicating with residents with various conditions)
- Resident rights
- Legal and ethical behavior
- Role and responsibilities of the nursing assistant as a member of the health care team

The test is made up of 50 to 75 multiple-choice questions that are given in a 90-minute time period. About one-third of the test is devoted to basic nursing skills.

The questions are not grouped by content area within the test booklet. Questions about basic nursing skills, for instance, appear throughout the test.

You will mark answers to test questions on the test booklet. A separate machine-readable information page is included to collect your name, sex, race, birth date, education level, work experience, and state of residence.

Multiple-Choice Format

Most standardized tests use multiple-choice items. This is because multiple-choice questions can measure a variety of learning outcomes, from simple to complex. They also provide the most consistent results. The multiple-choice item consists of a **stem,** which presents a problem situation, and four or five possible choices called **alternatives.** The alternatives include the correct answer and several wrong answers called **distractors.** The stem may be a question or an incomplete statement, as shown.

- Question form:

  Q. Which of the following people is responsible for taking care of a resident?

    Ⓐ janitor

    Ⓑ cook

    Ⓒ nurse aide

    Ⓓ dishwasher

- Incomplete-statement form:

  Q. The care of a resident is the responsibility of a

    Ⓐ janitor.

    Ⓑ cook.

    Ⓒ nurse aide.

    Ⓓ dishwasher.

Although worded differently, both stems present the same problem. The alternatives in the examples contain only one correct answer. All distractors are clearly incorrect.

Another type of multiple-choice item is the **best-answer** form. In this form, the alternatives are all partially correct. But one is clearly better than the others. Look at the following example.

- Best-answer form:

  Q. Which of the following ethical behaviors is the MOST important?

    Ⓐ Maintain a positive attitude.

    Ⓑ Act as a responsible employee.

    Ⓒ Be courteous to visitors.

    Ⓓ Promote quality of life for each resident.

Other variations of the best-answer form may ask you "what is the first thing to do," the "most helpful action," the "best response," or a similar kind of question. Whether the correct answer or best-answer form is used depends on the information given.

The examples use four alternatives. The chance of getting the correct answer by guessing is only one in four (25 percent).

MANAGING TEST ANXIETY

Test anxiety, or stress, is an emotional and physical response that the body makes to any demand made upon it. Stress may be good or bad. Its symptoms may be mild or severe. Mild stress may include feelings of anxiety, muscle tension, "butterflies" in the stomach, sweating, pounding of heart, dry mouth, and reduced ability to concentrate. You have probably had some of these feelings before.

Most stress, including test anxiety, does not last long. Once the stressful situation has passed, the symptoms disappear. You can learn to cope with test anxiety. The following guidelines will help you deal with test anxiety.

Understanding Stress

Two important characteristics to know about stress are that: (a) stress is normal, and (b) stress can be good. If you are anxious about taking a test, you are not alone. Almost everyone has some test anxiety. The person who does not feel anxious about taking a test is usually the abnormal one.

You may be surprised to learn that stress can be good. Studies have shown that mild stress is associated with improved performance in athletes, entertainers, public speakers, and yes, test-takers. Butterflies, breathing faster, sweating, and other symptoms are automatic bodily responses to stressful situations. Stress can sharpen your attention, keep you alert, and give you greater energy.

Controlling Negative Thoughts

Factors that increase test anxiety include negative thoughts and self-doubt. Perhaps you have thought such things as, "I am going to fail the exam," "I won't do well," or "What will my family and coworkers think when I don't pass?" You must stop thinking such thoughts. Instead, say to yourself, "I have done this job successfully for many years. I know what it takes to be a nurse assistant. I am prepared to take this exam." Think of the exam as a chance to show what you know and can do. Positive thinking comes before positive action and positive results.

Preparing Yourself Physically

Learning information and guidelines help you prepare mentally for an exam. Physical preparation is also important. Some stressful situations cannot be predicted. An exam, however, is known in advance. During the time before the exam, try not to schedule other stressful activities. Eat well and get plenty of rest. Combine studying with exercise and relaxation. Don't stay up late cramming the night before an exam. This is the time for reviewing studied material and getting a good night's sleep.

If you feel stressed during the period before the exam, try this deep-breathing method recommended by a stress management expert. Breathe deeply from your diaphragm. Do not move your chest and shoulders. You should feel your abdominal muscles expand as you breathe in and deflate when you breathe out. As you breathe out, your diaphragm and rib muscles relax, and your body may seem to sink down into the chair. Sixty seconds of deep breathing several times a day can help relieve stress.

GETTING READY FOR THE TEST

To prepare for a test, it is helpful to know whether it will contain **supply-type** or **selection-type** questions. Supply-type items are ones in which the test-taker supplies the answer. Essay and completion items are of this type. Selection-type items are ones in which the test-taker selects the answer from a number of possible answers. True-false, multiple-choice, and matching items are of this type. The exam you will take is a selection-type exam because it is made up of only multiple-choice questions. You must select the correct answer from four different choices.

Studying for a selection-type test is done differently than for a supply-type test. In studying for an essay exam (supply-type), you should be ready to explain major theories, principles, or ideas; look for ways to compare and contrast concepts; list pros and cons for important issues; and provide definitions of basic terms.

Whereas the essay test tends to measure one's ability to organize, integrate, and express ideas, the multiple-choice test more often measures word-for-word memory. The same subject matter should be studied for selection-type items as for supply-type items. But, for selection-type items, concentrate on learning specific facts and information.

Multiple-choice questions are used in standardized tests because they can be used to measure knowledge of facts and information as well as the application of facts and information. Knowledge items deal with such things as specific facts, common terms, methods and procedures, basic concepts and principles. Several examples of knowledge-level items follow.

Q. The most basic human need is for
   ① food.
   ② oxygen.
   ③ water.
   ④ elimination.

Q. Which of the following is NOT a psychological need?
   ① love
   ② belonging
   ③ exercise
   ④ identity

Application items measure a higher level of understanding. Here the test-taker must show that he or she not only understands the information but can also apply it to a situation. You must apply facts, concepts, principles, rules, methods, and theories to situations on the job. Following is an example of an application-level question.

Q. The self-actualization needs of a resident can be assisted by
   ① listening to the resident.
   ② calling the resident by name.
   ③ encouraging the resident to be independent.
   ④ praising accomplishments of the resident.

You should be prepared to answer both knowledge and application-level questions.

Studying and Reviewing

No matter what type of test you take, you must first learn the material. A good way to study for an exam is to use a system of index cards.

Obtain some 3 × 5 index cards or cut sheets of paper into a convenient size. On one side of the card, write the name of terms, methods and procedures, basic concepts and principles, and other specific facts. On the reverse side of the card, write the answer, definition, explanation, or whatever else is important. Here are several examples.

ethics	moral code that guides behavior of health care worker
Front	Back

Responsibilities of the nursing assistant	1. personal care of the resident 2. assisting with eating and hydration 3. care of the environment 4. infection control 5. observation and recording 6. assisting with movement, exercise, and ambulation 7. supporting resident's rights 8. assisting with mental and emotional needs
Front	Back

To study, look at the front of the card, and try to remember what is written on the back. Turn the card over to see whether you are correct. After going through all the cards once, shuffle them and review the cards again. You want to be sure you know the information in any order.

As you review the cards, begin to sort them into two piles. One pile will be those you know well and the other pile will be those you are having trouble remembering. Once you have two piles, try to learn the more difficult information. Continue reviewing the cards until you are sure you have learned the material. Review the cards several times a day during the time before the exam.

There are a number of advantages to using this system. First, preparing the cards is a learning experience. Second, the cards are easy to carry with you in a pocket or purse. You can study them during spare moments throughout the day. Another advantage is that you can use the cards with a friend to quiz each other.

Taking the Practice Test

Practicing what is required to get ready for a test is excellent preparation for taking an actual exam. Taking a practice test can get you used to the kinds of directions that are given, the types of questions you will be expected to answer, and the process of marking machine-readable test booklets. It can also help you learn your strengths and weaknesses.

Appendix C contains a practice test that you will take. Treat the practice test as a real test. The practice test will be given under conditions as similar as possible to the real test.

Practice working with time limits. Note specifically the average time it takes you to complete a question. If you work at a steady pace, you should have plenty of time to complete the exam in 90 minutes.

After finishing the practice test, you will have an opportunity to score it and discuss specific questions. Use this opportunity to ask questions about questions that you missed. Use the results of the practice test to identify those areas you need to study. The score does not indicate whether you will pass or fail the competency test. Different states use different passing scores.

TAKING THE TEST

To do well on a test, you should be at your best when you start. Eat a good breakfast or lunch. Try to avoid anything that will make you tense. Leave for the test site early enough to arrive on time. Be sure to allow for minor delays. Take a watch and two number two black lead pencils with erasers. Many states require you to bring an identification card with your picture on it to show the examiner. When you arrive, do not allow another person's last-minute questions or comments to disturb you. Follow these general rules for taking the test:

1. You will get verbal instructions before you take the test. You will complete an information page. Listen carefully to what the examiner tells you to

do. Remember that the examiner is required to read or give very specific directions. The rules and directions are designed to treat fairly everyone who takes the test.

2. Before the test begins, take a few seconds to pay attention. Close your eyes and take several deep breaths. Remind yourself that you have studied well. Think positive.

3. Once you get the test and are told to begin, carefully read the directions. Look at any sample questions. Make sure that you understand how to mark answers on the test booklet or answer sheet. The test probably will be machine-scored, so be careful in recording answers.

4. You will have 60 to 90 minutes to answer 50 to 75 questions. This is a very generous amount of time. If you work at a steady pace you should have no problem finishing the test on time. Pause to check time and make sure that you are working at about the right speed. The examiner will post the time remaining.

5. Read the stem of the question and answer it in your own words without looking at the choices or alternatives. Then search for the alternative that matches your answer. Always read all of the alternatives. Answer "A" may be right, but answer "C" may be a better answer.

6. Some questions may ask you to analyze a situation or use what you have learned to solve a problem. If you do not know the answer immediately, it is often helpful to cross out unnecessary information. Distracting or extra information has been crossed out in the following example.

Q. A resident ~~who~~ wears a wig ~~understands that the nurse aide will not talk about this information outside the facility~~ because this information is

① legal.
② confidential.
③ negligent.
④ cultural.

7. If you do not know an answer, circle the question and move on. You can come back to it later. This will save you time and help prevent the anxiety that comes from trying to remember. More importantly, you may find a clue to the answer somewhere in a later question.

8. If you encounter a very difficult question, do not worry. The rest of the test-takers will probably have trouble with it also. Keep in mind that a perfect score is not expected on a standardized test.

9. Be alert to such words as *not* and *except* that can completely change the intent of the question. Words in the stem are often *italicized*, CAPITALIZED, or are within "quotation marks" or (parentheses). Pay attention to such words. They are usually important to answering the question.

10. Standardized tests are revised several times so that the questions are clearly worded. Do not read more into a question than is asked for. Do not look for trick questions or hidden meanings. If a question seems unclear, read it several times. Pay close attention to how it is worded. Try to relate the question to information and tasks with which you are familiar.

11. Avoid unfamiliar choices or alternatives. An alternative that you do not know, uses difficult words, or seems complicated is probably incorrect.

12. If you do not know an answer, try to determine what the answer is *not*. Begin by crossing out alternatives that you know or feel are incorrect. If you can cross out two choices, you now have a 50% chance of choosing the correct answer of the remaining two alternatives.

13. Your score on the exam will be based on the number of questions answered correctly. So, be sure and answer all questions. There is no penalty for guessing. This means that for those items that have you completely stumped, you should go ahead and guess. First, however, try to cross out choices that seem wrong.

14. As you near the end of the test, do not worry if some individuals have finished already. Studies have shown that those who complete a test early do not necessarily get better scores than those who finish later.

15. When you get to the end of the test, go back and complete those items that you skipped earlier. You may remember the answer or be able to narrow down the answer.

16. If you answer all of the questions and still have time remaining, review your answers. After rereading a question, you may have second thoughts about the answer. Should you change it? For those who have studied well for an exam, research shows that more of them are helped than hurt by changing answers. Do not change answers without a good reason. But go ahead and change any answers that are based on new insights or recall of new information.

17. Before turning in the test, review how you marked the answers. Check to see that you answered every question, that you marked only one answer per question, that you marked the

answer neatly and legibly, and that you completely erased any changes that were made. Erase any other marks you may have made on the test booklet.

THE SKILLS EXAMINATION

Part of the state test you will take is a skills examination or competency evaluation. This examination is administered differently in each state. Usually, a nurse who has no affiliation with your training program will administer the examination. You will be tested on the number of skills required by your state. The pass and fail criteria are also determined by your state. In some states, testing is done in a skills laboratory setting. In other states, testing is done on residents of a nursing facility.

Preparing for the Skills Examination

The only way to adequately prepare for the skills examination is to practice the procedures in sequence. The skills that you will be tested on are randomly chosen from the procedures you learned in class. If your nursing assistant program has a review day or a mock skills examination before you take the test, be sure to attend. This will be very helpful to you in preparing for the test. You should also review your vocabulary terms so that you are familiar with the various names of the procedures. For example, the skills examiner may direct you to "ambulate the resident." From your review of the vocabulary, you know that *ambulate* means *to walk*. When reviewing the procedures, pay attention to the list of equipment and supplies that you will need to gather before you perform the procedure.

There is no way to study for the skills examination except by practicing the procedures you have learned in class. The skills examiner will watch for some things during the examination. Some of these observations are very important and may be the deciding factor on whether you pass or fail a particular skill on the examination.

Observations Made During the Skills Examination

- The skills examiner will observe **handwashing.** He will look at your handwashing technique to be sure that you follow the accepted procedure. The examiner will also observe how often you wash your hands and if you wear gloves when necessary. The examiner may observe how and where you dispose of the gloves.
- You will be observed in how well you **communicate** with the resident. You must introduce

yourself and the skills examiner. Explain what you are going to do, even if the resident is confused. You may also be evaluated on whether you talk to the resident while you are performing the procedure.

- The skills examiner will observe how well you practice **safety.** For example, do you put the side rails up on the bed when you are not directly next to it? Do you lock the brakes on the wheelchair before you transfer the resident?
- **Infection control** is another area on which you are evaluated. The skills examiner will observe whether you keep clean items separated from dirty ones, and how well you practice medical asepsis.
- **Practicing resident rights is important.** Be sure to knock on doors. Use the bath blanket during the bathing procedure. Pull the privacy curtain, close the window curtains, and close the door to the room.

Gather all of the supplies you will need before you take each section of the skills test. If you will be making a bed, stack the linen in the order of use. The test will go more smoothly for you if you are well organized.

If your state uses skills checklists that note the automatic failures on the skills examination, pay close attention to them. For example, in many states if you fail to balance the scale before you weigh the resident, you will fail this skill. If you are assigned to do peri care on a female, and you wash the resident from **back to front,** you will fail the skill. If this information is available in your nursing assistant program, it will be very helpful to you. The automatic failure points on the skills examination are things that could potentially cause harm to a resident, so studying them will do more than help you pass the test. Knowing these things will help you feel more secure that you are providing quality care when you are working with your assigned residents!

AFTER THE TEST

When time is called, you can breathe a sigh of relief. Listen carefully, however, to instructions about what to do with the test booklet. Information may also be given about when and how you will find out the results. The examiner may not be allowed to give you the answers to test questions.

You may have to wait several weeks before you receive the test results. During this time, try not to worry. People tend to underestimate their performance on an exam. Thousands of people will take this exam. Be confident that you probably will score as well as or better than most of them.

Practice Exam

Choose the best answer for the following questions.

1. The moral code that guides the behavior of the health care worker is called
   - (A) etiquette.
   - (B) ethics.
   - (C) care plan.
   - (D) dignity.

2. When communicating with the resident who is hearing-impaired, it is important to
   - (A) gently touch the resident to get his or her attention.
   - (B) face the resident when talking.
   - (C) identify yourself to the resident.
   - (D) all of the above.

3. When you position a resident in lateral position, you will use pillows to support
   - (A) the lower arm.
   - (B) the upper arm.
   - (C) the lower leg.
   - (D) the upper arm and leg.

4. Which of the following is a developmental task of the elderly resident?
   - (A) increased social involvement
   - (B) adjusting to losses
   - (C) having a second career
   - (D) adjusting to middle age

5. Which of the following would be considered an example of a pressure-relieving device?
   - (A) quad cane
   - (B) walker
   - (C) gel mattress
   - (D) pulley

6. Before replacing dentures into a resident's mouth,
   - (A) apply gloves.
   - (B) rinse the dentures with mouthwash.
   - (C) store dentures in denture cup.
   - (D) floss the resident's teeth.

7. The electronic thermometer can be used for taking what kind of temperature?
   - (A) oral temperatures only
   - (B) oral and axillary
   - (C) oral and rectal
   - (D) oral, rectal, and axillary

8. When you have completed colostomy care for a resident, you will record any output as
   - (A) urinary output.
   - (B) a bowel movement.
   - (C) an emesis.
   - (D) homeostasis.

9. To properly give a bed bath,
   - (A) cover the resident and bathe the entire body one part at a time.
   - (B) uncover the resident, bathe the entire body, then cover again.
   - (C) cover the resident and bathe face, hands, underarms, back, and genital area, one part at a time.
   - (D) cover the resident and take him or her to the shower in a shower chair.

10. When personal mail is sent to a long-term care facility, who has the right to open it first?
    - (A) administrator
    - (B) director of nurses
    - (C) resident
    - (D) state inspectors

11. Mrs. Smith is an ambulatory resident. It would be most appropriate in a long-term care facility for her to have lunch in
    - (A) her bed.
    - (B) her room.
    - (C) the dining room.
    - (D) the lobby.

12. The nursing assistant is responsible for:
    - (A) cutting the fingernails and toenails of all residents.
    - (B) keeping the fingernails and toenails of residents clean.
    - (C) filing the toenails with a nail file to round the edges.
    - (D) all of the above.

13. When you are washing your hands, what part of the procedure removes the most germs?
    - Ⓐ using warm, running water
    - Ⓑ shaking water off your hands
    - Ⓒ using friction while washing your hands
    - Ⓓ drying hands thoroughly

14. Safety of the resident is the responsibility of
    - Ⓐ the nurse in charge.
    - Ⓑ the nursing assistant.
    - Ⓒ the maintenance staff.
    - Ⓓ all of the above.

15. In order for a fire to occur, there must be a spark or flame, oxygen, and material that will burn. In most fire situations, where would the oxygen come from?
    - Ⓐ oxygen tanks
    - Ⓑ the air itself
    - Ⓒ the air conditioning
    - Ⓓ the heating system

16. Why is it important to explain lifting procedures to residents before you do them?
    - Ⓐ to be polite
    - Ⓑ to enlist their cooperation and help
    - Ⓒ to prevent any arguments
    - Ⓓ to provide communication

17. When removing soiled linen from the bed,
    - Ⓐ shake linen gently to find lost items.
    - Ⓑ roll it into a ball and place it on the floor.
    - Ⓒ place the linen into the hamper.
    - Ⓓ all of the above.

18. A resident is waving one arm wildly, grabbing at the throat area and coughing. Your best response is to
    - Ⓐ get him a drink of water.
    - Ⓑ give him oxygen by mask immediately.
    - Ⓒ stay in the room and allow him to continue coughing.
    - Ⓓ slap his back four times firmly.

19. The charge nurse asks you to check vital signs on Mrs. Jones. You will check her
    - Ⓐ blood pressure and pulse.
    - Ⓑ temperature and pulse.
    - Ⓒ temperature, pulse, and respirations.
    - Ⓓ blood pressure, temperature, pulse, and respirations.

20. When a resident with a paralyzed side wants to brush his own teeth, you should
    - Ⓐ brush his teeth for him anyway.
    - Ⓑ set out the supplies and allow him to do it.
    - Ⓒ explain that you are happy to help him and do it for him.
    - Ⓓ guide his toothbrush through the procedure.

21. Pressure ulcers are:
    - Ⓐ prevented by good skin care.
    - Ⓑ caused by pressure.
    - Ⓒ also called bedsores.
    - Ⓓ all of the above.

22. When communicating with a resident who has a hearing impairment, you should:
    - Ⓐ yell loudly in the resident's ear.
    - Ⓑ place a bright light behind your back so the resident can see you.
    - Ⓒ speak slowly and clearly.
    - Ⓓ always use sign language.

23. The correct positioning of the resident's body is called
    - Ⓐ muscle development.
    - Ⓑ body mechanics.
    - Ⓒ body alignment.
    - Ⓓ adaptive positioning.

24. What kind of problems exist for a resident who needs elastic stockings (TED hose)?
    - Ⓐ musculoskeletal
    - Ⓑ respiratory
    - Ⓒ circulatory
    - Ⓓ digestive

25. The nurse tells you to ambulate Mrs. Black in Room 202. This means to
    - Ⓐ sit her in the wheelchair.
    - Ⓑ sit her on the edge of the bed.
    - Ⓒ assist her to the bathroom.
    - Ⓓ walk the resident.

26. To properly wash the eyes while giving a bed bath, you would
    - Ⓐ wipe from outer side of eye to inner side.
    - Ⓑ wipe from inner side of eye to outer side.
    - Ⓒ use a back-and-forth motion.
    - Ⓓ use plenty of soap and water.

27. An example of meeting the spiritual needs of a resident would be to assist with
    - Ⓐ eating supper.
    - Ⓑ going to sleep.
    - Ⓒ saying prayers.
    - Ⓓ getting dressed.

28. Microorganisms are completely destroyed by
    - Ⓐ sterilization.
    - Ⓑ handwashing.
    - Ⓒ disinfection.
    - Ⓓ medical asepsis.

29. When you find a resident who appears to have fallen on the floor, your first action is
    - Ⓐ run to get help.
    - Ⓑ put the resident in bed.
    - Ⓒ stay with the resident.
    - Ⓓ call the paramedics.

30. The skin of the elderly resident becomes
    - Ⓐ thicker.
    - Ⓑ fatter.
    - Ⓒ thinner.
    - Ⓓ brittle.

31. Standard equipment in the resident's unit is the
    - Ⓐ television, electric bed, and telephone.
    - Ⓑ wheelchair, stretcher, and mechanical lift.
    - Ⓒ hopper, sink, table, and work counter.
    - Ⓓ bedside stand, bed, chair, and overbed table

32. Your resident's care plan states to check BP q.i.d. This means to check the blood pressure
    - Ⓐ every day.
    - Ⓑ four times a day.
    - Ⓒ every other day.
    - Ⓓ six times a day.

33. You have taken a resident's rectal temperature and the thermometer reads 100 degrees. From your knowledge about body temperature, the oral temperature on this resident is
    - Ⓐ 101.
    - Ⓑ 99.
    - Ⓒ 98.
    - Ⓓ 97.

34. Mrs. Gree is a 70-year-old resident who has been on bed rest with pneumonia for three days. You note a reddened area on her back. Your response is to
    - Ⓐ encourage her to get up and move about.
    - Ⓑ apply a dressing to the area.
    - Ⓒ massage the area with lotion.
    - Ⓓ report the area to the nurse.

35. If you are assisting a resident with ADLs, you are helping with
    - Ⓐ activities of daily living.
    - Ⓑ activities during leisure.
    - Ⓒ proper alignment.
    - Ⓓ AM care.

36. When residents are helpless and lie in one position for too long, there is a risk of developing
    - Ⓐ contractures.
    - Ⓑ atrophy.
    - Ⓒ bedsores.
    - Ⓓ all of the above.

37. When you take a resident's pulse, you are using a/an
    - Ⓐ artery.
    - Ⓑ vein.
    - Ⓒ capillary.
    - Ⓓ all of the above.

38. After completing the care for a resident who required isolation procedures, what is your *first* step in removing your gown, gloves, and mask?

Ⓐ Remove mask, touching only ties.
Ⓑ Untie waist ties and tie in front of gown.
Ⓒ Untie neck ties and loosen gown at shoulders.
Ⓓ Grasp cuff of glove and pull off.

39. The strongest muscles you should use for lifting are in your
    - Ⓐ buttocks.
    - Ⓑ thighs.
    - Ⓒ back.
    - Ⓓ abdomen.

40. Restraints require a doctor's order and must be released every
    - Ⓐ half-hour.
    - Ⓑ hour.
    - Ⓒ two hours.
    - Ⓓ four hours.

41. When residents are admitted to a long-term care facility, they
    - Ⓐ no longer have the right to vote.
    - Ⓑ can continue to vote in elections.
    - Ⓒ cannot leave the facility.
    - Ⓓ can keep medicine on the overbed table.

42. Exposing a resident unnecessarily would be a threat to the right to
    - Ⓐ privacy.
    - Ⓑ security.
    - Ⓒ acceptance.
    - Ⓓ belonging.

43. Basic human needs are
    - Ⓐ different for each person.
    - Ⓑ varied in men and women.
    - Ⓒ the same for all people.
    - Ⓓ different, depending on age.

44. When a resident has a need for recognition, you can easily provide this by
    - Ⓐ calling the resident by name.
    - Ⓑ explaining procedures.
    - Ⓒ providing privacy.
    - Ⓓ turning on the television.

45. A resident who frequently wanders at night, becomes easily agitated, and cannot be calmed down is displaying symptoms of
    - Ⓐ mental retardation.
    - Ⓑ multiple sclerosis.
    - Ⓒ Alzheimer's disease.
    - Ⓓ delusions.

46. When giving a bed bath, always obtain clean bathwater after washing the
    - Ⓐ abdomen.
    - Ⓑ legs and feet.
    - Ⓒ armpits.
    - Ⓓ face.

47. An example of an adaptive device to help a resident in dressing and grooming tasks would be a
    Ⓐ handroll.
    Ⓑ transfer belt.
    Ⓒ long-handled shoe horn.
    Ⓓ four-pronged cane.

48. Mr. Brown's TPR is 96.8-104-30. Which, if any, are normal?
    Ⓐ temperature
    Ⓑ pulse
    Ⓒ respirations
    Ⓓ none are normal

49. Who is responsible for balancing the scale before taking a resident's weight?
    Ⓐ charge nurse
    Ⓑ nursing assistant
    Ⓒ maintenance staff
    Ⓓ administrator

50. An occupied bed is made with the
    Ⓐ resident in a chair.
    Ⓑ assistance of the nurse.
    Ⓒ resident in the bed.
    Ⓓ resident out of the room.

51. The food pyramid should be used to:
    Ⓐ plan the diet for residents who are receiving tube feedings.
    Ⓑ plan your meals each day.
    Ⓒ calculate the resident's height and weight.
    Ⓓ all of the above.

52. The term *edema* means
    Ⓐ abnormal swelling in the tissues.
    Ⓑ loss of fluid from the tissues.
    Ⓒ instilling fluid into the rectum.
    Ⓓ the same as dehydration.

53. When counting a resident's pulse, you notice it is weak and irregular. Proper technique would be to count
    Ⓐ for one full minute, report it to the nurse and record.
    Ⓑ for 30 seconds, double that number, and record.
    Ⓒ for 15 seconds, multiply by 4, and record.
    Ⓓ the pulse in two separate locations.

54. One of your residents wants to see the chaplain immediately, but the chaplain has left for the day. What should you do?
    Ⓐ Ignore the request. The chaplain will be back tomorrow.
    Ⓑ Tell the resident the chaplain has left for the day.
    Ⓒ Ask the resident, "Why do you want to see him?"
    Ⓓ Refer the request to the nurse in charge.

55. The charge nurse reports to you that Mrs. White has high blood pressure. Another word for this is
    Ⓐ hypotension.
    Ⓑ systolic.
    Ⓒ hypertension.
    Ⓓ diastolic.

56. When you logroll a resident, before placing him on a bedpan, place your hands on the resident's
    Ⓐ shoulder and hip.
    Ⓑ waist and hip.
    Ⓒ hip and leg.
    Ⓓ arm and leg.

57. When you take a resident's blood pressure, you are measuring
    Ⓐ the volume of blood.
    Ⓑ the force of the heart.
    Ⓒ how fast the heart is beating.
    Ⓓ the rhythm of the pulse.

58. It is important for the nursing assistant to know that the skin of the geriatric resident produces
    Ⓐ more oil.
    Ⓑ less oil.
    Ⓒ no oil.
    Ⓓ none of the above.

59. When a resident has an ongoing like or dislike for certain foods, it may be because of
    Ⓐ the surroundings in which it is served.
    Ⓑ your influence on the resident.
    Ⓒ family customs and cultural influence.
    Ⓓ a decrease in appetite.

60. You are assigned to take blood pressures on four residents. Mr. Keeley is the second resident you have taken vital signs on. Mr. Keeley's vital signs are: T 98.2, P 96, R 18, B/P 202/126. You should:
    Ⓐ finish taking the vital signs on the other residents you are assigned to.
    Ⓑ go to the nurses' station and record Mr. Keeley's vital signs in the chart.
    Ⓒ notify the nurse of Mr. Keeley's abnormal pulse rate.
    Ⓓ notify the nurse of Mr. Keeley's blood pressure.

61. During Mrs. Smith's bath, you observe that her face is very flushed and her skin feels warm to the touch. The best way to report this to the team leader is
    Ⓐ "Mrs. Smith has a fever."
    Ⓑ "I think Mrs. Smith is getting sick."
    Ⓒ "You should take Mrs. Smith's temperature."
    Ⓓ "Mrs. Smith's face is flushed and her skin feels warm."

62. Effective communication is a very important part of your job as a nursing assistant. When you smile at a resident, what kind of communication are you using?
    (A) sign language
    (B) body language
    (C) oral communication
    (D) verbal communication

63. "STAT" means
    (A) as desired.
    (B) as necessary.
    (C) at once.
    (D) at mealtime.

64. When a resident is on I&O, you will do your recording as
    (A) ounces.
    (B) cups
    (C) cubic centimeters.
    (D) centigrade.

65. When you sit a resident up on the edge of the bed and the resident becomes dizzy, your best action is to
    (A) sit the resident in the chair.
    (B) lay the resident down and call the nurse.
    (C) tell the resident it will be okay in a few minutes.
    (D) put the resident into a wheelchair and take her to the nurse.

66. The extent a person is capable of moving a joint is called
    (A) flexibility.
    (B) contractures.
    (C) restoration.
    (D) range of motion.

67. When a resident has died and you are doing postmortem care, the right to privacy is
    (A) no longer necessary.
    (B) still protected after death.
    (C) only for the family.
    (D) all of the above.

68. When you assist residents to get ready for mealtime, you would also include checking their
    (A) weight.
    (B) blood pressure.
    (C) need to use the toilet.
    (D) need to say grace.

69. If a resident leaves 1/4 of an 8-ounce glass of milk on the tray, how much would you record as taken?
    (A) 60 cc.
    (B) 120 cc.
    (C) 180 cc.
    (D) 240 cc.

70. Mrs. Smith's blood pressure is 142/88. You will record the systolic reading as
    (A) 230.
    (B) 142.
    (C) 88.
    (D) 54.

71. Mr. Jones, a bedridden resident, states he has to move his bowels. You would help him use the
    (A) bedpan.
    (B) urinal.
    (C) urinary bag.
    (D) colostomy bag.

72. When you communicate to residents in a therapeutic manner called "therapeutic communication," what specifically are you doing?
    (A) preparing them for a visit from their doctor
    (B) healing or improving an existing situation
    (C) planning to take them to physical therapy
    (D) encouraging them to get involved in activities

73. Helping residents reach their highest level of ability is the goal of
    (A) range of motion.
    (B) disease prevention.
    (C) rehabilitation.
    (D) contractures.

74. A good ethical practice as a nursing assistant would be to
    (A) share your problems with the resident.
    (B) use care with the resident's belongings.
    (C) discuss the resident's condition at break.
    (D) borrow items from the resident's dresser.

75. To properly practice what you have been taught about standard precautions, it is best to
    (A) always wear a mask.
    (B) dispose of trash first.
    (C) scrub your hands with a brush.
    (D) carry gloves at all times.

ANSWERS TO PRACTICE EXAM

1. B	11. C	21. D	31. D	41. B	51. B	61. D	71. A
2. D	12. B	22. C	32. B	42. A	52. A	62. B	72. B
3. D	13. C	23. C	33. B	43. C	53. A	63. C	73. C
4. B	14. D	24. C	34. D	44. A	54. D	64. C	74. B
5. C	15. B	25. D	35. A	45. C	55. C	65. B	75. D
6. A	16. B	26. B	36. D	46. B	56. A	66. D	
7. D	17. C	27. C	37. A	47. C	57. B	67. B	
8. B	18. C	28. A	38. B	48. D	58. B	68. C	
9. A	19. D	29. C	39. B	49. B	59. C	69. C	
10. C	20. B	30. C	40. C	50. C	60. D	70. B	

Procedure Review

PERFORMANCE REVIEW CHECKLIST

Procedure ___1___

Procedure <u>Postmortem Care</u>

Name of Nurse Aide _____Date of Program _____ to _____

Social Security Number of Nurse Aide _____

Program Code Number _____

S=Satisfactory Performance
U=Unsatisfactory Performance

Place a full signature to correspond with each set of initials appearing below:

Initials	Corresponding Signature of Instructor	Title

Procedure Guidelines	S/U	Date	Initials	S/U	Date	Initials
1. Wash your hands.						
2. Gather supplies: shroud kit with gown and identification tags, a basin of warm water, soap, washcloth, towels, swabs for oral care, linen, gown, and gloves.						
3. Pull the curtains and close the door for privacy.						
4. Treat the body gently and with respect.						

(continues)

continued

5.	Apply gloves.						
6.	Raise the bed to a comfortable working height.						
7.	Place the resident on her back, with a pillow beneath the head and shoulders in proper body alignment.						
8.	Close the eyes by gently pulling eyelids down.						
9.	Provide mouth care using moistened oral care swabs or sponges.						
10.	Place cleaned dentures in the mouth or in a labeled denture cup. The dentures should be sent to the funeral home with the body.						
11.	Close the mouth. A rolled-up washcloth may be placed under the chin to keep the jaw closed.						
12.	Remove all tubing from the body if this is your facility policy. In most facilities this is done by the nurse.						
13.	Bathe the body, comb hair, and straighten the arms and legs.						
14.	Apply clean dressings to wounds, if necessary.						
15.	Place a disposable pad under the buttocks.						
16.	Put a gown on the body.						
17.	Attach an identification tag to the body if indicated by facility policy.						
18.	Replace soiled linen and cover the body to the shoulders with a sheet.						
19.	Remove gloves and dispose according to facility policy.						
20.	Wash your hands.						
21.	Tidy the unit.						
22.	Wash your hands.						
23.	Provide privacy and allow family members to be alone with the resident.						
24.	Collect all belongings, place them in a bag, and label them correctly. Usually these are given to the family. If no family members are present,						

(continues)

continued

follow facility policy. Complete and sign the inventory sheet if this is your facility policy.						
25. After the family leaves, wash your hands and put the shroud on the body. Wear gloves if contact with blood, body fluid, secretions, or excretions is likely.						
26. Remove gloves, if worn, and dispose according to facility policy.						
27. Follow facility policy to take the body to the morgue, or close the door until the funeral home staff arrives.						
28. Notify the nurse when the funeral home staff arrives.						
29. Assist the funeral home staff to move the body if necessary.						
30. Strip and clean the unit according to your facility policy after the body has been removed.						

PERFORMANCE REVIEW CHECKLIST

Procedure ___2___

Procedure <u>Handwashing</u>

Name of Nurse Aide _____ Date of Program _____ to _____

Social Security Number of Nurse Aide _____

Program Code Number _____

S=Satisfactory Performance
U=Unsatisfactory Performance

Place a full signature to correspond with each set of initials appearing below:

Initials	Corresponding Signature of Instructor	Title

	Procedure Guidelines	S/U	Date	Initials	S/U	Date	Initials
1.	Stand away from the sink. Your uniform and hands must not touch the sink.						
2.	Turn on warm water with a dry paper towel. Adjust water to a comfortable temperature.						
3.	Wet hands, keeping your fingertips pointed down.						
4.	Apply soap over hands and wrists, working it into a lather.						
5.	Rub your hands together vigorously to create a lather. Rub the hands together in a circular motion for 10 to 15 seconds. Rub all surfaces of the hands. Pay particular attention to the area between your fingers. Keep your fingertips pointed down.						
6.	Rub the fingernails against the palm of the opposite hand. Clean the nails with a brush or an orange stick if they are soiled.						
7.	Rinse your hands from the wrist to the fingertips. Keep the fingers pointed down.						
8.	Do not shake water from hands.						

(continues)

continued

9.	Dry hands with a clean paper towel. Discard paper towel properly.						
10.	Use a clean, dry paper towel to turn off the faucet. Do not touch the faucet handle with your hand.						
11.	Discard the paper towel in the wastebasket.						

PERFORMANCE REVIEW CHECKLIST

Procedure ___3–4___

Procedure <u>Isolation Procedures</u>

Name of Nurse Aide _____Date of Program _____ to _____

Social Security Number of Nurse Aide _____

Program Code Number _____

S=Satisfactory Performance
U=Unsatisfactory Performance

Place a full signature to correspond with each set of initials appearing below:

Initials	Corresponding Signature of Instructor	Title

Procedure Guidelines	S/U	Date	Initials	S/U	Date	Initials
Putting on disposable gown, gloves, and mask						
1. Remove your watch and place it on a clean paper towel. You will carry your watch with you into the isolation room on the paper towel.						
2. Wash your hands and dry them thoroughly.						
3. Put a mask on, and adjust it over your nose and mouth. Tie the mask securely at the back of your head, or slip the elastic straps over your ears.						
4. Put on a gown.						
5. Tie the neck ties.						
6. Tie the waist ties of the gown, making certain the gown is overlapping and covering your uniform.						
7. Put on gloves, covering the cuffs of the gown with the top edge of the glove.						
Removing disposable gown, gloves, and mask						
1. Make sure that all jobs in the isolation unit are complete and that the resident is comfortable and safe. Place needed personal items and the call signal within the resident's reach.						

(continues)

continued

2.	Remove gloves by turning them inside out and dispose of them in the biohazardous waste receptacle.						
3.	Untie the waist ties of the gown.						
4.	Using a clean paper towel, turn on the faucet. Wash and dry your hands. Turn off the faucet with a clean paper towel.						
5.	Remove the mask by grasping only the ties. Untie the bottom tie first, then the top tie, or slip the elastic straps over your ears.						
6.	Discard the mask in the covered trash container.						
7.	Untie the neck ties of the gown and loosen the gown at the shoulders.						
8.	Slip the fingers of one hand under the cuff of the gown on the opposite arm. Do not touch the outside of the gown. Pull it down over your hand.						
9.	With your hand inside the gown, pull the gown off the other arm.						
10.	Fold and roll the gown away from your body, with the contaminated side facing in.						
11.	Dispose of the gown in the covered biohazardous waste container.						
12.	Remove a clean paper towel to turn on the faucet. Wash and dry your hands. Turn off the faucet with a clean paper towel.						
13.	Pick up your watch and put it on your wrist.						
14.	Holding the clean upper side of the paper towel, pick up the towel and discard it in the trash.						
15.	Obtain a clean paper towel from the dispenser and use it to open the door of the room.						
16.	Discard the towel inside the room.						
17.	Repeat handwashing if this is your preference or facility policy.						

PERFORMANCE REVIEW CHECKLIST

Procedure ___5___

Procedure <u>Applying a Vest Restraint</u>

Name of Nurse Aide _____Date of Program _____ to _____

Social Security Number of Nurse Aide _____

Program Code Number _____

S=Satisfactory Performance
U=Unsatisfactory Performance

Place a full signature to correspond with each set of initials appearing below:

Initials	Corresponding Signature of Instructor	Title

Procedure Guidelines	S/U	Date	Initials	S/U	Date	Initials
1. Obtain a restraint of the proper type and size.						
2. Get help if necessary.						
3. Perform your beginning procedure actions.						
4. Slip the resident's arms through the armholes of the vest.						
5. Make sure that the clothing under the restraint is not wrinkled and that the vest fits smoothly.						
6. Cross the vest in the front and thread the straps through the slots on the sides of the vest. If a vest is used on a female resident, be sure that the breasts are not under the straps.						

(continues)

continued

7.	Thread the straps **between** the seat and the armrest if the resident is in a wheelchair. Pull the straps back securely. If the resident is in bed, attach the straps to the moveable part of the bed frame. Follow your facility policy for the type of beds used. Many different types of beds are used in health care facilities. (This way, if the bed is raised, the resident will not be restricted or strangled by the restraint.)						
8.	Finish tying the restraint in a slip knot under the chair or to the bed frame. Refer to the specific manufacturer's directions for the restraint you are using.						
9.	Insert three fingers under the restraint and check to be sure that it is not too tight.						
10.	Perform your procedure completion actions.						

PERFORMANCE REVIEW CHECKLIST

Procedure __6__

Procedure <u>Applying a Belt Restraint</u>

Name of Nurse Aide _____ Date of Program _____ to _____

Social Security Number of Nurse Aide _____

Program Code Number _____

S=Satisfactory Performance
U=Unsatisfactory Performance

Place a full signature to correspond with each set of initials appearing below:

Initials	Corresponding Signature of Instructor	Title

	Procedure Guidelines	S/U	Date	Initials	S/U	Date	Initials
1.	Perform your beginning procedure actions.						
2.	Get help from another nursing assistant, if necessary.						
3.	If the resident is in a wheelchair, move the hips as far back as possible, position the footrests to support the feet, and lock the brakes.						
4.	Place the belt around the waist. Cross the straps through the loops behind the resident.						
5.	After the straps are threaded through the loops, tighten the belt securely around the waist.						
6.	Insert the straps between the seat and armrest, or between the seat and backrest, according to the manufacturer's recommendations for the type of restraint you are using.						

(continues)

continued

7.	Bring the straps down and tie them to the kickspurs of the wheelchair, using a quick-release knot, according to the manufacturer's directions.						
8.	Insert three fingers under the restraint and check to be sure that it is not too tight.						
9.	Perform your procedure completion actions.						

PERFORMANCE REVIEW CHECKLIST

Procedure ___7___

Procedure <u>Clearing an Obstructed Airway (Heimlich Maneuver)</u>

Name of Nurse Aide _____ Date of Program _____ to _____

Social Security Number of Nurse Aide _____

Program Code Number _____

S=Satisfactory Performance
U=Unsatisfactory Performance

Place a full signature to correspond with each set of initials appearing below:

Initials	Corresponding Signature of Instructor	Title

Procedure Guidelines		S/U	Date	Initials	S/U	Date	Initials
Clearing an Obstructed Airway in a Conscious Resident							
1.	Call for the nurse immediately.						
2.	Tell the resident that you will help. If the resident is sitting or standing, stand behind her.						
3.	Wrap your arms around the resident's waist, above the hips.						
4.	Make a fist with one hand.						
5.	Place the thumb side of your fist against the resident's abdomen, just above the navel and below the tip of the breastbone.						
6.	Grasp the fist with the other hand.						
7.	Push inward and upward on the abdomen with a quick thrust.						
8.	Repeat the thrusts until the foreign body comes out or the resident loses consciousness. If the resident begins to cough, wait and see if she can expel the object.						

(continues)

continued

Clearing an Obstructed Airway in an Unconscious Resident						
It is important that you know your facility's policy regarding this procedure. This procedure may be the responsibility of the nurse. The procedure is listed here for your general understanding only.						
1. Call for help, but do not leave the resident alone.						
2. Lower the resident to the floor and position her on her back.						
3. Open the airway by doing a tongue/jaw lift. Check for signs of breathing. Look at the chest to see if it is rising and falling. Listen and feel for breaths on your cheek and on your ear.						
4. If the resident is not breathing, insert your index finger along the cheek and toward the base of the tongue. If an object is felt, try to remove it. Do not push the object farther down the throat.						
5. Attempt to ventilate. If the breath does not go in, reposition the head and attempt to ventilate again. Use a pocket mask or other barrier, according to facility policy.						
6. If your breath meets resistance, straddle the resident.						
7. Place the heel of one hand above the navel. Place the other hand on top. Keeping your elbows locked and shoulders straight, give five abdominal thrusts.						
8. Open the airway by doing a tongue-jaw lift. Check the resident's mouth and use your finger as a hook to remove any objects that you can see.						
9. Attempt to ventilate.						
10. Repeat steps 3 through 7 until the object is expelled.						
11. Assist the charge nurse, code team, or emergency medical services (EMS), as appropriate.						

(continues)

continued

12.	Discard gloves and face shield, or disinfect reusable ventilation device according to facility policy.						
13.	Perform your procedure completion actions.						
14.	Observe and report to the charge nurse: • exact time the choking and unconsciousness started and stopped. • the procedures done and the time that you started and stopped. • the resident's response. • factors related to the cause of choking, if known.						

PERFORMANCE REVIEW CHECKLIST

Procedure __8__

Procedure <u>Making the Unoccupied Bed</u>

Name of Nurse Aide _____ Date of Program _____ to _____

Social Security Number of Nurse Aide _____

Program Code Number _____

S=Satisfactory Performance
U=Unsatisfactory Performance

Place a full signature to correspond with each set of initials appearing below:

Initials	Corresponding Signature of Instructor	Title

Procedure Guidelines	S/U	Date	Initials	S/U	Date	Initials
1. Wash your hands. Gather supplies needed: two large sheets (or one flat and one fitted sheet), a linen draw sheet (if used), plastic or rubber draw sheet (if used), pillowcase, laundry bag or hamper, and clean bedspread, if needed. Stack the linen in the order in which it will be used. Obtain disposable gloves if the linen is soiled with blood or any moist body fluid.						
2. Perform your beginning procedure actions.						
3. Carry the clean linen away from your uniform.						
4. Place the linens on a clean area near the bed in the order of use, from bottom to top.						
5. Elevate the bed to a good working height for you.						
6. Position the bed so that it is flat.						
7. Remove and fold the bedspread if you are reusing it.						

(continues)

continued

8.	Apply gloves if linen is soiled.					
9.	Remove the linen from the bed by rolling it in a ball without letting it touch your uniform.					
10.	Place soiled linens in a laundry bag, or dispose of it according to facility policy. If gloves were used, remove them and dispose of them according to facility policy. Check the mattress to be sure it is in good repair. Wash your hands before handling clean linen, even if gloves were worn.					
11.	Follow your facility policy for wiping the mattress. Some facilities require that the mattress be wiped with disinfectant if the linen is soiled with excretions or secretions. (Wear gloves for this task.)					
12.	Place the bottom sheet on the bed, centering the lengthwise middle fold of the sheet in the middle of the bed.					
13.	Open the sheet.					
14.	Place the sheet with small hem even with the foot edge of the mattress.					
15.	Tuck the top of the sheet under the top of the mattress.					
16.	Miter the corner of the sheet at the head of the bed on the side where you are working. OR Secure upper and lower corners of fitted sheet.					
17.	Tuck in the bottom sheet on the side of bed, working from head to foot.					
18.	Place the plastic draw sheet, if used, over the middle one-third of the bed.					
19.	Place the linen draw sheet over the plastic sheet, covering the entire plastic sheet.					
20.	Tuck the edge of the plastic sheet and draw sheet under the mattress.					
21.	Place the top sheet on the bed, centering the lengthwise middle fold in the center of the bed.					

(continues)

continued

22.	Position the sheet with the top edge even with the top of the mattress.					
23.	Tuck the bottom of the sheet under the mattress at the foot of the bed.					
24.	Place the bedspread on the bed.					
25.	Position the bedspread about four inches above the top edge of the mattress.					
26.	Miter linens at the foot of the bed.					
27.	Move to the other side of the bed.					
28.	Pull and smooth out the bottom sheet.					
29.	Tuck the bottom sheet under the mattress at the head of the bed, pulling tight.					
30.	Miter the corner of the sheet at the head of the bed. OR Secure upper and lower corners of the fitted sheet.					
31.	Pull and tightly tuck the side of the bottom sheet under the mattress.					
32.	Pull the plastic sheet tightly.					
33.	Tuck the plastic sheet under the mattress, pulling and tucking from the middle of the plastic sheet first. Then pull and tuck the edges of the sheet.					
34.	Pull the linen draw sheet tightly.					
35.	Tuck the linen draw sheet under the mattress, pulling and tucking from the middle of the draw sheet first. Then pull and tuck the edges of the sheet.					
36.	Check the foundation of the bed. Make sure the bed is smooth and wrinkle-free.					
37.	Pull and smooth the top sheet.					
38.	Pull and smooth the spread.					
39.	Tuck the sheet and spread under the foot of the mattress.					
40.	Miter the top linens at the foot of the bed.					
41.	Fold the spread back about 30 inches.					

(continues)

continued

42.	Make a cuff on the top sheet by folding it back about four inches at the top edge of the sheet.						
43.	Place the pillow on the bed.						
44.	Fold the pillow in half and insert the zippered end of the pillow in the pillowcase toward the closed end.						
45.	Straighten the pillowcase on the pillow.						
46.	Place the pillow at the head of the bed with the open end facing away from the door.						
47.	Cover the pillow with the bedspread.						
48.	Perform your procedure completion actions.						

PERFORMANCE REVIEW CHECKLIST

Procedure ___9___

Procedure <u>Positioning the Resident in the Supine Position</u>

Name of Nurse Aide _____Date of Program _____ to _____

Social Security Number of Nurse Aide _____

Program Code Number _____

S=Satisfactory Performance
U=Unsatisfactory Performance

Place a full signature to correspond with each set of initials appearing below:

Initials	Corresponding Signature of Instructor	Title

Procedure Guidelines		S/U	Date	Initials	S/U	Date	Initials
1.	Perform your beginning procedure actions.						
2.	Position the resident so that she is lying on her back.						
3.	Place the resident's arms at her sides in a comfortable, functional position, supporting them with pillows if necessary.						
4.	Check for good body alignment.						
5.	Pad bony prominences of elbows and heels, if indicated.						
6.	Elevate the knees slightly for comfort, if desired.						
7.	Perform your procedure completion actions.						

PERFORMANCE REVIEW CHECKLIST

Procedure ___10___

Procedure Moving the Resident to the Side of the Bed

Name of Nurse Aide _____ Date of Program _____ to _____

Social Security Number of Nurse Aide _____

Program Code Number _____

S=Satisfactory Performance
U=Unsatisfactory Performance

Place a full signature to correspond with each set of initials appearing below:

Initials	Corresponding Signature of Instructor	Title

Procedure Guidelines	S/U	Date	Initials	S/U	Date	Initials
1. Perform your beginning procedure actions.						
2. Stand on the side of the bed opposite from the one on which the resident will lie.						
3. Use proper body mechanics to move the resident.						
4. Place the resident's arms across his chest. Cross the resident's legs at the ankles.						
5. Remove the pillow.						
6. Place one of your arms under the resident's shoulder. Place the other arm under the back.						
7. Move the upper part of the resident's body toward you.						
8. Place one of your arms under the resident's waist and the other arm under the resident's thighs.						
9. Move the resident's midsection toward you.						

(continues)

continued

10. Move the resident's legs toward you. Uncross the ankles. Straighten the resident's arms.						
11. Replace the pillow.						
12. Begin positioning or transferring the resident, or go to the next step of this procedure.						
13. If the resident is to be left in this position, straighten the linen and raise the side rails.						
14. Perform your procedure completion actions.						

PERFORMANCE REVIEW CHECKLIST

Procedure ___11___

Procedure Moving the Resident to the Side of the Bed Using a Draw Sheet

Name of Nurse Aide _____ Date of Program _____ to _____

Social Security Number of Nurse Aide _____

Program Code Number _____

S=Satisfactory Performance
U=Unsatisfactory Performance

Place a full signature to correspond with each set of initials appearing below:

Initials	Corresponding Signature of Instructor	Title

Procedure Guidelines	S/U	Date	Initials	S/U	Date	Initials
1. Perform your beginning procedure actions.						
2. Use proper body mechanics to move the resident.						
3. Place the resident's arms across her chest. Cross the resident's legs at the ankles.						
4. Remove the pillow.						
5. Roll the ends of the draw sheet toward the resident until they touch the body.						
6. Using an overhand grip, place one hand at the upper end of the draw sheet, by the resident's shoulders. Place the lower hand on the draw sheet in the hip area.						
7. The nursing assistant on the side of the bed to which the resident will be moved does most of the work and calls the signals.						

(continues)

continued

8.	Move one foot about 12 inches forward to give you a broad base of support. Place your weight on this foot.						
9.	Flex your knees and keep your back straight.						
10.	On the count of three, both nursing assistants lift and pull the sheet toward the side of the bed.						
11.	Uncross the resident's ankles and straighten her arms.						
12.	Replace the pillow and unroll the draw sheet.						
13.	Begin positioning or transferring the resident, or go to the next step of this procedure.						
14.	If the resident is to be left in this position, straighten the linen and raise the side rails.						
15.	Perform your procedure completion actions.						

PERFORMANCE REVIEW CHECKLIST

Procedure ___12___

Procedure <u>Assisting the Resident to Move Up in Bed</u>

Name of Nurse Aide _____ Date of Program _____ to _____

Social Security Number of Nurse Aide _____

Program Code Number _____

S=Satisfactory Performance
U=Unsatisfactory Performance

Place a full signature to correspond with each set of initials appearing below:

Initials	Corresponding Signature of Instructor	Title

	Procedure Guidelines	S/U	Date	Initials	S/U	Date	Initials
1.	Perform your beginning procedure actions.						
2.	Lower the head of the bed.						
3.	Remove the pillow and lean it against the headboard.						
4.	Stand next to the bed.						
5.	Ask the resident to bend her knees and put her feet flat on the mattress.						
6.	If the resident is able, ask her to bend her arms at her sides, place her hands on the bed, and ask her to push when told to do so.						
7.	Slide one hand and arm under the resident's upper back and shoulders.						
8.	Slide the other arm under the resident's hips and buttocks.						
9.	Instruct the resident to push with her hands and feet on the count of three.						

(continues)

continued

10.	On the count of three, move the resident to the head of the bed.						
11.	Replace the pillow.						
12.	Check to see if the resident is in good alignment.						
13.	Perform your procedure completion actions.						

PERFORMANCE REVIEW CHECKLIST

Procedure ___13___

Procedure Moving the Resident to the Head of the Bed Using a Draw Sheet

Name of Nurse Aide _____ Date of Program _____ to _____

Social Security Number of Nurse Aide _____

Program Code Number _____

S=Satisfactory Performance
U=Unsatisfactory Performance

Place a full signature to correspond with each set of initials appearing below:

Initials	Corresponding Signature of Instructor	Title

Procedure Guidelines	S/U	Date	Initials	S/U	Date	Initials
1. Perform your beginning procedure actions.						
2. Place the resident's arms across his chest.						
3. Remove the pillow.						
4. Roll the ends of the draw sheet toward the resident until they touch his body.						
5. Using an overhand grip, place one hand at the upper end of the draw sheet, by the resident's shoulders. Place the lower hand on the draw sheet in the hip area.						
6. Both nursing assistants should stand with their feet apart, one foot ahead of the other.						
7. Bend your knees and keep your back straight.						

(continues)

continued

8. On the count of three, both nursing assistants should shift their weight from one foot to the other while lifting the draw sheet and moving it toward the head of the bed.						
9. Straighten the resident's arms.						
10. Replace the pillow and unroll the draw sheet.						
11. Straighten the linen and leave the resident comfortable.						
12. Perform your procedure completion actions.						

PERFORMANCE REVIEW CHECKLIST

Procedure ___14___

Procedure <u>Using a Transfer (Gait) Belt</u>

Name of Nurse Aide _____Date of Program _____ to _____

Social Security Number of Nurse Aide _____

Program Code Number _____

S=Satisfactory Performance
U=Unsatisfactory Performance

Place a full signature to correspond with each set of initials appearing below:

Initials	Corresponding Signature of Instructor	Title

	Procedure Guidelines	S/U	Date	Initials	S/U	Date	Initials
1.	Perform your beginning procedure actions.						
2.	Assist the resident to sit on the side of the bed.						
3.	Assist the resident to put on clothing and shoes or other footwear with non-slip soles.						
4.	Explain to the resident that the transfer belt is a safety device that will prevent pulling and tugging on the resident. Explain that it will be removed when the resident has been transferred.						
5.	Always apply the belt over the resident's clothing.						
6.	Place the belt around the resident's waist and buckle it in the front. Take care with female residents to ensure that the breasts are not under the belt.						

(continues)

continued

7.	Thread the belt through the teeth side first. Place the end of the belt through both openings so that it is double locked.					
8.	The belt should fit snugly, but you should check it by slipping your fingers comfortably underneath to be sure it is not too tight. Monitor female residents to be sure that the breasts are not under the belt.					
9.	Using an underhand grasp, insert your hands under the belt on each side and assist the resident to stand.					
10.	Complete the transfer or ambulation procedure.					
11.	Perform your procedure completion actions.					

PERFORMANCE REVIEW CHECKLIST

Procedure ___15___

Procedure Transferring the Resident from Bed to Wheelchair—One Person

Name of Nurse Aide _____Date of Program _____ to _____

Social Security Number of Nurse Aide _____

Program Code Number _____

S=Satisfactory Performance
U=Unsatisfactory Performance

Place a full signature to correspond with each set of initials appearing below:

Initials	Corresponding Signature of Instructor	Title

	Procedure Guidelines	S/U	Date	Initials	S/U	Date	Initials
1.	Perform your beginning procedure actions.						
2.	Position the wheelchair so the resident's stronger side will be closest to the wheelchair when the resident is sitting on the edge of the bed. Place the wheelchair within one foot of the bed at a slight angle.						
3.	Raise or remove the wheelchair footrests.						
4.	Lock the wheelchair brakes.						
5.	Raise the head of the bed.						
6.	Lock the wheels of the bed.						
7.	Lower the bed to the lowest position. Lower the side rail.						
8.	Assist the resident to sit on the side of the bed.						
9.	Assist the resident to put on clothing and shoes or other footwear with non-slip soles.						

(continues)

continued

10.	Place the transfer belt around the resident's waist and buckle it in the front.						
11.	Thread the belt through the teeth side first. Place the end of the belt through both openings so that it is double locked.						
12.	Check the fit of the belt by inserting your fingers underneath it.						
13.	Make sure that the resident's feet are flat on the floor. If not, use the transfer belt to move the resident to the side of the bed until his feet touch the floor.						
14.	Instruct the resident to push off the bed with his hands on the count of three.						
15.	Using an underhand grasp, insert your hands under the belt on each side, count to three, and assist the resident to stand.						
16.	Support the resident's weaker side.						
17.	Pivot and turn the resident with his back to the wheelchair.						
18.	Continue to hold the transfer belt and guide the resident backward until he can feel the edge of the wheelchair seat with the back of his legs.						
19.	Tell the resident to place his hands on the wheelchair arms. Seat the resident in the chair.						
20.	Remove the transfer belt.						
21.	Adjust the wheelchair footrests.						
22.	Cover the resident's lap with a lap blanket or other covering. Be sure the blanket does not become caught in the wheels.						
23.	Perform your procedure completion actions.						

PERFORMANCE REVIEW CHECKLIST

Procedure ___16___

Procedure <u>Transferring the Resident from Bed to Wheelchair—Two Persons</u>

Name of Nurse Aide _____Date of Program _____ to _____

Social Security Number of Nurse Aide _____

Program Code Number _____

S=Satisfactory Performance
U=Unsatisfactory Performance

Place a full signature to correspond with each set of initials appearing below:

Initials	Corresponding Signature of Instructor	Title

Procedure Guidelines	S/U	Date	Initials	S/U	Date	Initials
1. Perform your beginning procedure actions.						
2. Position the wheelchair so the resident's stronger side will be closest to the wheelchair when the resident is sitting on the edge of the bed. Place the wheelchair within one foot of the bed at a slight angle.						
3. Raise or remove the wheelchair footrests.						
4. Lock the wheelchair brakes.						
5. Raise the head of the bed.						
6. Lock the wheels of the bed.						
7. Lower the bed to the lowest position. Lower the side rail.						
8. Assist the resident to sit on the side of the bed.						
9. Assist the resident to put on clothing and shoes or other footwear with non-slip soles.						

(continues)

continued

10.	Place the transfer belt around the resident's waist and buckle it in the front.					
11.	Thread the belt through the teeth side first. Place the end of the belt through both openings so that it is double locked.					
12.	Check the fit of the belt by inserting your fingers underneath it.					
13.	Use the transfer belt to move the resident to the edge of the bed until his feet are flat on the floor. Each nursing assistant places the hand closest to the resident at the back of the belt and the other hand at the front of the belt and slides the resident forward.					
14.	On the count of three, both nursing assistants will move the resident at the same time. Coordination of movement is very important.					
15.	Each nursing assistant places the hand closest to the resident through the belt with an underhand grasp behind the resident.					
16.	The nursing assistant closest to the chair, on the resident's right side, stands in a position so that she can pivot and move away, allowing the resident access to the chair. This nursing assistant should stand with the left leg further back than her right leg.					
17.	The other nursing assistant should use her left knee to support the resident's weaker left leg. This nursing assistant's right leg is positioned further back than the left one.					
18.	Instruct the resident to lean forward and push off the bed, using the palms of his hands, on the count of three.					
19.	The resident's knees should be spread apart. Tell the resident to put both feet back with the stronger foot behind the weaker foot.					
20.	Both nursing assistants should bend their knees, squat slightly, and spread their feet to provide a broad base of support.					

(continues)

continued

21.	On the count of three, the resident stands. The nursing assistants pivot the resident slowly and smoothly by pivoting their feet, legs, and hips toward the left until the resident can feel the wheelchair with the back of his legs.						
22.	Tell the resident to place both hands on the armrests of the chair and lean forward slightly.						
23.	Both nursing assistants should bend their knees and lower the resident into the chair.						
24.	Remove the transfer belt.						
25.	Adjust the wheelchair footrests.						
26.	Cover the resident's lap with a lap blanket or other covering. Be sure that the blanket does not become caught in the wheels.						
27.	Perform your procedure completion actions.						

PERFORMANCE REVIEW CHECKLIST

Procedure   __17__

Procedure <u>Ambulating the Resident with a Gait Belt</u>

Name of Nurse Aide _____ Date of Program _____ to _____

Social Security Number of Nurse Aide _____

Program Code Number _____

S=Satisfactory Performance
U=Unsatisfactory Performance

Place a full signature to correspond with each set of initials appearing below:

Initials	Corresponding Signature of Instructor	Title

Procedure Guidelines	S/U	Date	Initials	S/U	Date	Initials
1. Perform your beginning procedure actions.						
2. Assist the resident to sit on the side of the bed.						
3. Assist the resident to put on shoes or other footwear with nonslip soles.						
4. Explain to the resident that the gait belt is a safety device that will prevent pulling and tugging on the resident. It allows you to guide and support the resident during the ambulation procedure.						
5. Always apply the belt over the resident's clothing.						
6. Place the belt around the resident's waist and buckle it in the front.						
7. Thread the belt through the teeth side first. Place the end of the belt through both openings so that it is double locked.						

(continues)

continued

#							
8.	The belt should fit snugly, but you should check it by slipping your fingers comfortably underneath to be sure it is not too tight. Monitor female residents to be sure that the breasts are not under the belt.						
9.	Using an underhand grasp, insert your hands under the belt on each side and assist the resident to stand.						
10.	Walk behind and slightly to one side of the resident during ambulation. Maintain a firm, underhand grasp at the center back of the gait belt.						
11.	Encourage the resident to use handrails in the hallway.						
12.	Walk the distance recommended by the care plan or the nurse's instructions.						
13.	Monitor the resident for signs of fatigue. If this occurs, assist the resident to sit in a chair.						
14.	After ambulating the resident, return to the resident's room.						
15.	Assist the resident to sit in the chair or return to bed.						
16.	Remove the gait belt.						
17.	Perform your procedure completion actions.						

PERFORMANCE REVIEW CHECKLIST

Procedure ___18___

Procedure <u>Ambulating the Resident with a Cane or Walker</u>

Name of Nurse Aide _____Date of Program _____ to _____

Social Security Number of Nurse Aide _____

Program Code Number _____

S=Satisfactory Performance
U=Unsatisfactory Performance

Place a full signature to correspond with each set of initials appearing below:

Initials	Corresponding Signature of Instructor	Title

Procedure Guidelines	S/U	Date	Initials	S/U	Date	Initials
1. Perform your beginning procedure actions.						
2. Assist the resident to sit on the side of the bed.						
3. Assist the resident to put on shoes or other footwear with nonslip soles.						
4. Check the tips of the cane and walker for safety.						
5. Place the gait belt around the resident's waist and check the fit.						
6. Place the cane in the resident's hand or the walker in front of the resident.						
7. Help the resident stand. Grasp the gait belt underhand at the resident's sides.						
8. When the resident is standing and is balanced, ask her if she feels dizzy or weak.						
9. Walk behind and slightly to one side of the resident during ambulation. Maintain a firm, underhand grasp at the center back of the gait belt.						

(continues)

continued

10.	Walk the distance recommended by the care plan or the nurse's instructions.					
11.	Monitor the resident for signs of fatigue. If this occurs, assist the resident to sit in a chair.					
12.	After ambulating the resident, return to the resident's room.					
13.	Assist the resident to sit in the chair or return to bed.					
14.	Remove the gait belt.					
15.	Perform your procedure completion actions.					

PERFORMANCE REVIEW CHECKLIST

Procedure ___19___

Procedure <u>Transferring the Resident from Wheelchair to Toilet</u>

Name of Nurse Aide _____ Date of Program _____ to _____

Social Security Number of Nurse Aide _____

Program Code Number _____

S=Satisfactory Performance
U=Unsatisfactory Performance

Place a full signature to correspond with each set of initials appearing below:

Initials	Corresponding Signature of Instructor	Title

Procedure Guidelines		S/U	Date	Initials	S/U	Date	Initials
1.	Perform your beginning procedure actions.						
2.	Make sure the bathroom is empty.						
3.	Bring the resident in a wheelchair to the bathroom.						
4.	Close the bathroom door.						
5.	Position the wheelchair at right angles to the toilet.						
6.	Place the transfer belt around the resident's waist.						
7.	Lock the wheelchair brakes.						
8.	Tell the resident to push up from the wheelchair while you lift her with the transfer belt. Count to three to match movements.						
9.	Ask the resident to hold the bathroom grab bar.						
10.	Help the resident stand, giving her time to get balanced.						

(continues)

continued

11.	Pivot the resident so she is standing in front of the toilet, facing you.						
12.	Lower the resident's underwear.						
13.	Help the resident sit on the toilet.						
14.	Be sure the call light is close to the resident. Instruct the resident to call when she is finished.						
15.	Wash your hands and leave the bathroom if doing so is safe for the resident. Close the door behind you.						
16.	Return when the resident calls.						
17.	Put on gloves if helping the resident wipe excess urine or bowel movement is necessary.						
18.	Remove the gloves and discard according to facility policy.						
19.	Wash your hands.						
20.	Assist the resident to stand by using the gait belt. Tell the resident to hold onto the bathroom grab bar and pull herself up. Match movements on the count of three.						
21.	Pull the resident's underwear up.						
22.	Smooth the resident's clothing.						
23.	Pivot and seat the resident in the locked wheelchair. Flush the toilet. If abnormalities are noted in the urine or stool, do not flush. Save the specimen for the nurse to see.						
24.	Help the resident wash her hands.						
25.	Remove the resident from the bathroom.						
26.	Remove the transfer belt.						
27.	Perform your procedure completion actions.						

PERFORMANCE REVIEW CHECKLIST

Procedure ___20___

Procedure <u>Transferring the Resident Using a Mechanical Lift</u>

Name of Nurse Aide _____Date of Program _____ to _____

Social Security Number of Nurse Aide _____

Program Code Number _____

S=Satisfactory Performance
U=Unsatisfactory Performance

Place a full signature to correspond with each set of initials appearing below:

Initials	Corresponding Signature of Instructor	Title

Procedure Guidelines	S/U	Date	Initials	S/U	Date	Initials
1. Perform your beginning procedure actions.						
2. Place the wheelchair at right angles to the foot of the bed, facing the head. Lock the wheelchair and elevate or remove the footrests.						
3. Elevate the bed to a good working height for you. Lock the wheels of the bed.						
4. Lower the side rail on the side nearest you.						
5. Roll the resident on her side.						
6. Position the lift seat under the resident's body so that it supports the resident's shoulders, buttocks, and thighs. Smooth out the sling.						
7. Roll the resident back onto the sling and properly position it on the other side.						

(continues)

continued

8. Position the frame of the lift over the bed. Spread the legs of the lift to the widest open position to maintain a broad base of support.						
9. Attach the suspension straps or chains to the sling. The "S" hook should face *away* from the resident's body, to prevent injury.						
10. Position the resident's arms comfortably inside the sling.						
11. Attach the straps or chains to the lift frame.						
12. While talking to and reassuring the resident, slowly raise the boom of the lift until the resident is above the bed.						
13. Slowly guide the lift away from the bed.						
14. Position the lift over the chair.						
15. The second nursing assistant holds the sling and helps lower the resident slowly into the chair, keeping the hips back while the first nursing assistant slowly lowers the lift.						
16. Monitor the location of the resident's feet and arms to prevent injury.						
17. Unhook the straps or chains and remove the lift.						
18. Support the resident's feet with footrests.						
19. Perform your procedure completion actions.						

PERFORMANCE REVIEW CHECKLIST

Procedure ___21___

Procedure Giving Passive Range-of-Motion Exercises

Name of Nurse Aide _____ Date of Program _____ to _____

Social Security Number of Nurse Aide _____

Program Code Number _____

S=Satisfactory Performance
U=Unsatisfactory Performance

Place a full signature to correspond with each set of initials appearing below:

Initials	Corresponding Signature of Instructor	Title

Procedure Guidelines	S/U	Date	Initials	S/U	Date	Initials
1. Perform your beginning procedure actions.						
2. Position the resident in the supine position.						
3. Exercise the extremities as indicated on the care plan, supporting the extremity at the closest joints.						
Head and neck. Perform range of motion in this area only if it is your facility policy or if you have a physician's order.						
1. Lean the head forward, bringing the chin to the chest.						
2. Lean the head backward, with the chin up.						
3. Turn the head from side to side.						
4. Turn the head back and forth in a circular motion.						

(continues)

continued

Shoulders, arms, and elbows						
1. Move the arm over the head, with arm touching the top of head.						
2. Return the arm to the side.						
3. Move the arm across the chest.						
4. Return the arm to the side.						
5. Move the arm straight up.						
6. Return the arm to the side.						
7. Bring the arm away from body at the side to the shoulder level.						
8. Return the arm to the side.						
9. With the arm straight out at the side, bend at the elbow and rotate the shoulder.						
10. Return the arm to the side.						
11. Bend at the elbow and bring hand to chin.						
12. Return the arm to the side.						
Wrists, fingers, and forearms						
1. Bend the hand backward at the wrist.						
2. Bend the hand forward at the wrist.						
3. Clench the fingers and thumb slightly, as if making a fist.						
4. Extend the fingers and thumb.						
5. Move fingers and thumb together and then apart.						
6. Flex and extend joints in the thumb and fingers.						
7. Move each finger in a circular motion.						
8. Extend the arm along the side of the body with the palm facing upward.						
9. Rotate the forearm with the palm facing upward, then downward.						
Legs, hips, and knees						
1. Stretch the leg out from the body. Return the leg to the other leg, crossing over the other leg only at the ankle.						
2. Bend and straighten the knee.						

(continues)

continued

3. Roll the knees inward and outward.						
Ankles, feet, and toes						
1. With one leg straight on the bed, push foot and toes toward front of the leg.						
2. Push the foot and toes out straight. Point toward the foot of the bed.						
3. With the leg straight, turn the foot and ankle from side to side.						
4. Curl toes downward and upward.						
5. Spread the toes and move each toe away from the second toe, then toward the second toe.						
6. Repeat each exercise as indicated on the care plan.						
7. Note the resident's response to exercise.						
8. Perform your procedure completion actions.						

PERFORMANCE REVIEW CHECKLIST

Procedure ___22___

Procedure <u>Brushing the Resident's Teeth</u>

Name of Nurse Aide _____Date of Program _____ to _____

Social Security Number of Nurse Aide _____

Program Code Number _____

S=Satisfactory Performance
U=Unsatisfactory Performance

Place a full signature to correspond with each set of initials appearing below:

Initials	Corresponding Signature of Instructor	Title

Procedure Guidelines	S/U	Date	Initials	S/U	Date	Initials
1. Perform your beginning procedure actions.						
2. Place a towel across the resident's chest.						
3. Help the resident in self-care, if possible.						
4. Moisten the toothbrush. Apply toothpaste.						
5. Brush the resident's teeth using a circular motion on all surfaces. Brush gums, tongue, sides, and roof of the mouth.						
6. Let the resident rinse the mouth with water or mouthwash.						
7. Hold the emesis basin while the resident spits.						
8. Wipe the mouth with a towel.						
9. Check the mouth for sores, redness, or irritation.						
10. Perform your procedure completion actions.						

PERFORMANCE REVIEW CHECKLIST

Procedure __23__

Procedure <u>Special Oral Hygiene</u>

Name of Nurse Aide _____Date of Program _____ to _____

Social Security Number of Nurse Aide _____

Program Code Number _____

S=Satisfactory Performance
U=Unsatisfactory Performance

Place a full signature to correspond with each set of initials appearing below:

Initials	Corresponding Signature of Instructor	Title

	Procedure Guidelines	S/U	Date	Initials	S/U	Date	Initials
1.	Perform your beginning procedure actions.						
2.	Cover the pillow with a towel and turn the resident's head to the side. Position the head forward so that any fluid and secretions will not run down the resident's throat.						
3.	Place the emesis basin against the resident's chin.						
4.	Gently open the resident's mouth.						
5.	Dip the premoistened applicators into water, mouthwash, or solution used by the facility.						
6.	Wipe the gums, teeth, and inside of the mouth with applicators.						
7.	Discard the used applicators in the plastic bag.						
8.	Apply lubricant to the resident's lips.						
9.	Perform your procedure completion actions.						

PERFORMANCE REVIEW CHECKLIST

Procedure __24__

Procedure <u>Giving a Bed Bath</u>

Name of Nurse Aide _____Date of Program _____ to _____

Social Security Number of Nurse Aide _____

Program Code Number _____

S=Satisfactory Performance
U=Unsatisfactory Performance

Place a full signature to correspond with each set of initials appearing below:

Initials	Corresponding Signature of Instructor	Title

	Procedure Guidelines	S/U	Date	Initials	S/U	Date	Initials
1.	Perform your beginning procedure actions.						
2.	Remove the bedspread and blanket. Fold them and place on the chair.						
3.	Place the bath blanket over the top sheet. Remove the sheet without exposing the resident. Place the soiled sheet in the hamper or dispose of it according to facility policy.						
4.	Remove the resident's gown.						
5.	Raise the side rail.						
6.	Fill the basin with warm water. Check the temperature with a thermometer. It should be 105°F. Changing the water during the procedure may be necessary. Add more hot water if it becomes too cool.						
7.	Return to the bedside and lower the side rail.						
8.	Place a towel under the resident's chin.						

(continues)

continued

9.	Offer the resident the washcloth to wash his own face, if possible.						
10.	Make a mitten by folding the washcloth around your hand.						
11.	Wash the resident's eyelids from the inner side of the eye to the outer side of the eye, using plain water without soap. The eyes have a mucous membrane, so you should wear gloves during this part of the procedure.						
12.	Rinse the washcloth.						
13.	Dry the washed area.						
14.	Wash the remainder of the resident's face, neck, and ears. Ask the resident if he prefers to use soap. Some elderly residents do not use soap on the face.						
15.	Place a towel under the resident's arm farthest from you.						
16.	Hold the resident's arm up. Wash the whole arm from the shoulder to the wrist and fingertips.						
17.	Rinse and dry the arm.						
18.	Wash, rinse, and dry the axilla, or armpit.						
19.	Repeat for the other arm.						
20.	If possible, place the resident's hands in water. Wash, rinse, and dry hands, fingers, and nails.						
21.	Place the towel across the chest. Pull the bath blanket down to the abdomen.						
22.	Move the towel to expose half of the chest.						
23.	Wash, rinse, and dry the chest. In the female resident, dry the area under the breasts well. Repeat for the other side of the chest.						
24.	Cover the chest with the towel.						
25.	Pull the bath blanket down to expose the abdomen.						
26.	Wash, rinse, and dry the abdomen.						
27.	Return the bath blanket to the resident's shoulders.						

(continues)

continued

28.	Remove the towel from under the blanket.						
29.	Uncover the leg farthest from you. Place the towel under the leg.						
30.	Wash, rinse, and dry the leg from the groin area to the toes.						
31.	Repeat for the other leg.						
32.	If possible, place feet in a basin one at a time.						
33.	Wash, rinse, and dry the feet. Make sure that you dry well between the toes.						
34.	Cover the legs with the bath blanket.						
35.	Raise the side rail.						
36.	Empty the basin and refill with clean water.						
37.	Lower the side rail.						
38.	Ask the resident to turn with his back toward you. Assist if necessary.						
39.	Wash, rinse, and dry the back.						
40.	Put lotion on back, massaging the entire back.						
41.	Use gloves to wash the genital area. Wash from the front of the genital area to the rectal area.						
42.	Dispose of soiled linen according to facility policy.						
43.	Remove gloves and dispose of them according to facility policy.						
44.	Put the side rail up.						
45.	Wash your hands.						
46.	Return to the bedside and put the side rail down.						
47.	Help the resident into a clean gown or other clothing of choice.						
48.	Comb the resident's hair. Help with other grooming requests.						
49.	Replace bed linens, if indicated, or straighten the bed.						
50.	Perform your procedure completion actions.						

PERFORMANCE REVIEW CHECKLIST

Procedure ___25___

Procedure <u>Giving a Partial Bath</u>

Name of Nurse Aide _____Date of Program _____ to _____

Social Security Number of Nurse Aide _____

Program Code Number _____

S=Satisfactory Performance
U=Unsatisfactory Performance

Place a full signature to correspond with each set of initials appearing below:

Initials	Corresponding Signature of Instructor	Title

	Procedure Guidelines	S/U	Date	Initials	S/U	Date	Initials
1.	Perform your beginning procedure actions.						
2.	Place a towel under the chin.						
3.	Offer the resident the washcloth to wash her own face, if possible.						
4.	Make a mitten by folding the washcloth around your hand.						
5.	Wash the resident's eyelids from the inner side of the eye to the outer side of the eye, using plain water without soap. Wash the eye on the opposite side first, then the eye closest to you. The eyes have mucous membranes, so you should wear gloves for this part of the procedure.						
6.	Rinse the washcloth.						
7.	Dry the washed area.						
8.	Wash the remainder of the resident's face, neck, and ears. Ask the resident if she prefers to use soap. Some elderly residents do not use soap on the face.						

(continues)

continued

9.	Dry the washed area.						
10.	Place the towel under the hand farthest from you.						
11.	If possible, place resident's hand in the basin. Wash, rinse, and dry hand.						
12.	Repeat for other hand.						
13.	Wash, rinse, and dry axilla (armpit).						
14.	Repeat for the other axilla.						
15.	Ask the resident to turn with her back toward you. Assist if necessary.						
16.	Wash, rinse, and dry the back.						
17.	Put lotion on back, massaging the entire back lightly.						
18.	Use gloves when washing the genital area. Wash from the front of the genital area to the rectal area.						
19.	Put side rail up.						
20.	Remove gloves and dispose of them according to facility policy.						
21.	Wash your hands.						
22.	Return to the bedside and put side rail down.						
23.	Help the resident into a clean gown or other clothing of choice.						
24.	Comb the resident's hair. Help with other grooming requests.						
25.	Replace bed linens, if indicated, or straighten the bed.						
26.	Perform your procedure completion actions.						

PERFORMANCE REVIEW CHECKLIST

Procedure ___26___

Procedure <u>Female Perineal Care</u>

Name of Nurse Aide _____Date of Program _____ to _____

Social Security Number of Nurse Aide _____

Program Code Number _____

S=Satisfactory Performance
U=Unsatisfactory Performance

Place a full signature to correspond with each set of initials appearing below:

Initials	Corresponding Signature of Instructor	Title

Procedure Guidelines	S/U	Date	Initials	S/U	Date	Initials
1. Perform your beginning procedure actions.						
2. Remove the bedspread and blanket. Fold them and place on the chair.						
3. Place the bath blanket over the top sheet. Fanfold the sheet to the foot of the bed without exposing the resident. If the sheet is soiled, dispose of it according to facility policy.						
4. Ask the resident to raise her hips while you place a bed protector under her buttocks. Remove the soiled bed protector, if present. (Apply the principles of standard precautions during this activity.)						
5. Raise the side rail.						
6. Fill the basin with warm water.						
7. Return to the bedside and lower the side rail.						
8. Position the bath blanket so that only the area between the legs is exposed.						

(continues)

continued

9.	Ask the resident to separate and bend her knees.						
10.	Put on disposable gloves.						
11.	Wet the washcloth and make a mitten out of it.						
12.	Apply soap to the washcloth. Use caution. Too much soap can be irritating.						
13.	With one hand, separate the labia.						
14.	With the other hand:						
	a. Wash the far side of the labia from top to bottom, using a single downward stroke.						
	b. Rinse the washcloth.						
	c. Wash the near side of the labia from top to bottom, using a single downward stroke.						
	d. Rinse the washcloth.						
	e. Wash the center of the labia from top to bottom, using a single downward stroke.						
	f. Rinse the area well with the washcloth.						
	g. Gently dry the area with a towel.						
15.	Turn the resident away from you. Flex the upper leg slightly, if possible.						
16.	Wet washcloth and make a mitt. Apply soap.						
17.	Expose the anus.						
18.	Wash the area, stroking from the perineum to the coccyx.						
19.	Rinse the area well with the washcloth.						
20.	Gently dry the area with a towel.						
21.	Return the resident to her back.						
22.	Remove and dispose of the bed protector according to facility policy.						
23.	Raise the side rail.						
24.	Dispose of soiled linen according to facility policy.						
25.	Remove gloves and dispose of them according to facility policy.						

(continues)

continued

26.	Wash your hands.						
27.	Lower the side rail. Replace the top covers and remove the bath blanket.						
28.	Help the resident into a clean gown or other clothing of choice.						
29.	Perform your procedure completion actions.						

PERFORMANCE REVIEW CHECKLIST

Procedure ___27___

Procedure <u>Male Perineal Care</u>

Name of Nurse Aide _____Date of Program _____ to _____

Social Security Number of Nurse Aide _____

Program Code Number _____

S=Satisfactory Performance
U=Unsatisfactory Performance

Place a full signature to correspond with each set of initials appearing below:

Initials	Corresponding Signature of Instructor	Title

Procedure Guidelines	S/U	Date	Initials	S/U	Date	Initials
1. Perform your beginning procedure actions.						
2. Remove the bedspread and blanket. Fold them and place on the chair.						
3. Place the bath blanket over the top sheet. Fanfold the sheet to the foot of the bed without exposing the resident. If the sheet is soiled, dispose of it according to facility policy.						
4. Ask the resident to raise his hips while you place a bed protector under his buttocks. Remove the soiled bed protector, if present. Apply the principles of standard precautions during this activity.						
5. Raise the side rail.						
6. Fill the basin with warm water.						
7. Return to the bedside and lower the side rail.						

(continues)

continued

8.	Position the bath blanket so that only the area between the legs is exposed.						
9.	Ask the resident to separate and bend his knees.						
10.	Put on disposable gloves.						
11.	Wet the washcloth and make a mitten out of it.						
12.	Apply soap to the washcloth. Use caution. Too much soap can be irritating.						
13.	With one hand, grasp the penis gently and wash. Begin washing at the urinary meatus and wash the penis in a circular motion toward the base of the penis.						
14.	If the resident is not circumcised, pull the foreskin back to wash it. Rinse the penis, dry, and replace the retracted foreskin.						
15.	Wash the scrotum, then gently lift it and wash the perineum.						
16.	Rinse the washcloth, make a mitten, and rinse the entire area, beginning with the penis.						
17.	Gently dry the area with a towel.						
18.	Ask the resident to turn so his back is facing you. Assist if necessary.						
19.	Expose the anus.						
20.	Wash the area, stroking from the perineum to the coccyx.						
21.	Rinse the area well with the washcloth.						
22.	Gently dry the area with a towel.						
23.	Return the resident to his back.						
24.	Remove and dispose of the bed protector according to facility policy.						
25.	Raise the side rail.						
26.	Dispose of soiled linen according to facility policy.						
27.	Remove gloves and dispose of them according to facility policy.						
28.	Wash your hands.						
29.	Return to the bedside and lower the side rail.						

(continues)

continued

30. Replace the top covers and remove the bath blanket.						
31. Help the resident into a clean gown or other clothing of choice.						
32. Perform your procedure completion actions.						

PERFORMANCE REVIEW CHECKLIST

Procedure ___28___

Procedure Giving a Back Rub

Name of Nurse Aide _____Date of Program _____ to _____

Social Security Number of Nurse Aide _____

Program Code Number _____

S=Satisfactory Performance
U=Unsatisfactory Performance

Place a full signature to correspond with each set of initials appearing below:

Initials	Corresponding Signature of Instructor	Title

Procedure Guidelines	S/U	Date	Initials	S/U	Date	Initials
1. Perform your beginning procedure actions.						
2. Place the bottle of lotion in the basin of water to warm it.						
3. Expose the resident's back and upper buttocks.						
4. Wash, rinse, and dry.						
5. Pour a small amount of lotion into one hand.						
6. Warm the lotion by holding it between your hands, if necessary.						
7. Apply lotion to the back.						
8. Rub the back with gentle but firm strokes with both hands in a circular motion from buttocks to shoulders:						
a. Begin at the base of the spine and rub up the center of the back with long, soothing strokes.						

(continues)

continued

	b. Use a circular motion with your hands as you bring them down from the shoulders back to the buttocks.						
	c. Repeat this procedure for three to five minutes.						
9.	Remove excess lotion from the back.						
10.	Straighten and tighten the bottom sheet and draw sheet.						
11.	Change the resident's gown, if necessary.						
12.	Perform your procedure completion actions.						

PERFORMANCE REVIEW CHECKLIST

Procedure ___29___

Procedure <u>Combing the Resident's Hair</u>

Name of Nurse Aide _____ Date of Program _____ to _____

Social Security Number of Nurse Aide _____

Program Code Number _____

S=Satisfactory Performance
U=Unsatisfactory Performance

Place a full signature to correspond with each set of initials appearing below:

Initials	Corresponding Signature of Instructor	Title

	Procedure Guidelines	S/U	Date	Initials	S/U	Date	Initials
1.	Perform your beginning procedure actions.						
2.	Cover the pillow with a towel. If the resident is sitting in a chair, place the towel over the shoulders.						
3.	Section the resident's hair with one hand between the scalp and the ends of the hair.						
4.	Brush the hair thoroughly.						
5.	Have the resident turn so that you can comb and brush the back of the hair.						
6.	If the hair is tangled, use the comb to separate it. Take a small section of hair. Beginning at the end, comb downward. Support the hair above where you are combing with the fingers of your other hand so that you do not pull on the resident's scalp. Continue working upward until you reach the scalp.						

(continues)

continued

7.	Style the hair attractively and in a style appropriate for the resident's age. If the resident has long hair, consider braiding it or putting it up. Coarse, tightly curled hair may require special treatment.					
8.	Perform your procedure completion actions.					

PERFORMANCE REVIEW CHECKLIST

Procedure ___30___

Procedure <u>Shaving the Resident</u>

Name of Nurse Aide _____Date of Program _____ to _____

Social Security Number of Nurse Aide _____

Program Code Number _____

S=Satisfactory Performance
U=Unsatisfactory Performance

Place a full signature to correspond with each set of initials appearing below:

Initials	Corresponding Signature of Instructor	Title

Procedure Guidelines	S/U	Date	Initials	S/U	Date	Initials
1. Perform your beginning procedure actions.						
2. Cover the resident's chest with the towel.						
3. Soften the resident's beard by placing a warm washcloth over it for two to three minutes. Moisten the face with water and apply shaving cream.						
4. Put on disposable gloves.						
5. Beginning in front of the ear, hold the skin taut.						
6. Bring the razor down from the cheek to the chin in one-half- to one-inch increments. Continue until the entire cheek has been shaved. Rinse the razor between strokes.						
7. Repeat with other cheek.						
8. Ask the resident to tighten his upper lip. Shave from the nose to the upper lip in short, downward strokes.						

(continues)

continued

9. Ask the resident to tighten his chin. Shave the chin in downward strokes in one-half- to one-inch increments.						
10. Ask the resident to tip his head back.						
11. Apply shaving cream to the neck area.						
12. Hold the skin taut. Shave the neck area in smooth, upward strokes in one-half- to one-inch increments.						
13. Wash the resident's face and neck. Dry the area well.						
14. Apply aftershave lotion if resident prefers.						
15. Perform your procedure completion actions.						

PERFORMANCE REVIEW CHECKLIST

Procedure ____31____

Procedure <u>Hand and Fingernail Care</u>

Name of Nurse Aide _____Date of Program _____ to _____

Social Security Number of Nurse Aide _____

Program Code Number _____

S=Satisfactory Performance
U=Unsatisfactory Performance

Place a full signature to correspond with each set of initials appearing below:

Initials	Corresponding Signature of Instructor	Title

Procedure Guidelines	S/U	Date	Initials	S/U	Date	Initials
1. Perform your beginning procedure actions.						
2. Adjust the height of the overbed table and place it in front of the resident. Cover the overbed table with the bed protector.						
3. Place the basin of water on the table.						
4. Instruct the resident to place hands in the water.						
5. Soak the hands for approximately 10 minutes. Cover the resident's hands and the basin with a towel to keep the water warm. Add more warm water if necessary.						
6. Wash the resident's hands. Push the cuticles back gently with the washcloth or an orange stick.						
7. Lift the resident's hands out of the water and dry them with the towel.						

(continues)

continued

8. Clip the nails if permitted by facility policy.						
a. Cut the nails straight across.						
b. Do not trim the nails below the fingertips.						
c. Keep the nail clippings on the bed protector to be discarded later.						
9. Shape the nails with the nail file or emery board. Apply fingernail polish if requested by a female resident.						
10. Pour a small amount of lotion into your hands and rub it into the resident's hands.						
11. Perform your procedure completion actions.						

PERFORMANCE REVIEW CHECKLIST

Procedure ___32___

Procedure <u>Applying Support Hosiery</u>

Name of Nurse Aide _____Date of Program _____ to _____

Social Security Number of Nurse Aide _____

Program Code Number _____

S=Satisfactory Performance
U=Unsatisfactory Performance

Place a full signature to correspond with each set of initials appearing below:

Initials	Corresponding Signature of Instructor	Title

Procedure Guidelines	S/U	Date	Initials	S/U	Date	Initials
1. Perform your beginning procedure actions.						
2. Expose one leg at a time.						
3. Grasp the stocking with both hands at the top opening and roll or gather toward the toe end.						
4. Apply the stocking to the leg by rolling or pulling upward over the leg.						
5. Make sure the stocking is on evenly. Be sure there are no wrinkles.						
6. Expose the other leg.						
7. Grasp the stocking with both hands at the top opening and roll or gather toward the toe end.						
8. Apply the stocking to the leg by rolling or pulling upward over the leg.						
9. Make sure the stocking is on evenly. Be sure there are no wrinkles.						
10. Perform your procedure completion actions.						

PERFORMANCE REVIEW CHECKLIST

Procedure ___33___

Procedure <u>Making the Occupied Bed</u>

Name of Nurse Aide _____Date of Program _____ to _____

Social Security Number of Nurse Aide _____

Program Code Number _____

S=Satisfactory Performance
U=Unsatisfactory Performance

Place a full signature to correspond with each set of initials appearing below:

Initials	Corresponding Signature of Instructor	Title

	Procedure Guidelines	S/U	Date	Initials	S/U	Date	Initials
1.	Perform your beginning procedure actions.						
2.	Remove the bedspread and blanket. Fold them and place on the chair.						
3.	Place the bath blanket over the top sheet. Remove the sheet without exposing the resident. Place the soiled sheet in the hamper, or dispose of it according to facility policy.						
4.	Help the resident to turn on the side away from you.						
5.	Loosen bottom linens.						
6.	Roll the soiled draw sheet and rubber sheet, and tuck along resident's back.						
7.	Place the clean sheet on the bed with the center fold at the center of the bed.						
8.	Unfold one-half of the sheet.						

(continues)

continued

9.	Place the bottom hem of the sheet even with the edge of the mattress, or fit the corner of the fitted sheet.						
10.	Tuck the top of the sheet under half of the head end of the mattress.						
11.	Miter the corner.						
12.	Tuck the sheet under the side of the entire mattress, working from the head to the foot of the bed.						
13.	Roll the remaining half sheet and tuck it under the soiled sheet.						
14.	Place the rubber draw sheet in the middle of the bed. Tuck in at the side.						
15.	Place a clean linen draw sheet over the rubber draw sheet. Tuck in at the side. If a bed protector is used, place it on top of the draw sheet and roll it inside the draw sheet.						
16.	Roll the remaining halves of draw sheets and tuck them along resident's back under the soiled sheets.						
17.	Help the resident roll over the linen pile on his side facing you.						
18.	Raise the side rail.						
19.	Go to the other side of the bed.						
20.	Lower the side rail.						
21.	Loosen and remove soiled linens from under the mattress.						
22.	Raise the side rail if leaving the bedside.						
23.	Dispose of soiled linens according to facility policy. *Do not put soiled linen on the floor. Hold soiled linen away from your uniform.*						
24.	Remove gloves and dispose according to facility policy.						
25.	Wash your hands.						
26.	Return to the bedside and lower the side rail.						
27.	Pull the clean bottom sheet over the mattress.						
28.	Tuck the bottom sheet tightly under the head of the mattress.						

(continues)

continued

29.	Miter the corner of the sheet at the head of the bed, or fit the corner of the fitted sheet.						
30.	Pull the bottom sheet tight and tuck under the side of the mattress, working from head to foot.						
31.	Pull the rubber sheet tight and tuck over the bottom sheet at the side of the mattress.						
32.	Pull the draw sheet tight and tuck over the rubber sheet at the side of the mattress. If a bed protector is used, smooth and straighten it.						
33.	Help the resident to roll on his back. Cover the resident with the bath blanket.						
34.	Place the clean sheet over the bath blanket, centering the center fold of the sheet.						
35.	Pull the bath blanket from under the clean sheet.						
36.	Place the blanket and bedspread over the sheet.						
37.	Fold the top sheet over the edge of the blanket. Spread to make a cuff with the sheet.						
38.	Tuck the top linens under the foot of the mattress, allowing room for the resident's toes. Follow the care plan instructions for special devices, such as bed cradles and footboards.						
39.	Miter the corner of top linens at the foot of the bed.						
40.	Raise the side rail.						
41.	Go to the other side of the bed.						
42.	Lower the side rail.						
43.	Miter the corner of the top linens at the foot of the bed.						
44.	Remove the pillow and soiled pillowcase.						
45.	Place a clean pillowcase on the pillow.						
46.	Perform your procedure completion actions.						

PERFORMANCE REVIEW CHECKLIST

Procedure ___34___

Procedure <u>Feeding the Resident</u>

Name of Nurse Aide _____Date of Program _____ to _____

Social Security Number of Nurse Aide _____

Program Code Number _____

S=Satisfactory Performance
U=Unsatisfactory Performance

Place a full signature to correspond with each set of initials appearing below:

Initials	Corresponding Signature of Instructor	Title

Procedure Guidelines		S/U	Date	Initials	S/U	Date	Initials
1.	Perform your beginning procedure actions.						
2.	Check the name on the tray and the diet served.						
3.	Check the meal tray for silverware and spilled foods.						
4.	Place the tray on the table. Remove food covers.						
5.	Sit near the resident.						
6.	Explain what is on the tray.						
7.	Ask the resident what foods she would like to eat first.						
8.	Encourage the resident to feed herself, if able, by using finger foods or adaptive equipment.						
9.	Use hand-over-hand technique to help the resident feed herself, if consistent with the care plan.						

(continues)

continued

10. Fill the fork or spoon only half full or less, according to the resident's ability to swallow.						
11. Use a straw for liquids.						
12. Encourage the resident to eat. Talk pleasantly. Do not rush.						
13. Wipe the resident's mouth.						
14. Offer liquids between bites of solid food.						
15. Remove the tray when the resident is finished.						
16. Wash the resident's hands, if necessary.						
17. Perform your procedure completion actions.						

PERFORMANCE REVIEW CHECKLIST

Procedure ___35___

Procedure Recording Intake and Output

Name of Nurse Aide _____ Date of Program _____ to _____

Social Security Number of Nurse Aide _____

Program Code Number _____

S=Satisfactory Performance
U=Unsatisfactory Performance

Place a full signature to correspond with each set of initials appearing below:

Initials	Corresponding Signature of Instructor	Title

Procedure Guidelines	S/U	Date	Initials	S/U	Date	Initials
1. Perform your beginning procedure actions.						
2. Check to identify equivalents used in your facility.						
3. Identify foods considered to be liquid as taken by the resident.						
4. Estimate liquid food taken.						
5. Record how much liquid is taken by the resident in cubic centimeters.						
6. Record amounts under the intake column.						
7. Apply the principles of standard precautions when measuring output.						
8. Measure output by pouring the contents of the bedpan, urinal, or emesis basin into the graduate. Remove one glove. Flush contents down the toilet after they are measured by holding graduate with gloved hand and pushing flush lever on toilet with ungloved hand.						

(continues)

continued

9.	Rinse and disinfect the graduate and bedpan, urinal, or emesis basin according to facility policy.					
10.	Perform your procedure completion actions.					

PERFORMANCE REVIEW CHECKLIST

Procedure ___36___

Procedure <u>Giving a Bedpan</u>

Name of Nurse Aide _____ Date of Program _____ to _____

Social Security Number of Nurse Aide _____

Program Code Number _____

S=Satisfactory Performance
U=Unsatisfactory Performance

Place a full signature to correspond with each set of initials appearing below:

Initials	Corresponding Signature of Instructor	Title

Procedure Guidelines	S/U	Date	Initials	S/U	Date	Initials
1. Perform your beginning procedure actions.						
2. Ask the resident to flex his knees and rest weight on his heels, if able.						
3. Help the resident to raise his buttocks:						
a. Put one hand under the small of the resident's back, and gently lift while the resident pushes with his feet.						
b. With the other hand, insert the bed protector under the resident.						
4. If the resident is unable to lift his buttocks:						
a. Help the resident to turn on his side, with his back toward you.						
b. Place the bed protector on the bed.						
c. Place the bedpan flat against the resident's buttocks.						
d. Roll the resident on his back, while holding the bedpan in place.						

(continues)

continued

5.	Cover the resident with the top sheet.						
6.	Raise the head of the bed slightly for comfort.						
7.	Remove the disposable gloves.						
8.	Raise the side rail.						
9.	Dispose of gloves according to facility policy.						
10.	Wash your hands.						
11.	Give the resident the call signal and toilet tissue. Instruct him to use the signal when he is done. Leave the room.						
12.	Return immediately when the resident calls.						
13.	Put on disposable gloves.						
14.	Lower the side rail.						
15.	Remove the bedpan by asking the resident to raise his hips.						
16.	If the resident is unable to raise hips, hold the bedpan securely while the resident rolls to his side with back facing you. Remove the bedpan. Cover the pan with a bedpan cover or other cover according to facility policy.						
17.	Place the bedpan on a bed protector on the chair in the room, or according to facility policy. It is usually not placed on the overbed table or bedside stand.						
18.	Fill the washbasin with water (105°F). Help the resident to clean his perineal area, if necessary. Dispose of toilet tissue in the bedpan. Cover the bedpan.						
19.	Wash the resident's perineal area with soap and water. Rinse and dry.						
20.	Remove one glove and raise the side rail with the ungloved hand.						
21.	Take the covered bedpan to the bathroom. Empty and disinfect it according to facility policy. Use the ungloved hand to turn on faucets and flush the toilet. Store the bedpan in its proper location.						
22.	Remove the other glove and dispose according to facility policy.						

(continues)

continued

23.	Wash your hands.						
24.	Help the resident to wash his hands. Clean and return the basin to its proper location.						
25.	Perform your procedure completion actions.						

PERFORMANCE REVIEW CHECKLIST

Procedure ___37___

Procedure <u>Giving a Urinal</u>

Name of Nurse Aide _____Date of Program _____ to _____

Social Security Number of Nurse Aide _____

Program Code Number _____

S=Satisfactory Performance
U=Unsatisfactory Performance

Place a full signature to correspond with each set of initials appearing below:

Initials	Corresponding Signature of Instructor	Title

1. Perform your beginning procedure actions.							
2. Lift the top covers and hand the resident the urinal under the covers. If the resident is unable to take the urinal, place the urinal in the bed and insert the resident's penis into the opening.							
3. Remove the disposable gloves and dispose according to facility policy.							
4. Raise the side rail.							
5. Wash your hands.							
6. Give the resident the call signal and instruct him to use it when he is done. Leave the room.							
7. Return immediately when the resident calls.							
8. Put on one disposable glove.							

(continues)

continued

9.	Ask the resident to hand you the urinal. Remove it if he is unable.						
10.	Take the urinal to the bathroom, and empty and disinfect it according to facility policy. Use the ungloved hand to turn on faucets and flush the toilet. Store the urinal in its proper location.						
11.	Remove the glove and dispose according to facility policy.						
12.	Wash your hands.						
13.	Fill the washbasin with water (105°F).						
14.	Lower the side rail.						
15.	Help the resident to wash his hands.						
16.	Raise the side rail.						
17.	Lower the height of the bed.						
18.	Clean and return the basin to its proper location.						
19.	Perform your procedure completion actions.						

PERFORMANCE REVIEW CHECKLIST

Procedure ___38___

Procedure <u>Giving Catheter Care</u>

Name of Nurse Aide _____ Date of Program _____ to _____

Social Security Number of Nurse Aide _____

Program Code Number _____

S=Satisfactory Performance
U=Unsatisfactory Performance

Place a full signature to correspond with each set of initials appearing below:

Initials	Corresponding Signature of Instructor	Title

	Procedure Guidelines	S/U	Date	Initials	S/U	Date	Initials
1.	Perform your beginning procedure actions.						
2.	Cover the resident with a bath blanket.						
3.	Fanfold the upper linen down to the foot of the bed.						
4.	Ask the resident to raise hips and place the bed protector under the resident.						
5.	Position the bath blanket to expose the resident's catheter.						
6.	Wash the urethra area around the catheter entrance.						
7.	Wash the genital area from front to back. Rinse well.						
8.	Dry the area well.						
9.	Secure the catheter with a catheter strap or tape.						
10.	Place the drainage tubing over the resident's leg.						

(continues)

continued

11. Place the rubber band around the tubing and pin it to the sheet at the edge of the mattress to make sure that the tubing stays on the bed.						
12. Cover the resident. Replace the bedding and remove the bath blanket.						
13. Perform your procedure completion actions.						

PERFORMANCE REVIEW CHECKLIST

Procedure ___39___

Procedure Emptying a Catheter Bag

Name of Nurse Aide _____Date of Program _____ to _____

Social Security Number of Nurse Aide _____

Program Code Number _____

S=Satisfactory Performance
U=Unsatisfactory Performance

Place a full signature to correspond with each set of initials appearing below:

Initials	Corresponding Signature of Instructor	Title

	Procedure Guidelines	S/U	Date	Initials	S/U	Date	Initials
1.	Perform your beginning procedure actions.						
2.	Place a paper towel on the floor and place the graduate on top of it.						
3.	Remove the drainage spout from the bag and center it over the graduate. Be careful not to touch the tip of the drainage spout. Do not let the tip or the sides of the drainage spout touch the graduate.						
4.	Open the clamp on the drainage spout and allow the urine to drain into the graduate.						
5.	After the urine has drained into the graduate, wipe the spout with the alcohol sponge, if this is your facility policy. Some facilities do not wipe the tip of the spout unless it has contacted your hands or the graduate.						

(continues)

continued

#	Step						
6.	Replace the drainage spout into the holder on the side of the catheter bag. Pick up the graduate. Dispose of the paper towel.						
7.	Note the amount, color, and character of urine.						
8.	Discard urine and disinfect the graduate according to facility policy. Store the graduate in its proper location.						
9.	Perform your procedure completion actions.						

PERFORMANCE REVIEW CHECKLIST

Procedure ___40___

Procedure Taking the Oral Temperature with a Glass Thermometer

Name of Nurse Aide _____ Date of Program _____ to _____

Social Security Number of Nurse Aide _____

Program Code Number _____

S=Satisfactory Performance
U=Unsatisfactory Performance

Place a full signature to correspond with each set of initials appearing below:

Initials	Corresponding Signature of Instructor	Title

Procedure Guidelines	S/U	Date	Initials	S/U	Date	Initials
1. Perform your beginning procedure actions.						
2. Rinse the thermometer with cold water, and wipe with tissue from stem to the mercury bulb end, if the thermometer has been in disinfectant.						
3. Read the thermometer. Shake down to 96°F.						
4. Ask the resident if he has had hot or cold liquids or smoked a cigarette. If so, wait 15 minutes and return.						
5. Cover the thermometer with a disposable sheath if this is your facility policy.						
6. Apply gloves if contact with oral secretions is likely or if this is your facility policy.						
7. Place the bulb of the thermometer under the resident's tongue.						
8. Ask the resident to close his lips and breathe through his nose.						

(continues)

continued

9.	Note the time of insertion and remove the thermometer after three minutes, or time interval specified by your facility. Take pulse, respiration, and blood pressure.						
10.	Apply gloves if you are not already wearing them.						
11.	Remove the disposable sheath from the thermometer and dispose according to facility policy. OR Wipe the thermometer from stem to the bulb end with a tissue if a sheath was not used.						
12.	Read the thermometer to the nearest two-tenths of a degree.						
13.	Clean the thermometer, if indicated, or replace in container at bedside.						
14.	Perform your procedure completion actions.						

PERFORMANCE REVIEW CHECKLIST

Procedure ___41___

Procedure Taking the Pulse and Respiration

Name of Nurse Aide _____Date of Program _____ to _____

Social Security Number of Nurse Aide _____

Program Code Number _____

S=Satisfactory Performance
U=Unsatisfactory Performance

Place a full signature to correspond with each set of initials appearing below:

Initials	Corresponding Signature of Instructor	Title

Procedure Guidelines	S/U	Date	Initials	S/U	Date	Initials
1. Perform your beginning procedure actions.						
2. Position the resident's arm on a flat surface. Ask the resident to relax.						
3. Place the tips of two or three fingers on the palm and thumb side of the resident's wrist. Do not use your thumb.						
4. Find the pulse with your fingers.						
5. Press lightly with your fingers to feel the pulse.						
6. Look at the position of the second hand on your watch.						
7. Count and remember the pulse beats for 60 seconds. Note volume and rhythm.						
8. Continue to hold the resident's wrist as if you are still taking the pulse count.						
9. Observe the rising and falling of the resident's chest.						

(continues)

continued

10.	Count for 60 seconds or according to facility policy. Note regularity.						
11.	Perform your procedure completion actions.						

PERFORMANCE REVIEW CHECKLIST

Procedure ___42___

Procedure <u>Taking the Blood Pressure</u>

Name of Nurse Aide _____Date of Program _____ to _____

Social Security Number of Nurse Aide _____

Program Code Number _____

S=Satisfactory Performance
U=Unsatisfactory Performance

Place a full signature to correspond with each set of initials appearing below:

Initials	Corresponding Signature of Instructor	Title

Procedure Guidelines	S/U	Date	Initials	S/U	Date	Initials
1. Perform your beginning procedure actions.						
2. Clean the ear pieces and bell or diaphragm of the stethoscope with alcohol wipes.						
3. Remove or loosen clothing from the resident's arm. If the resident is wearing long sleeves, push the sleeve up to expose the brachial area.						
4. Place the arm in a comfortable position on a flat surface.						
5. Locate the brachial artery.						
6. Make sure that the cuff is decompressed.						
7. Wrap the cuff snugly and smoothly around the upper arm. Place it about one to one-and-one-half inches above the bend of the elbow. The inflatable portion of the cuff must be over the brachial artery.						

(continues)

continued

8.	Make sure the tubing from the cuff is centered. An arrow or marking on the cuff will indicate exactly where to place it.					
9.	Find the radial artery at the wrist and palpate it as you quickly inflate the cuff to 50mm Hg.					
10.	Continue to inflate the cuff in 10mm Hg increments until the radial pulse cannot be felt. When you can no longer feel the pulse, this number is known as the palpated pressure.					
11.	Deflate the cuff quickly. Ask the resident to raise his arm and flex his fingers.					
12.	Find the brachial artery inside the elbow area with your fingers.					
13.	Place the ear pieces of the stethoscope in your ears. Place the diaphragm or bell of the stethoscope over the brachial artery.					
14.	Reinflate the blood pressure cuff to 20mm Hg above the palpated pressure.					
15.	Slowly release the valve in the cuff and let the air escape slowly.					
16.	Listen carefully with the stethoscope until the first sound is heard. Remember this number. This is the systolic blood pressure.					
17.	Continue to release the air until the sound changes abruptly from very loud to soft and muffled. In some facilities, this number is recorded as the diastolic blood pressure. In other facilities, the diastolic blood pressure is recorded as the last sound that you hear before the sound completely disappears. Know and follow your facility policy.					
18.	Remember the diastolic reading while you rapidly deflate the blood pressure cuff.					
19.	Remove the stethoscope from your ears and wipe the ear pieces and bell or diaphragm with the alcohol sponges.					
20.	Perform your procedure completion actions.					

Procedure Guidelines	S/U	Date	Initials	S/U	Date	Initials

_____   _____
Instructor Signature   Date

_____   _____
Student Signature   Date

Practice Exam Answer Sheets

1. Ⓐ Ⓑ Ⓒ Ⓓ	41. Ⓐ Ⓑ Ⓒ Ⓓ		1. Ⓐ Ⓑ Ⓒ Ⓓ	41. Ⓐ Ⓑ Ⓒ Ⓓ
2. Ⓐ Ⓑ Ⓒ Ⓓ	42. Ⓐ Ⓑ Ⓒ Ⓓ		2. Ⓐ Ⓑ Ⓒ Ⓓ	42. Ⓐ Ⓑ Ⓒ Ⓓ
3. Ⓐ Ⓑ Ⓒ Ⓓ	43. Ⓐ Ⓑ Ⓒ Ⓓ		3. Ⓐ Ⓑ Ⓒ Ⓓ	43. Ⓐ Ⓑ Ⓒ Ⓓ
4. Ⓐ Ⓑ Ⓒ Ⓓ	44. Ⓐ Ⓑ Ⓒ Ⓓ		4. Ⓐ Ⓑ Ⓒ Ⓓ	44. Ⓐ Ⓑ Ⓒ Ⓓ
5. Ⓐ Ⓑ Ⓒ Ⓓ	45. Ⓐ Ⓑ Ⓒ Ⓓ		5. Ⓐ Ⓑ Ⓒ Ⓓ	45. Ⓐ Ⓑ Ⓒ Ⓓ
6. Ⓐ Ⓑ Ⓒ Ⓓ	46. Ⓐ Ⓑ Ⓒ Ⓓ		6. Ⓐ Ⓑ Ⓒ Ⓓ	46. Ⓐ Ⓑ Ⓒ Ⓓ
7. Ⓐ Ⓑ Ⓒ Ⓓ	47. Ⓐ Ⓑ Ⓒ Ⓓ		7. Ⓐ Ⓑ Ⓒ Ⓓ	47. Ⓐ Ⓑ Ⓒ Ⓓ
8. Ⓐ Ⓑ Ⓒ Ⓓ	48. Ⓐ Ⓑ Ⓒ Ⓓ		8. Ⓐ Ⓑ Ⓒ Ⓓ	48. Ⓐ Ⓑ Ⓒ Ⓓ
9. Ⓐ Ⓑ Ⓒ Ⓓ	49. Ⓐ Ⓑ Ⓒ Ⓓ		9. Ⓐ Ⓑ Ⓒ Ⓓ	49. Ⓐ Ⓑ Ⓒ Ⓓ
10. Ⓐ Ⓑ Ⓒ Ⓓ	50. Ⓐ Ⓑ Ⓒ Ⓓ		10. Ⓐ Ⓑ Ⓒ Ⓓ	50. Ⓐ Ⓑ Ⓒ Ⓓ
11. Ⓐ Ⓑ Ⓒ Ⓓ	51. Ⓐ Ⓑ Ⓒ Ⓓ		11. Ⓐ Ⓑ Ⓒ Ⓓ	51. Ⓐ Ⓑ Ⓒ Ⓓ
12. Ⓐ Ⓑ Ⓒ Ⓓ	52. Ⓐ Ⓑ Ⓒ Ⓓ		12. Ⓐ Ⓑ Ⓒ Ⓓ	52. Ⓐ Ⓑ Ⓒ Ⓓ
13. Ⓐ Ⓑ Ⓒ Ⓓ	53. Ⓐ Ⓑ Ⓒ Ⓓ		13. Ⓐ Ⓑ Ⓒ Ⓓ	53. Ⓐ Ⓑ Ⓒ Ⓓ
14. Ⓐ Ⓑ Ⓒ Ⓓ	54. Ⓐ Ⓑ Ⓒ Ⓓ		14. Ⓐ Ⓑ Ⓒ Ⓓ	54. Ⓐ Ⓑ Ⓒ Ⓓ
15. Ⓐ Ⓑ Ⓒ Ⓓ	55. Ⓐ Ⓑ Ⓒ Ⓓ		15. Ⓐ Ⓑ Ⓒ Ⓓ	55. Ⓐ Ⓑ Ⓒ Ⓓ
16. Ⓐ Ⓑ Ⓒ Ⓓ	56. Ⓐ Ⓑ Ⓒ Ⓓ		16. Ⓐ Ⓑ Ⓒ Ⓓ	56. Ⓐ Ⓑ Ⓒ Ⓓ
17. Ⓐ Ⓑ Ⓒ Ⓓ	57. Ⓐ Ⓑ Ⓒ Ⓓ		17. Ⓐ Ⓑ Ⓒ Ⓓ	57. Ⓐ Ⓑ Ⓒ Ⓓ
18. Ⓐ Ⓑ Ⓒ Ⓓ	58. Ⓐ Ⓑ Ⓒ Ⓓ		18. Ⓐ Ⓑ Ⓒ Ⓓ	58. Ⓐ Ⓑ Ⓒ Ⓓ
19. Ⓐ Ⓑ Ⓒ Ⓓ	59. Ⓐ Ⓑ Ⓒ Ⓓ		19. Ⓐ Ⓑ Ⓒ Ⓓ	59. Ⓐ Ⓑ Ⓒ Ⓓ
20. Ⓐ Ⓑ Ⓒ Ⓓ	60. Ⓐ Ⓑ Ⓒ Ⓓ		20. Ⓐ Ⓑ Ⓒ Ⓓ	60. Ⓐ Ⓑ Ⓒ Ⓓ
21. Ⓐ Ⓑ Ⓒ Ⓓ	61. Ⓐ Ⓑ Ⓒ Ⓓ		21. Ⓐ Ⓑ Ⓒ Ⓓ	61. Ⓐ Ⓑ Ⓒ Ⓓ
22. Ⓐ Ⓑ Ⓒ Ⓓ	62. Ⓐ Ⓑ Ⓒ Ⓓ		22. Ⓐ Ⓑ Ⓒ Ⓓ	62. Ⓐ Ⓑ Ⓒ Ⓓ
23. Ⓐ Ⓑ Ⓒ Ⓓ	63. Ⓐ Ⓑ Ⓒ Ⓓ		23. Ⓐ Ⓑ Ⓒ Ⓓ	63. Ⓐ Ⓑ Ⓒ Ⓓ
24. Ⓐ Ⓑ Ⓒ Ⓓ	64. Ⓐ Ⓑ Ⓒ Ⓓ		24. Ⓐ Ⓑ Ⓒ Ⓓ	64. Ⓐ Ⓑ Ⓒ Ⓓ
25. Ⓐ Ⓑ Ⓒ Ⓓ	65. Ⓐ Ⓑ Ⓒ Ⓓ		25. Ⓐ Ⓑ Ⓒ Ⓓ	65. Ⓐ Ⓑ Ⓒ Ⓓ
26. Ⓐ Ⓑ Ⓒ Ⓓ	66. Ⓐ Ⓑ Ⓒ Ⓓ		26. Ⓐ Ⓑ Ⓒ Ⓓ	66. Ⓐ Ⓑ Ⓒ Ⓓ
27. Ⓐ Ⓑ Ⓒ Ⓓ	67. Ⓐ Ⓑ Ⓒ Ⓓ		27. Ⓐ Ⓑ Ⓒ Ⓓ	67. Ⓐ Ⓑ Ⓒ Ⓓ
28. Ⓐ Ⓑ Ⓒ Ⓓ	68. Ⓐ Ⓑ Ⓒ Ⓓ		28. Ⓐ Ⓑ Ⓒ Ⓓ	68. Ⓐ Ⓑ Ⓒ Ⓓ
29. Ⓐ Ⓑ Ⓒ Ⓓ	69. Ⓐ Ⓑ Ⓒ Ⓓ		29. Ⓐ Ⓑ Ⓒ Ⓓ	69. Ⓐ Ⓑ Ⓒ Ⓓ
30. Ⓐ Ⓑ Ⓒ Ⓓ	70. Ⓐ Ⓑ Ⓒ Ⓓ		30. Ⓐ Ⓑ Ⓒ Ⓓ	70. Ⓐ Ⓑ Ⓒ Ⓓ
31. Ⓐ Ⓑ Ⓒ Ⓓ	71. Ⓐ Ⓑ Ⓒ Ⓓ		31. Ⓐ Ⓑ Ⓒ Ⓓ	71. Ⓐ Ⓑ Ⓒ Ⓓ
32. Ⓐ Ⓑ Ⓒ Ⓓ	72. Ⓐ Ⓑ Ⓒ Ⓓ		32. Ⓐ Ⓑ Ⓒ Ⓓ	72. Ⓐ Ⓑ Ⓒ Ⓓ
33. Ⓐ Ⓑ Ⓒ Ⓓ	73. Ⓐ Ⓑ Ⓒ Ⓓ		33. Ⓐ Ⓑ Ⓒ Ⓓ	73. Ⓐ Ⓑ Ⓒ Ⓓ
34. Ⓐ Ⓑ Ⓒ Ⓓ	74. Ⓐ Ⓑ Ⓒ Ⓓ		34. Ⓐ Ⓑ Ⓒ Ⓓ	74. Ⓐ Ⓑ Ⓒ Ⓓ
35. Ⓐ Ⓑ Ⓒ Ⓓ	75. Ⓐ Ⓑ Ⓒ Ⓓ		35. Ⓐ Ⓑ Ⓒ Ⓓ	75. Ⓐ Ⓑ Ⓒ Ⓓ
36. Ⓐ Ⓑ Ⓒ Ⓓ			36. Ⓐ Ⓑ Ⓒ Ⓓ	
37. Ⓐ Ⓑ Ⓒ Ⓓ			37. Ⓐ Ⓑ Ⓒ Ⓓ	
38. Ⓐ Ⓑ Ⓒ Ⓓ			38. Ⓐ Ⓑ Ⓒ Ⓓ	
39. Ⓐ Ⓑ Ⓒ Ⓓ			39. Ⓐ Ⓑ Ⓒ Ⓓ	
40. Ⓐ Ⓑ Ⓒ Ⓓ			40. Ⓐ Ⓑ Ⓒ Ⓓ	

Vocabulary Puzzles

CHAPTERS 1, 2, AND 3
WORD SEARCH PUZZLE

Directions: Circle the vocabulary words from the following list in the puzzle.

ABUSE	DIGNITY	INTERDISCIPLINARY	PSYCHOLOGICAL
ACTUALIZATION	DISEASE	LPN	REHABILITATION
ADAPTIVE	ESTEEM	LVN	REPRISAL
ATTITUDE	ETHICS	NEGLECT	RESIDENT
CHARGE	ETIQUETTE	OBRA	RESTORATIVE
CLIENT	GERIATRICS	OMBUDSMAN	RESTRAINTS
CONFIDENTIALITY	GRIEVANCE	PATIENT	RN
CONTINUITY	GRIEVING	PHYSIOLOGICAL	SECLUSION
DEPENDABILITY	HEALTH	PLAN	SPIRITUAL
DESCRIPTION	INFRINGE	POSTMORTEM	THERAPEUTIC

```
R T L A C I G O L O I S Y H P R S R S I E
G E N N O I T P I R C S E D E E F P A T P
N R P E E T H I C S M W N S G E I N I O Y
G Y I R I B H H N A L P I N D R A Q S T I
Z E T E I T U H H Y I D I U I M U T I N R
E S R I V S A L R J E R T T S E M U T P E
N C T I L I A P M N F I U D T O N E E S H
Y C N N A A N L T N T A U T R I R H V Y A
T I I A I T I G I T L B E T T D O E I C B
I T T L V A R T A L M V E N I C R A T H I
L U G V H E R I N O I M O S I W A L A O L
I E M N D N I T C E B C C D E N D T R L I
B P E R Z Q O R S S D I D G R P N H O O T
A A S C V I E I G E P I A I D K P K T G A
D R U A K S T Y S L R D F D G T L D S I T
N E B V T C T E I U K T I N A N N N E C I
E H A E E I G N Z Y L P C S O P I E R A O
P T E L N R A U J X W C Y M E C T T I L N
E M G G A R J C R S N R E M P A T I Y L Q
D E I H Y O B R A F H K H S H K S G V F C
N D C H N O I T A Z I L A U T C A E H E P
```

CHAPTERS 4 AND 5
KRISS-KROSS

Directions: Complete the following puzzle using the words found in Chapters 4 and 5.

3 Letters
AID

4 Letters
PAIN
SKIN

5 Letters
NEEDS
SIGNS

6 Letters
MENTAL
MODIFY
SENDER
VERBAL
VISION

7 Letters
BARRIER
HEARING
LEGIBLE
MEDICAL
MESSAGE
REALITY
URINARY

8 Letters
ABNORMAL
AGITATED
BEHAVIOR
DEMENTIA
IMPAIRED

LETHARGY
RECEIVER
SYMPTOMS

9 Letters
CONFUSION
DIGESTIVE
EFFECTIVE
NONVERBAL
REINFORCE
REPORTING

10 Letters
ALZHEIMERS
MANAGEMENT
VALIDATION

11 Letters
OBSERVATION
ORIENTATION
RESPIRATORY
RETARDATION
THERAPEUTIC

12 Letters
OBSERVATIONS
PSYCHOSOCIAL

13 Letters
ABBREVIATIONS
COMMUNICATION

14 Letters
DISORIENTATION

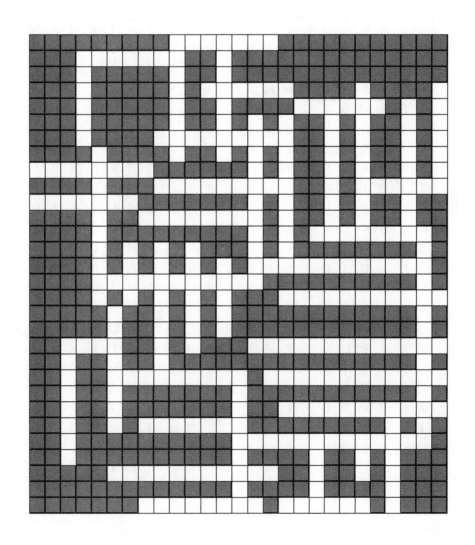

CHAPTERS 6 AND 7
WORD SEARCH PUZZLE

Directions: Circle the vocabulary words from the following list in the puzzle.

AIDS	GERIATRIC	MATERIAL	SOURCE
AIRBORNE	GERMS	MICROBE	SPARK
AIRWAY	GLOVES	MICROORGANISM	STANDARD
ASEPTIC	GOWN	MITE	STERILE
BACTERIA	HAZARD	MRSA	SUSCEPTIBILITY
BIOHAZARDOUS	HEPA	OBSTRUCTED	SWEAT
CARRIER	HIV	OXYGEN	TB
COMMUNICABLE	IMMOBILE	PATHOGEN	TRANSFER
CONTACT	IMPAIRMENT	PORTAL	TRANSMISSION
CONTAMINATED	INCIDENT	PROTECTIVE	VIRUS
CPR	INDIRECT	RESERVOIR	VRE
DROPLET	INFECTION	RESISTANT	
EMERGENCY	ISOLATION	RESTRAINT	
GAIT	MASK	SCABIES	

```
A O R C a G B A D Q Q T I A G S I A N A R S M
P I D E I i E K J E S R P C E G S D I E T I K
R S R U I R r R P P O W N V V E I R S A C R P
O W N B Y R T w M R L J O X P N E T N R A T A
Z E V M O T R A a S G L M T F T R D O P B B X
E A V R Z R I A I y G I I E C A A B S I D B J
V T H S X T N L C R C C A I R E L A Z G J Z
I M N A Z H S E I R E T B N D D S D A K V U K
T I S I G V I H O B I G T L F T R E R T R D S
C Q S T J D E O E O I S Z O D N R O I A R Q A
E E D K K N R M N R I T U E T T E A P B Z O M
T Q I B E G E M E M C M P O N N C G N L A A P
O U A G A R A S N O S I M E D O A E O S E C H
R M Y N G T E T N T A C D O C R I T R H F T S
P X I E E R N T E I H P X Q B S A T S I T E Y
O S N R V E A R M B N G E R V I U Z A I D A R
M C I O D C I K Z U I S N W O G L S A L S N P
Y A I I T L E B Y H Q Y S U R I V E P H O E I
L R C B E C O B S T R U C T E D A L O D O S R
W N B X R M S L J F J T N E M R I A P M I I I
I J Q U T R A N S M I S S I O N Z Y Q Q U J B
G O O C O N T A M I N A T E D M I T E Z X F Z
S S H E P A I L R A N E L B A C I N U M M O C
```

CHAPTERS 8 AND 9
KRISS-KROSS

Directions: Complete the following puzzle using the words found in Chapters 8 and 9.

3 Letters
ADL

4 Letters
FLEX
UNIT

5 Letters
EDEMA
GATCH
PRONE
RANGE

6 Letters
EXTEND
SUPINE

7 Letters
ATROPHY
BEDSIDE
FOWLERS
LATERAL
OVERBED

8 Letters
AMBULATE

FRICTION
PRESSURE
SHEARING

9 Letters
ALIGNMENT
MECHANICS
PARALYSIS

10 Letters
HEMIPLEGIA
IMMOBILITY
PROSTHESIS

11 Letters
CONTRACTURE
RESTORATIVE

14 Letters
REHABILITATION

15 Letters
CONTRAINDICATED

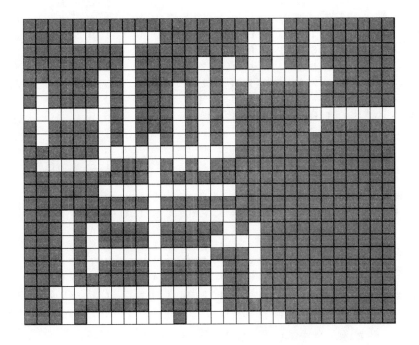

CHAPTERS 10 AND 11
WORD SEARCH PUZZLE

Directions: Circle the vocabulary words from the following list in the puzzle.

ABRASION	DIGESTION	GRADUATE	PERINEAL
ANUS	EDEMA	INCONTINENT	PRESSURE
ASPIRATION	EMBOLISM	INFUSION	PROSTHESIS
AXILLA	EMESIS	INTAKE	PYRAMID
CENTIMETER	FLUIDS	INTRAVENOUS	RESTRICT
DECUBITUS	FOOD	MILLILITER	THERAPEUTIC
DEHYDRATION	FORCE	NUTRIENTS	
DENTURES	GASTROSTOMY	OUNCE	
DIET	GENITAL	OUTPUT	

```
Y S E D S F O R C E F A H O X F G I N A
G M T T I I F O O D A W C O L E N O N M
W M O N A M S L Q Y U I P U N F I O F K
Z I U T E U A E J Z Q T I I U T I V S O
L L P S S I D R M I H D T S S T X A O F
L L Z H T O R A Y E S A I E A B G Y S C
N I A X K J R T R P L O G R X V D U I I
O L N Y N Z G T U G N I D H D W Q O S T
I I T D N A O T S N D Y D N U Z H G E U
T T U S J Q U A P A H P R Z B F T A H E
A E P U Z X K R A E G B E E A S E M T P
R R T N X A E M D I P D S R S T I E S A
I B U A L S S A J X G U E E I T D D O R
P H O L S I B J O M B H E C R N R E R E
S I I U L R U K J K R C A H U U E I P H
A X R O A S U N X V E C N U O B T A C T
A E B S N Z K N S F E K A T N I I N L T
Q M I C E N T I M E T E R R W X V T E H
E O I N T R A V E N O U S A R L V O U D
N I N C O N T I N E N T D B N X I F A S
```

CHAPTER 12
KRISS-KROSS

Directions: Complete the following puzzle using the words found in Chapter 12.

4 Letters
ANUS
VOID

5 Letters
BOWEL
COLON
ENEMA
FECES

STOMA
STOOL

6 Letters
BEDPAN
OSTOMY
URINAL

7 Letters
COMMODE

URETHRA
URINATE

8 Letters
CATHETER
DEFECATE

9 Letters
COLOSTOMY
IMPACTION

11 Letters
HOMEOSTASIS
INCONTINENT
INVOLUNTARY

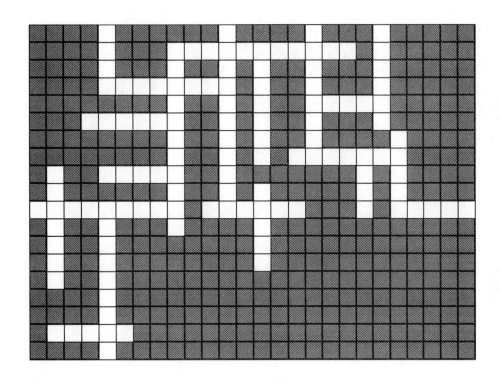

CHAPTER 13
WORD SEARCH PUZZLE

Directions: Circle the vocabulary words from the following list in the puzzle.

AURAL	DYSPNEA	OXYGEN	SPHYGMOMANOMETER
AXILLARY	EXHALATION	PALPATED	SYSTOLIC
BLOOD	EXPIRATION	PRESSURE	TACHYCARDIA
BODY	HEIGHT	PULSE	TEMPERATURE
BRACHIAL	HYPERTENSION	RATE	VOLUME
BRADYCARDIA	HYPOTENSION	RECTAL	WEIGHT
CYANOSIS	INHALATION	RESPIRATION	
DIASTOLIC	ORAL	RHYTHM	

```
Y A R E X P I R A T I O N S V J C C B
R R E H B N N I E S L U P O F I L C R
E N A N Y B R S D L K J L Y L A I M A
S R E L P T T F J N R U N O I L A Q D
P Y E G L S H A X C M O T H O O U B Y
I R W T Y I Y M C E I S C T W R R A C
R D M O E X X D I S A A S H W A A I A
A P B K L M O A N I R Y I X H L L D R
T I C Q L X O E D B S J A W Z Y Q R D
I D E V E T T N N C P W S O K P F A I
O O T I R R I P A O Y E E Z C D V C A
N O A Q E L A Q R M I A R I Z U E Y A
G L R P A L V H V Z O T N U G O N H W
Y B Y T P T Q D E V N M A O S H L C M
H H C A H U S F V M V R G L S S T A R
P E T G Z P Z N Q Y D O B Y A I E T O
R E I I N H A L A T I O N W H H S R Q
D E X V E R U T A R E P M E T P X V P
H H Y P O T E N S I O N A E S B S E Z
```

VOCABULARY PUZZLE SOLUTIONS

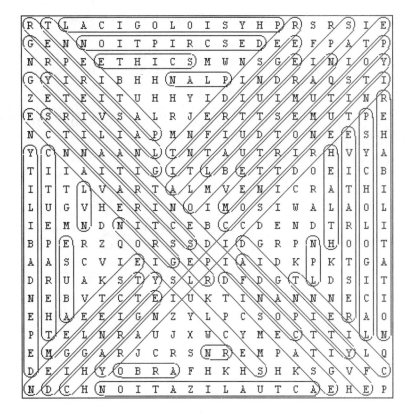

**CHAPTERS 1, 2, AND 3
WORD SEARCH SOLUTION**

**CHAPTERS 4 AND 5
KRISS-KROSS SOLUTION**

**CHAPTERS 6 AND 7
WORD SEARCH
SOLUTION**

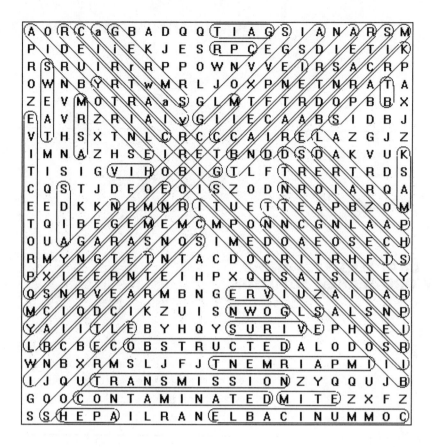

**CHAPTERS 8
AND 9
KRISS-KROSS
SOLUTION**

CHAPTERS 10 AND 11
WORD SEARCH SOLUTION

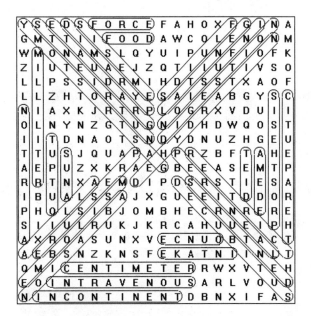

CHAPTER 12
KRISS-KROSS SOLUTION

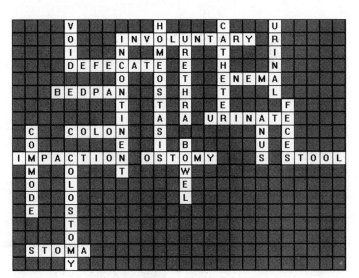

CHAPTER 13
WORD SEARCH SOLUTION

Answer Keys to Chapter Review Quizzes and Crossword Puzzles

CHAPTER 1 KEY

1. b	6. d	10. d	14. a	18. d
2. c	7. a	11. a	15. c	19. c
3. d	8. c	12. d	16. b	20. b
4. a	9. c	13. b	17. c	21. c
5. b				

CHAPTER 1 PUZZLE SOLUTION

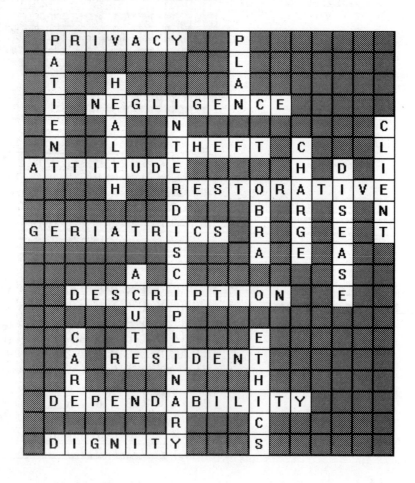

CHAPTER 2 KEY

1. a	6. c	10. d	14. d	18. a
2. b	7. a	11. a	15. b	19. d
3. d	8. c	12. b	16. b	20. b
4. b	9. b	13. c	17. c	21. c
5. d				

CHAPTER 2
PUZZLE SOLUTION

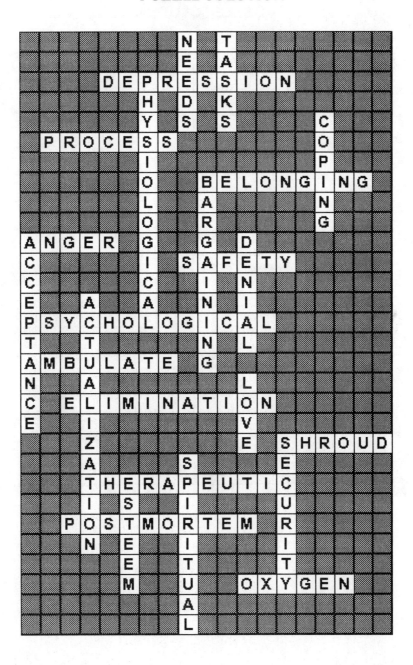

CHAPTER 3 KEY

1. c	7. a	13. a	19. d	25. a
2. d	8. b	14. d	20. a	26. d
3. a	9. c	15. a	21. d	
4. c	10. d	16. c	22. a	
5. b	11. c	17. b	23. c	
6. d	12. b	18. c	24. b	

CHAPTER 3
PUZZLE SOLUTION

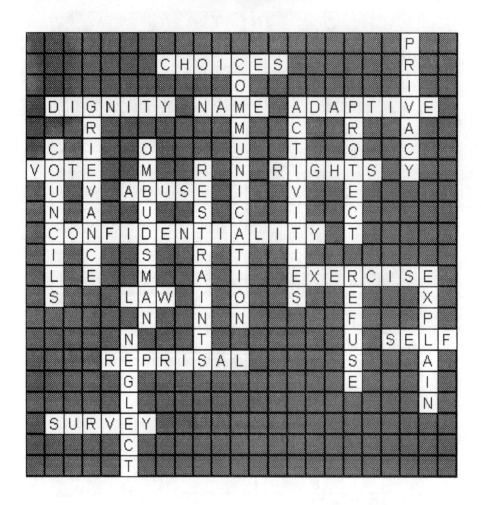

CHAPTER 4 KEY

1. b	5. b	9. c	13. a	17. d
2. d	6. d	10. d	14. c	18. a
3. a	7. b	11. a	15. d	19. b
4. c	8. a	12. c	16. b	20. c

CHAPTER 4
PUZZLE SOLUTION

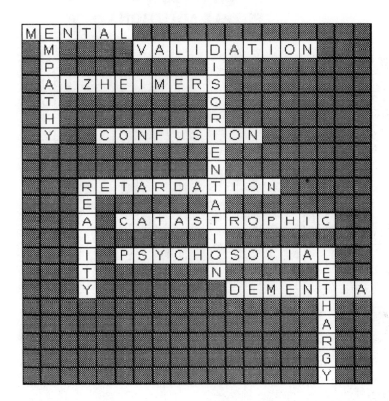

CHAPTER 5 KEY

1. b	7. c	13. d	19. d	25. d
2. d	8. a	14. a	20. a	26. c
3. a	9. c	15. d	21. a	27. a
4. d	10. b	16. b	22. a	28. b
5. b	11. c	17. d	23. b	29. a
6. d	12. c	18. c	24. c	

CHAPTER 5
PUZZLE SOLUTION

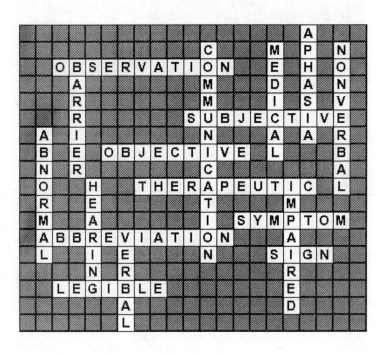

CHAPTER 6 KEY

1. c	7. a	13. b	19. d	25. d
2. a	8. c	14. d	20. b	26. c
3. c	9. a	15. b	21. c	27. b
4. d	10. b	16. c	22. a	
5. b	11. c	17. d	23. c	
6. d	12. d	18. a	24. a	

CHAPTER 6
PUZZLE SOLUTION

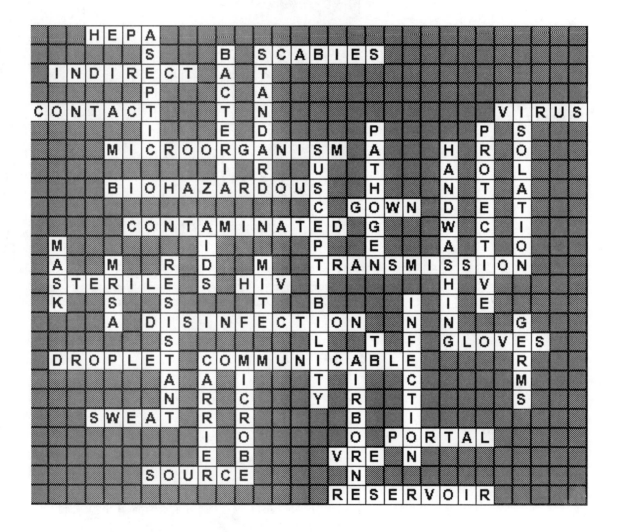

CHAPTER 7 KEY

1. d	5. a	9. c	13. c	17. d
2. c	6. d	10. b	14. c	18. b
3. b	7. b	11. a	15. a	19. d
4. a	8. d	12. b	16. d	20. b

**CHAPTER 7
PUZZLE SOLUTION**

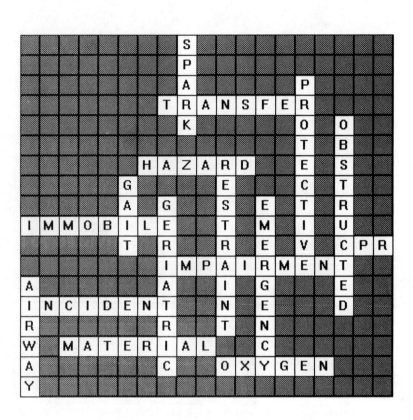

CHAPTER 8 KEY

1. c	4. b	7. c	9. d	11. c
2. d	5. b	8. d	10. a	12. d
3. a	6. a			

**CHAPTER 8
PUZZLE SOLUTION**

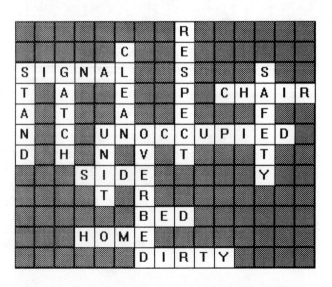

CHAPTER 9 KEY

1. b	6. a	11. a	16. a	21. b
2. c	7. d	12. d	17. d	22. c
3. d	8. b	13. b	18. d	23. d
4. c	9. b	14. a	19. c	24. c
5. a	10. c	15. b	20. b	25. b

CHAPTER 9
PUZZLE SOLUTION

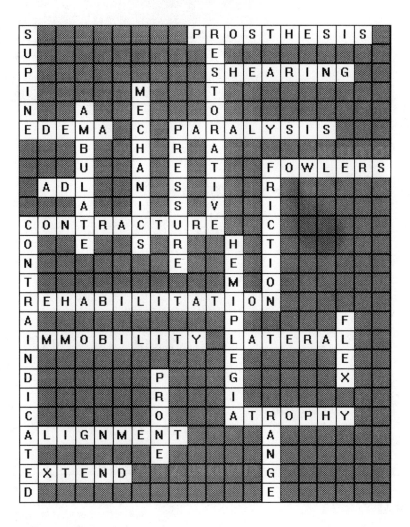

CHAPTER 10 KEY

1. a	5. b	9. d	13. b	17. b
2. d	6. a	10. b	14. c	18. d
3. d	7. b	11. a	15. b	19. a
4. b	8. c	12. c	16. c	20. b

CHAPTER 10
PUZZLE SOLUTION

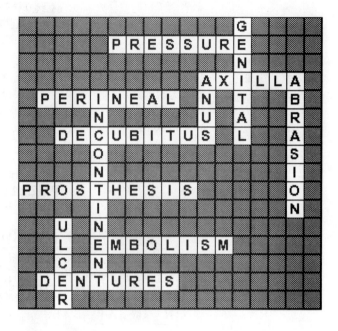

CHAPTER 11 KEY

1. a	5. d	9. b	13. d	17. c
2. c	6. a	10. c	14. c	18. a
3. b	7. d	11. a	15. b	19. d
4. d	8. b	12. b	16. b	20. b

CHAPTER 11
PUZZLE SOLUTION

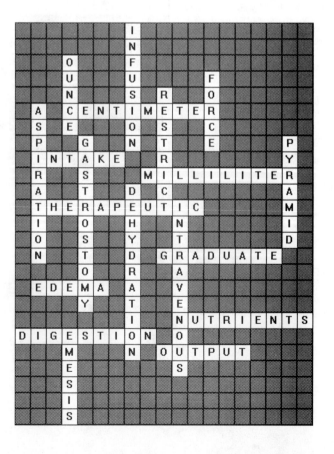

CHAPTER 12 KEY

1. c	5. a	9. b	13. b	17. d
2. b	6. d	10. d	14. c	18. b
3. a	7. c	11. c	15. b	19. a
4. b	8. c	12. a	16. c	20. c

**CHAPTER 12
PUZZLE SOLUTION**

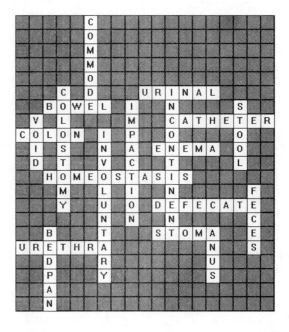

CHAPTER 13 KEY

1. b	5. c	9. d	13. c	17. d
2. d	6. b	10. b	14. b	18. a
3. a	7. c	11. c	15. a	19. d
4. b	8. d	12. a	16. c	20. a

**CHAPTER 13
PUZZLE SOLUTION**

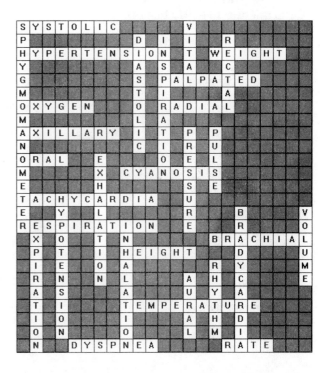

Index

Confusion, 51–52
Constipation, 176
Contact precautions, 79, 91
Contact transmission, 79
  of pathogen, 83
Contaminated, 79
  linen, 81
Continuity of care, 1, 6
  resident's rights and, 43
Contracture, 128, 130
Contraindicated, 128
Convalescent homes, 2
Coping mechanisms, 18, 29–30
CPR, *See* Cardiopulmonary
  resuscitation
Cubic centimeter (cc), 176
  in measuring intake, 186
Culture, 18
  influences on health care, 22–27
Cyanosis, 206, 212

D

Death and dying, 30–34
  cultural beliefs affecting care at time
    of, 31–34
  cultural beliefs surrounding, 30
  physical signs of approaching, 30
Decubitus ulcer, 153, 154–156
  See also Pressure ulcer
Defecate, 191
  help to, 193
Dehydration, 176
  dehydration and, 181
  signs of, 180–181
Dementia, 51
Denial, 18
  stage of grief, 29
Denture care, 157, 160
Dentures, 153
  nutrition and, 179
Dependability, 2
  of nursing assistants, 5
Depression, 18
  stage of grief, 29
Developmental tasks, 18, 28
Diabetic diet, 180
Diarrhea, 191
  medications and, 193
Diastolic pressure, 206, 212
Diets, special, 179–180
Digestion, 176
  fluid balance and, 180
Digestive system, 8
  main organs of, 192
  normal aging of, 10, 12
Dignity, 2, 4
  maintaining resident's, 45
Disabilities and communication,
  65–69
Disease, 2, 8
  common, 83–85
Disinfection, 79, 81
Disorientation, 51–52
Draw sheet, moving resident using, 135
Droplet precautions, 80, 91
Droplet transmission, 80
  of pathogen, 83
Droplets, 80, 83

Drug-resistant pathogens, 80, 84
Dycem, 109
Dying, 30–34
  See also Death and dying
Dyspnea, 206, 212

E

Edema, 128, 181
Electronic thermometers, 208–209
Elimination
  help with, 193
  interference with normal, 192–193
  normal, 192
Emergency, 99
Emergency measures, 111
Emesis, 176, 186
Empathy, 51
  behavior management and, 54
Endocrine system, 8
  normal aging of, 12
Enema, 191, 200
  guidelines for giving, 201
Enteral feeding, 176, 184
Essential nutrients, 176
  balanced diet and, 177
Ethics, 2
  for nursing assistant, 5–6
Etiquette, 2
  of nursing assistant, 6
Exhalation, 206, 212
Expiration, 206, 212
Extension, 128, 144
Eye contact and culture, 23

F

Fahrenheit, 206
  thermometers measuring in, 208
False imprisonment, 2, 6
Feces, 191
  characteristics of normal, 192
  observing and measuring output,
    197
Feeding techniques, 182–183
  by tube, 184
Fingernail care, procedure for, 169
Fire
  actions to take in, 110–111
  causes of, 110
  safety, 110–111
Flexion, 128, 144
Fluid balance, 180–181
  reasons for, 180
Fluids
  forcing, 181
  restricting, 181
Foley, 198
  See also Catheter
Food choice, cultural influences on,
  23
Food groups, 177–178
Food pyramid, 176
  as guide to proper nutrition,
    177–178
Foot care of resident, 168
Force fluids, 176
Fowler's position, 128
  using the, 131–132
Friction, 128, 134

G

Gait belt, 99
  ambulating resident with, 134–135,
    140–141
  procedure for using, 137
  See also Transfer belt
Gastrostomy (G) tube, 176, 184
Gatch handles, 118
  safe use of, 119
Genital area, 153
  washing the, 160
Genitourinary system, 192
Geri chair, *See also* Geriatric chair
Geriatric aide, 3
Geriatric chair, 99–100
Geriatrics, 2–3
Germs, 80
Gestures and culture, 23
Gloves
  discarding used, 88
  when to use, 87–88
Graduate, 176
  measuring output with, 186
Grief, stages of, 29
Grievance, 41
  filing a, 44
Grieving process, 18, 28–30
Gripper, 109
Grooming resident, 166–167

H

Hand care, procedure for, 169
Handwashing, 85, 87
  guidelines for, 88
  procedure for, 89
Hazard, 99
  fire, 110
  in long-term care facility, 100
HBV (hepatitis B virus), 80, 84
Health, 2, 8
Health care facilities, 2–3
Health practices, cultural influences
  on, 23
Hearing aid
  care of, 64–65
  troubleshooting problems with, 65
Hearing impairment, communication
  and, 64
Height
  abbreviations for, 207
  guidelines for measurements, 218
  measuring and recording, 214–215
  methods of measuring, 215, 217
Heimlich maneuver, 99, 111
  procedure for performing, 113
Hemiplegia, 128
  moving residents with, 136
HEPA filter, *See also* High-efficiency
  particulate air filter respirator
Hepatitis B virus, *See also* HBV
High Fowler's position, 128
  using the, 131–132
High-efficiency particulate air (HEPA)
  filter respirator, 80
  and airborne precautions, 91
  and tuberculosis, 84
HIV (human immunodeficiency virus),
  80, 8

of feces, 197
of urine, 196–197
Overbed table, 118
use of, 119
Oxygen, 99
as fire hazard, 110

P

Pain, cultural influences on, 23
Palpated pressure, 206, 216
Paralysis, 128, 142
Pathogen, 80, 81, 82
Patient, 2
Perineal (peri) care, 153, 160
procedure for female, 163–164
procedure for male, 165
Personal care of residents, 156–157
guidelines for providing, 158
Personal hygiene, cultural influences
on, 23, 24–27
Personal protective equipment, 80, 82
Personal space, 18
cultural influences on, 23
PFR95 respirator, 80
and airborne precautions, 91
and tuberculosis, 84
Physiological needs, 18, 19
meeting resident's, 19–20
Portal of entry of germ, 83
Postmortem care, 18, 34–35
Pressure ulcers, 128, 130
nursing measures and, 156
observing and reporting, 155–156
stages of, 155
See also Decubitus ulcer
Prioritize, 61, 69
Prone position, 128
using the, 132–133
Prosthesis, 129
care of, 167–168
following care plan for, 130
Protective device, 99
use of, 101
Protective eyewear, use of, 88–90
guidelines for putting on, 90
guidelines for removing, 90
Psychological needs (psychosocial
needs), 18, 19
Psychosocial needs (psychological
needs), 18, 19
Pulse, 206, 210–211
guidelines for measurement of, 211
procedure for taking, 216
Pulse location, 211
Pulse rate, 210–211
measuring, 211
Pulse volume, 211
measuring, 211
Pureed diet, 180

R

Radial pulse, 206, 211
Range-of-motion (ROM) exercises,
129
encouraging, 130
giving passage, 145–147
guidelines for doing, 145
purpose of, 144–145

Rate, 207
measuring pulse, 211
Recordkeeping, 71
Rectal, 207
Rectal temperature, measuring, 209
Registered nurse (RN), 2, 3–4
Rehabilitation, 129–130
principles of, 129–130
Rehabilitation center, 2, 3
Rehabilitation team, 129
Religion, 18, 28
meeting needs of resident, 22
Reprisal, 41
resident's rights and fear of, 43
Reproductive system, 8
normal aging of, 10, 12
Reservoir of germ, 83
Resident, 2, 3
moving to side of bed, 133
using draw sheet, 134
Resident's Bill of Rights, 41–43
Resident's rights
making choices and, 43–44
nursing assistants responsibility for,
43
Resident's unit, 118–120
Respiration, 207, 212
guidelines for counting, 212
normal, 212
procedure for taking, 216
Respiratory system, 8
normal aging of, 10–11, 12
Restorative care, 2, 8
Restorative nursing care, 129–130
principles of, 129–130
Restraints, 41
alternatives to, 104–109
guidelines for using, 103–104
reasons for using, 101
resident's rights and, 43
side effects of, 103
types of, 101–103
Restrict fluids, 177
Rhythm, 207
measuring pulse, 211
ROM exercises, *See also* Range-of-
motion exercises

S

Safety in resident's unit, 118–120
Safety needs of resident, 21
Safety of residents, 99–100
Scabies, 80
contact precautions for, 91
mite, 84
Security needs of resident, 21
Self-actualization, 18
meeting needs of resident, 22
Self-esteem, 18
meeting needs of resident, 22
Semi-Fowler's position, 129
using the, 131–132
Semiprone position, 129
using the, 132
Semisupine position, 129
using the, 132, 133
Senses, normal aging of, 11

Sensory impairments and
communication, 65–69
Shaving residents, procedure for, 168
Shearing, 129, 134
Sign, 62
of disease, 70
Sims' position, 129
using the, 132
Skeletal system, 8
normal aging of, 12
Skin, age-related changes in, 153–154
Skin care, 153
goals of, 154
Soft diet, 179–180
Speaking problems and
communication, 68
Sphygmomanometer, 207, 213
Spiritual needs, 19
meeting for resident, 22
Spirituality, 19, 28
meeting needs of resident, 22
Standard precautions, 80, 86
against spread of infection, 85
airborne precautions and, 91
tranmission-based precautions
and, 91
State tested nurse assistant (STNA), 2
See also Nursing assistant (NA)
Stereotyping, 19
avoiding, 22–23
Sterile, 80–81
Sterilization, 80–81
Stethoscope, 207, 211
sphygmomanometer and, 213
Stoma, 191, 198
Stool, 191–192
Subacute care, 2–3
Subjective, 62
finding, 70
Supine position, 129
positioning in, 133
using the, 132
Support hosiery, applying, 168, 170
Surgical mask, use of, 90
guidelines for wearing, 90
Susceptibility to germs, 83
Symptom, 62, 70
Systolic pressure, 207, 212

T

Tachycardia, 207, 211
Tape measure for measuring height, 217
TB (tuberculosis), 80, 84
and airborne precautions, 91
and HEPA filters, 84
Telephone communication, 69
Temperature, 207
body, 207
guidelines for taking, 210
measuring aural, 210
measuring axillary, 210
measuring oral, 209
measuring rectal, 209
Theft, 2
and nursing assistant, 6
Therapeutic, 19
Therapeutic communication, 30,
62–63